# Therapeutic Modalities for Musculoskeletal Injuries

## Second Edition

### Athletic Training Education Series

**Craig R. Denegar, PhD, ATC, PT**
Penn State University

**Ethan Saliba, PhD, ATC, PT**
University of Virginia

**Susan Saliba, PhD, ATC, PT**
University of Virginia

**David H. Perrin, PhD, ATC**
Series Editor
University of North Carolina at Greensboro

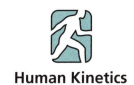

Human Kinetics

**Library of Congress Cataloging-in-Publication Data**

Denegar, Craig R.
  Therapeutic modalities for musculoskeletal injuries / Craig R. Denegar, Ethan Saliba, Susan Saliba.-- 2nd ed.
      p. ; cm. -- (Athletic training education series)
  Rev. ed. of: Therapeutic modalities for athletic injuries / Craig R. Denegar. c2000.
  Includes bibliographical references and index.
  ISBN 0-7360-5582-7 (hard cover)
  1. Sports injuries--Treatment. 2. Musculoskeletal system--Wounds and injuries--Treatment. 3. Sports medicine.
  [DNLM: 1. Athletic Injuries--therapy. 2. Musculoskeletal System--injuries. 3. Pain--prevention & control. 4. Rehabilitation--methods. QT 261 D392t 2006] I. Saliba, Ethan, 1956- II. Saliba, Susan Foreman, 1963- III. Denegar, Craig R. Therapeutic modalities for athletic injuries. IV. Title. V. Series.
  RD97.D46 2006
  617.1'027--dc22
                                                                           2005013423

ISBN-10: 0-7360-5582-7

ISBN-13: 978-0-7360-5582-6

Copyright © 2006 by Craig R. Denegar, Ethan Saliba, and Susan Saliba
Copyright © 2000 by Craig R. Denegar

Permission notices for material reprinted in this book from other sources can be found on page(s) xv-xvi.

This book is a revised edition of *Therapeutic Modalities for Athletic Injuries,* published in 2000 by Human Kinetics.

The Web addresses cited in this text were current as of September 2005, unless otherwise noted.

**Acquisitions Editor:** Loarn D. Robertson, PhD; **Developmental Editor:** Maggie Schwarzentraub; **Assistant Editors:** Amanda M. Eastin, Scott Hawkins, and Maureen Eckstein; **Copyeditor:** Joyce Sexton; **Proofreader:** Joanna Hatzopoulus Portman; **Indexer:** Sharon Duffy; **Permission Manager:** Dalene Reeder; **Graphic Designer:** Fred Starbird; **Graphic Artist:** Angela K. Snyder; **Photo Manager:** Sarah A. Ritz; **Cover Designer:** Keith Blomberg; **Photographer (cover):** Kelly Huff; **Photographer (interior):** Tom Roberts, except photos on pages 13, 16, 27, 43, 69, 71, 76, 83, 93, 149, 177, 241, 265, © Human Kinetics; **Art Manager:** Kelly Hendren; **Illustrators:** Argosy and Brian McElwain; **Printer:** Edwards Brothers

Printed in the United States of America          10  9  8  7  6  5  4  3

**Human Kinetics**
Web site: www.HumanKinetics.com

*United States:* Human Kinetics
P.O. Box 5076
Champaign, IL 61825-5076
800-747-4457
e-mail: humank@hkusa.com

*Canada:* Human Kinetics
475 Devonshire Road, Unit 100
Windsor, ON N8Y 2L5
800-465-7301 (in Canada only)
e-mail: orders@hkcanada.com

*Europe:* Human Kinetics
107 Bradford Road
Stanningley
Leeds LS28 6AT, United Kingdom
+44 (0)113 255 5665
e-mail: hk@hkeurope.com

*Australia:* Human Kinetics
57A Price Avenue
Lower Mitcham, South Australia 5062
08 8372 0999
e-mail: liaw@hkaustralia.com

*New Zealand:* Human Kinetics
Division of Sports Distributors NZ Ltd.
P.O. Box 300 226 Albany
North Shore City, Auckland
0064 9 448 1207
e-mail: info@humankinetics.co.nz

To my wife, Sue, for her love, support, and sacrifices made so I can work, write, and play. And to our sons, Charlie and Cody, who bring joy to our lives and provide a daily reminder of what is really important.

—Craig R. Denegar

# Contents

# Introduction to the Athletic Training Education Series

The five textbooks of the Athletic Training Education Series—*Introduction to Athletic Training*, *Examination of Musculoskeletal Injuries* (formerly *Assessment of Athletic Injuries*), *Therapeutic Exercise for Musculoskeletal Injuries* (formerly *Therapeutic Exercise for Athletic Injuries*), *Therapeutic Modalities for Musculoskeletal Injuries* (formerly *Therapeutic Modalities for Athletic Injuries*), and *Management Strategies in Athletic Training*—were written for athletic training students and as a reference for practicing certified athletic trainers. Other allied health care professionals, such as physical therapists, physician's assistants, and occupational therapists, will also find these texts to be an invaluable resource in the prevention, examination, treatment, and rehabilitation of injuries to physically active people.

The rapidly evolving profession of athletic training necessitates a continual updating of the educational resources available to educators, students, and practitioners. The authors of the five new editions in the series have made key improvements and have added important information. *Introduction to Athletic Training* includes a revised and simplified chapter on pharmacology. A new part I in *Examination of Musculoskeletal Injuries* makes this text one of the most comprehensive presentations of the foundational techniques for each assessment tool used in injury examination. Updated information on proprioceptive neuromuscular facilitation and sacroiliac joint evaluation and treatment is included in *Therapeutic Exercise for Musculoskeletal Injuries*, and a section on Pilates has been added. In *Therapeutic Modalities for Musculoskeletal Injuries*, a new chapter on evidence-based practice has been added, and the FDA's approval of laser treatment for selected injuries has led to a new chapter on this topic. Finally, the impact of the Health Insurance Portability and Accountability Act and the appropriate medical coverage model of the National Athletic Trainers' Association (NATA) are now addressed in *Management Strategies in Athletic Training*.

The Athletic Training Education Series offers a coordinated approach to the process of preparing students for the NATA Board of Certification examination. If you are a student of athletic training, you must master the material in each of the content areas delineated in the NATA publication *Competencies in Athletic Training*. The Athletic Training Education Series addresses these competencies comprehensively and sequentially while avoiding unnecessary duplication.

The series covers the educational content areas developed by the Education Council of the National Athletic Trainers' Association for accredited curriculum development. These content areas and the texts that address each content area are as follows:

- Risk management and injury prevention (*Introduction* and *Management Strategies*)
- Pathology of injury and illnesses (*Introduction*, *Examination*, *Therapeutic Exercise*, and *Therapeutic Modalities*)
- Assessment and evaluation (*Examination* and *Therapeutic Exercise*)
- Acute care of injury and illness (*Introduction*, *Examination*, and *Management Strategies*)
- Pharmacology (*Introduction* and *Therapeutic Modalities*)
- Therapeutic exercise (*Therapeutic Exercise*)
- General medical conditions and disabilities (*Introduction* and *Examination*)
- Nutritional aspects of injury and illness (*Introduction*)
- Psychosocial intervention and referral (*Introduction*, *Therapeutic Modalities*, and *Therapeutic Exercise*)
- Health care administration (*Management Strategies*)
- Professional development and responsibilities (*Introduction* and *Management Strategies*)

The authors for this series—Craig Denegar, Susan Hillman, Peggy Houglum, Richard Ray, Ethan Saliba, Susan Saliba, Sandra Shultz, and I—are eight certified athletic trainers with well over a century of collective experience as clinicians, educators, and leaders in the athletic training profession. The clinical experience of the authors spans virtually every setting in which athletic trainers practice, including the high school, sports medicine clinic, college, professional sport, hospital, and industrial settings. The professional positions of the authors include undergraduate and graduate curriculum director, head athletic trainer, professor, clinic director, and researcher. The authors have chaired or served on the NATA's most important committees, including the Professional Education Committee, Education Task Force, Education Council, Research Committee of the Research and Education Foundation, Journal Committee, Appropriate Medical Coverage for Intercollegiate Athletics Task Force, and Continuing Education Committee.

This series is the most progressive collection of texts and related instructional materials currently available to athletic training students and educators. Several elements are present in all the books in the series:

- Chapter objectives and summaries are tied to one another so that students will know and achieve their learning goals.
- Chapter-opening scenarios illustrate the importance and relevance of the chapter content.
- Cross-referencing among texts offers a complete education on the subject.
- Thorough reference lists allow for further reading and research.

To enhance instruction, each text includes an instructor guide and test bank. *Therapeutic Exercise for Musculoskeletal Injuries*, *Therapeutic Modalities for Musculoskeletal Injuries*, and *Examination of Musculoskeletal Injuries* each include a presentation package. Presentation packages (formerly known as graphics packages) are provided in Microsoft® PowerPoint format and delivered on CD-ROM. They contain selected illustrations, photos, and tables from the text. Instructors can use these presentation packages to enhance lectures and demonstration sessions. Other features vary from book to book, depending on the subject matter; but all include various aids for assimilation and review of information, extensive illustrations, and material to help students apply the facts in the text to real-world situations. For more information about the series, visit the Web site at www.HumanKinetics.com/Athletic EducationTrainingSeries.

Beyond the introductory text by Hillman, the order in which the books should be used is determined by the philosophy of each curriculum director. In any case, each book can stand alone so that a curriculum director does not need to revamp an entire curriculum in order to use one or more parts of the series.

When I entered the profession of athletic training over 25 years ago, one text—*Prevention and Care of Athletic Injuries* by Klafs and Arnheim—covered nearly all the subject matter required for passing the NATA Board of Certification examination and practice as an entry-level athletic trainer. Since that time we have witnessed an amazing expansion of the information and skills one must master in order to practice athletic training, along with an equally impressive growth of practice settings in which athletic trainers work. You will find these updated editions of the Athletic Training Education Series textbooks to be invaluable resources as you prepare for a career as a certified athletic trainer, and you will find them to be useful references in your professional practice.

David H. Perrin, PhD, ATC
Series Editor

# Preface

Times they are a-changing, especially in health care! Change is also reflected in the second edition of this book. We, the authors of the original text and laboratory manual, have joined forces to provide the most contemporary review possible of the use of therapeutic modalities in the management of athletic injuries.

Preparing the second edition of this text has permitted a more leisurely reflection on the subject of therapeutic modalities and treatment of injured athletes. Since the beginning of work on the first edition there has been little change in some respects. Certified athletic trainers generally apply the same modalities to treat the same types of problems as they did 10 years ago. Athletic training students must gain an understanding of the injury and recovery process, acquire knowledge of the principles and applications of therapeutic modalities, and learn to make decisions about the care of real people in the context of a 3- or 4-year educational experience. Injured athletes need skilled care to recover from injuries. The first edition was written to prepare students to apply contemporary therapeutic modalities in athletic training in order to facilitate achievement of the rehabilitation goals of the athletes they will care for. Like the first edition, this text is organized to provide an overview of the rehabilitation process before introducing the physiology of inflammation and the phenomenon of pain and neuromuscular control. With a foundation expanded from the first edition, the text progresses to discuss each of the contemporary therapeutic modalities prior to summarizing the issues of clinical management in the concluding three chapters.

The primary goal of this second edition is the same as for the original. Why is a second edition needed? While many aspects of athletic health care in general, and modality application in particular, have not changed, the health care system in which we practice has. Furthermore, new research related to therapeutic modalities is continually being published, and government regulation has responded to new evidence. For example, due to the accumulated research evidence, the FDA has approved the use of therapeutic laser for the treatment of carpal tunnel syndrome. Thus, we have added in this edition a chapter devoted to laser.

Relman (1988) stated that health care has entered into an "era of assessment and accountability" (page 1220) and evidence-based health care has emerged as the newest initiative to improve patient care across several medical and allied medical disciplines. The clinician of tomorrow will practice in a different health care world than previously has been experienced. The revisions in this text, it is hoped, will better prepare the reader—student or practicing clinician—for the challenges of the new health care setting.

Evidence-based practice has more than one facet. In a new chapter, the basic concepts of evidence-based practice are introduced. On a case-by-case basis, evidence-based practice calls upon the clinician to search the literature to identify an optimal treatment strategy. On a more global level, evidence-based practice guidelines are being developed to synthesize the literature and define standards of practice. This text goes beyond the "how" of modality application to ask about the "why" and "when." Specific treatments for specific problems are not prescribed, but reference is made to specific guidelines and summary papers as well as selected research papers. Individual clinicians must seek evidence to support the clinical decisions they make, and this text better prepares the student to search the literature and apply the vast amount of information related to modality application and health care.

Efficacy studies involving control groups provide the strongest evidence for or against particular interventions. True efficacy studies are very difficult to conduct in general and are especially challenging in an athletic health care environment, where the return of highly skilled athletes to competition is the goal of treatment. Effectiveness studies involve the assessment of treatment outcomes in the daily practice of health care. Effectiveness studies are unfortunately rare in athletic health care. It is through quality studies, however, that certified athletic trainers will likely gain the most insight into the inventions that provide the optimal treatment outcomes. Moreover, such studies also help clinicians decide how often and for how long treatments are necessary.

Although higher expectations for accountability can be intimidating, the opportunities to develop as an individual health care provider and render care based upon evidence, rather than tradition, have never been greater. We are hopeful that this text will help you in your journey toward your professional goals.

## CITED SOURCES

Relman A: Assessment and accountability: The third revolution in medical care. *N Engl J Med* 319:1220-1222, 1988.

# Acknowledgments

As the final touches come together for this second edition, we would first like to thank two individuals who were not recognized in the rush to complete the first edition. Loarn Robertson, PhD, Human Kinetics acquisitions editor, guided the development of the Athletic Training Series from the beginning. His vision, skill, and patience have made both editions of *Therapeutic Modalities for Musculoskeletal Injuries* possible. Ted Worrell, EdD, PT, ATC, provided considerable assistance in preparing the second chapter of both editions and offered valuable recommendations incorporated into the second edition. Without Loarn and Ted, as well as those recognized in the first edition, neither book could have been completed.

A special thank you is deserved by everyone at Human Kinetics who had a part in this book. Publication is a team effort, and we have had a great team behind us. We have worked most closely with developmental editor Maggie Schwarzentraub in the preparation of this new edition. Maggie's touch is evident throughout the text. Thank you, Maggie.

I (CRD) truly appreciate the support of the athletic training graduate students and faculty from Penn State. All have been willing to review a draft or offer constructive criticism when called upon. I most appreciate the undergraduate athletic training students who helped in the development of the first edition and those who have read and critiqued it since. My greatest reward for the labor of writing this book has been the opportunity to use it in my classes. Positions taken and statements made in print often provide for meaningful discussion and debate. The practice of health care is ever challenging and changing. I only hope that this book better prepares those who take up the challenge of the practice of athletic training.

# Credits

**Text on page 6**
Adapted from Professional ethics: A guide for rehabilitation professionals, R.W. Scott, pgs. 53-55, Copyright 1998, with permission from Elsevier.

**Figure 1.3** Reprinted, by permission, from J. Hertel and C.R. Denegar, 1998, "A rehabilitation paradigm for restoring neuromuscular control following athletics injury, "*Athletic therapy today* September 3(5): 13.

**Figure 1.5**
Adapted, by permission, from J.H. Gieck and E.N. Saliba, 1988, The athletic trainer and rehabilitation. In *Injured athlete*, 2nd edition, edited by D.N. Kulund (Philadelphia, PA: Lippincott, Williams, and Wilkins), 230.

**Figure 1.6**
Reprinted, by permission, from P.A. Houglum, 2005, *Therapeutic exercises for musculoskeletal injuries*, 2nd ed. (Champaign, IL: Human Kinetics), 168.

**Figure 1.7**
Reprinted, by permission, from R. Ray, 1994, *Management strategies in athletic training* (Champaign, IL: Human Kinetics), 147.

**Figure 3.6**
Adapted from L.L. Langley, J.B. Christensen, and I.R. Telford, 1974, Dynamic anatomy and physiology,_ 4th ed. (McGraw-Hill Companies), 389-391.

**Figure 4.1**
Reprinted, by permission, from C.R. Denegar and D.H. Perrin, 1992, "Effect of transcentaneous electrical nerve stimulation, cold and a combined treatment on pain, decreased range of motor and strength loss associated with delayed onset muscle soreness," *Journal of Athletic Training* 27(3): 202.

**Figure 4.2**
Reprinted, by permission, from M.S. Margolis, 1994, Spatial properties of pain. In *Pin measurement and assessment*, edited by R. Melzack (Philadelphia, PA: Lippincott, Williams, and Wilkins), 216.

**Figure 4.3**
Pollard, C.A. Preliminary validity study of the Pain Disability Index. *Perceptual and Motor Skills*, 1984, 59, 974. © Perceptual and Motor Skills 1984.

**Figure 4.4**
Reprinted, by permission, from J.J. Bonica, 1990, *The management of pain*, (Lippincott, Williams, and Wilkins), 89.

**Figure 4.5**
Reprinted, by permission, from J.J. Bonica, 1990, *The management of pain*, (Lippincott, Williams, and Wilkins), 89.

**Figure 4.6**
Reprinted, by permission, from J.H. Wilmore and D.L. Costill, 1999, *Physiology of sport and exercise*, 2nd ed. (Champaign, IL: Human Kinetics), 67 and 72.

**Table 4.3**
Reprinted from *Athletic Training Sport Health Care Perspective*, vol. 2(2), "Electrotherapy in the treatment of athletic injuries," pgs. 108-115, Copyright 1996, with permission from Elsevier.

**Figure 4.8**
Adapted, by permission, from E.R. Kandel, J.H. Schwartz, and T.M. Jessell, 2000, *Anatomy of the somatic sensory system* (New York: McGraw-Hill Companies), 1414. © McGraw-Hill Companies.

**Figure 5.2**
Reprinted, by permission, from C.R. Denegar and A. Peppard, 1997, "Evaluation and treatment of persistent pain and myofascial pain syndrome," *Athletic Therapy Today*, September 2(4): 40.

**Figure 5.3**
Reprinted, by permission, from C.R. Denegar and A. Peppard, 1997, "Evaluation and treatment of persistent pain and myofascial pain syndrome," *Athletic Therapy Today*, September 2(4): 42.

**Figure 5.4**

Reprinted, by permission, from C.R. Denegar and A. Peppard, 1997, "Evaluation and treatment of persistent pain and myofascial pain syndrome," *AthleticTherapy Today*, September 2(4): 42.

**Figure 6.2**

Reprinted, by permission, from J. Hertel and C.R. Denegar, 1998, "A rehabilitation paradigm for restoring neuromuscular control following athletics injury," *Athletic therapy today* September 3(5): 13.

**Figure 6.3**

Reprinted, by permission, from J. Hertel and C.R. Denegar, 1998, "A rehabilitation paradigm for restoring neuromuscular control following athletics injury," *Athletic therapy today* September 3(5): 14.

**Figure 6.4**

Reprinted, by permission, from Human Kinetics, *Progressive rehabilitation of lower extremity sport injury* (Champaign, IL: Human Kinetics), 52.

**Figure 7.1**

Reprinted, by permission, from J. Lysholm, and J. Gillquist, 1982, "Evaluation of knee ligament surgery results with special emphasis on use of a scoring  scale," *American Journal of Sports Medicine* 10: 150-154.

**Figure 7.2**

Reprinted from Spine Research Institute of San Diego.

**Figure 9.1**

Adapted, by permission, from J.H. Wilmore and D.L. Costill, 2004 *Physiology of sport and exercise*, 3rd ed. Champaign, IL: Human Kinetics), 94.

**Figure 10.7**

Reprinted, by permission, from Dynatronics Corporation.

**Figure 11.3**

Courtesy of Brigham Young University Sports Injury Research Center.

**Figure 11.10**

Reprinted from *Electrotherapy Explained: Principles and Practice*, 2nd Edition, J. Low and A. Reed, pg. 230, Copyright 1994, with permission from Elsevier.

**Figure 12.1**

Reprinted, by permission, from Georgia State University. Available: www.hyperphysics.phy-astr.gsu.edu/hbase/ems1.html. Assessed 3/8/05.

**Figure 12.7**

Image courtesy of the Lawrence Berkeley National Laboratory.

**Figure 13.2**

Adapted, by permission, from J.H. Wilmore and D.L. Costill, *Physiology of sport and exercise*, 3rd ed. (Champaign, IL: Human Kinetics), 67, 74, 79.

**Figure 13.10**

Reprinted, by permission, from C.D. Clemente, 1981, *Anatomy-A regional atlas of the human body*, 2nd ed. (München, Germany: Urban & Fischer Verlag GmbH & Co.), 465.

**Figure 13.11**

Reprinted, by permission, from C.D. Clemente, 1981, *Anatomy-A regional atlas of the human body*, 2nd ed. (München, Germany: Urban & Fischer Verlag GmbH & Co.), 471.

**Figure 13.12**

Reprinted, by permission, from W.H. Hollinshead and C. Rosse, 1985, *Textbook of anatomy*, 4th ed. (Philadelphia, PA: Lippincott, Williams, and Wilkins), 928.

**Figure 16.3**

Reprinted, by permission, from C.R. Denegar and A. Peppard, 1997, "Evaluation and treatment of persistent pain and myofascial pain syndrome," *Athletic Therapy Today* September 2(4): 40.

# The Contemporary Use of Therapeutic Modalities

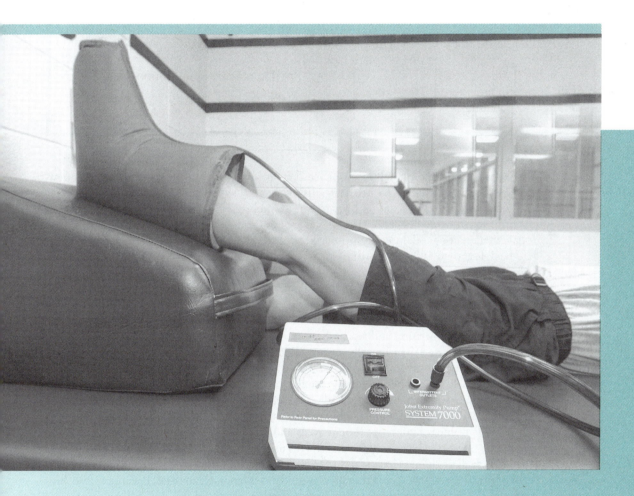

## Objectives

After reading this chapter, the student will be able to

1. discuss how state regulation of athletic training may influence the use of therapeutic modalities in the care of physically active individuals;

2. identify the hierarchy of components in a progressive rehabilitation plan; and

3. discuss guidelines for progressing an athlete through a comprehensive plan of care.

I

t is your first day working as a certified athletic trainer for a sports medicine clinic. Your position primarily involves service to a local high school but also involves a few hours in the clinic each morning. A varsity football player for the local high school sprained his ankle on the first day of practice yesterday. The team physician has evaluated the injury and referred the athlete to the clinic for treatment.

Questions arise, and the answers lead to more questions. What will be the plan of care for this injured athlete (i.e., short- and long-term treatment goals)? Can therapeutic modalities be used to achieve any of these goals? You identify pain control, restoration of range of motion, and return to full weight bearing as goals to be achieved within 7 to 10 days, and you choose therapeutic modalities including cold and transcutaneous electrical nerve stimulation (TENS). Can you, as a certified athletic trainer, administer these modalities to this athlete in the sports medicine clinic? Who has the answers?

Chapter 1 introduces a progressive rehabilitation paradigm from which treatment goals can be developed. In addition, the chapter discusses medical-legal issues affecting modality application, including regulation of practice and negligence. These issues are basic to the practice of athletic training and the use of therapeutic modalities.

The use of therapeutic modalities or physical agents in treating human ailments is not new. Massage, "cupping" (applying heated shells over painful areas), and the use of electric eels are mentioned in archives dating back to early Greek and Roman cultures. However, there was little scientific evidence to support the treatments administered by early practitioners. Today, therapeutic modalities are primarily applied by providers whose professional origins date back less than 100 years. Although several medical and allied medical care providers, including physicians, chiropractors, podiatrists, and dentists, may administer or apply therapeutic modalities, this practice is undertaken primarily by physical therapists and certified athletic trainers. Athletic trainers have applied therapeutic modalities since the beginnings of the profession (figure 1.1) and have contributed to the collective knowledge of therapeutic modalities through writing and research.

**Therapeutic modality** literally means a device or apparatus having curative powers. Heat, cold, massage, ultrasound, and diathermy have been used by athletic trainers since the profession's early days. These treatments may be better classified as **physical agents,** treatments that cause some change to the body. The scientific basis for the use of these therapeutic modalities has grown, providing a greater understanding of how modality applications may help athletic trainers achieve treatment goals and return injured athletes to sport.

Athletic trainers' educational preparation to use these modalities, however, has been challenged. As athletic trainers have sought recognition through state credentialing and establishment of practice acts, the use of therapeutic modalities has been an issue. Because internships are no longer the route to athletic training certification, all athletic trainers will receive formal preparation in the safe use of therapeutic modalities based on the best available science.

To effectively use therapeutic modalities to treat physically active individuals and other patients, we must cooperate and share knowledge. Our collective understanding of the physics of therapeutic modalities, physiological responses to therapeutic modalities, and clinical benefits of these modalities is evolving. Over the last 70 years, therapeutic ultrasound, diathermy, and the therapeutic use of electricity have been developed. Researchers are exploring how to best use these and other therapeutic modalities. As we learn more, our practices change, which is critical to our profession. The health care system is changing, and all providers are under increasing scrutiny to demonstrate improved patient outcomes and cost-effectiveness.

More athletic trainers than ever are working outside the traditional setting of the professional, college, and high school athletic training room. The profession is seeking greater recognition of the certified athletic trainer as a care provider to physically active individuals. Thus, although some athletic trainers practice in settings sheltered from some of the changes in health care, such as capitated services, these issues touch all in the profession.

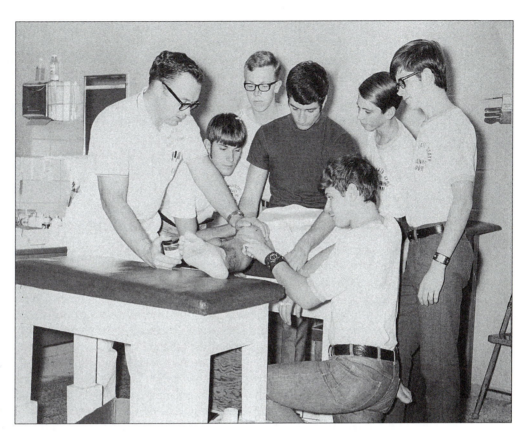

**Figure 1.1** An early athletic training room.

Photo courtesy of Minnesota State University Mankato.

Much has been learned about how therapeutic modalities affect the body. The theoretical basis for the application of therapeutic modalities following musculoskeletal injuries continues to evolve, and the rationale for the use of therapeutic modalities is often based upon "logical argument." In the last two decades, however, a model of evidence-based practice in health care has emerged. Databases have been developed to provide clinicians rapid access to reports of clinical trials, including the applications of therapeutic modalities for the treatment of several musculoskeletal disorders. Most of the revisions in this text are the result of a shift to evidence-based health care. This topic is discussed in greater detail in chapter 7.

An evidence-based approach to clinical practice, as described by Sacket (Sacket et al. 2000, 1), is the "integration of best research evidence with clinical expertise and patient values." Evidence that application of a therapeutic modality improves treatment outcomes or hastens the return to athletic competition, however, is often lacking. Until more is discovered through research, certified athletic trainers and other health care providers must integrate theory and clinical observations and research evidence to guide their use of therapeutic modalities in clinical practice.

## LEGAL ASPECTS OF THERAPEUTIC MODALITY APPLICATION: PRACTICE ACTS AND NEGLIGENT TREATMENT

Athletic training has been recognized as a distinct allied medical profession in many states through the development of **practice acts** and state credentialing. Recognition of the profession and higher educational standards influence the practice of athletic training. The certified athletic trainer must comply with regulations set forth by the state in which he or she practices, including regulations that affect the therapeutic modalities an athletic trainer may apply, whom the athletic trainer may administer treatment to, and the setting in which the athletic trainer may render treatment. The agency responsible for regulating athletic training practice can provide you with copies of the relevant practice act; these materials are also often available through state athletic trainers' associations or societies.

Changes in athletic training regulation and the education of athletic trainers also have elevated the standard of care expected from certified athletic trainers. Before the days of certification by the National Athletic Trainers' Association (NATA), there was no standard by which to judge athletic trainers' actions. Today, certification by the Board of Certification (BOC) for the NATA, recognition of athletic training as a profession by individual states through licensure or certification, and higher educational standards have defined the standards of athletic training and elevated levels of practice. Failure to practice according to these standards, including causing injury by therapeutic modality application, may constitute negligence.

## State Regulation of Athletic Training

Athletic trainer certification by the BOC for the NATA is determined by an examination that tests the applicant's knowledge and skills in preventing, recognizing, treating, and rehabilitating athletic injuries as well as performing administrative aspects of athletic training. A standard of preparation for the certified athletic trainer has been established through the examination.

Therapeutic modalities are addressed in a subsection of *Athletic Training Educational Competencies for Health Care of the Physically Active* (NATA 1999). Through education and supervised clinical experience, the athletic trainer learns how and when to apply therapeutic modalities and then demonstrates the associated knowledge and skills during the certification examination. The certified athletic trainer has met established standards to practice athletic training and to use therapeutic modalities. One might then assume that a certified athletic trainer's practice is governed by the National Athletic Trainers' Association's *Code of Ethics* (NATA 2005), the *Role Delineation Study* (NATA 2004), and the *Athletic Training Educational Competencies* (NATA 1999).

Such an assumption should never be made. The Joint Review Committee for Athletic Training has established criteria for accreditation of educational programs including preparation in the use of therapeutic modalities. The examination administered by the BOC for the NATA assesses this preparation. The BOC for the NATA further requires evidence of continuing education to maintain certification. The practice of athletic training was, however, governed by the state in which the athletic trainer practiced in 37 states of the United States in 2002. Thus, although a certified athletic trainer may be well qualified to use a specific therapeutic modality or administer a particular treatment, state laws specify what the athletic trainer may legally do. Moreover, in states that do not regulate the practice of athletic training, the application of a modality may infringe upon the practice of other disciplines as defined in that state. The certified athletic trainer must understand and practice within the boundaries of the state's practice act. Failure to do so may lead to revocation of a state license or certification and loss of practice privileges or charges of practicing another discipline without proper credentials.

It is not possible here to review the regulations of all states. In addition, regulations may change. This text and the instruction you receive are intended to develop your knowledge and skills related to the clinical competencies established by the profession. It is your responsibility to learn how the laws of your state affect what you can do and whom you can treat.

## Consent to Treat and Tort

Other medical and legal considerations relate to athletic training in general and the use of therapeutic modalities. This text is not intended to cover the legal and administrative aspects of athletic training and sports medicine in detail. However, two issues closely related to the application of therapeutic modalities are covered: informed consent and liability in tort.

### Informed Consent

*Informed consent* refers to the right of physically active individuals to receive information about their diagnosis and treatment options and consent to treatment. Informed consent has received little attention from certified athletic trainers. Schools and community youth athletic programs receive parental consent to provide immediate treatment of injuries. However, few athletic training rooms have policies regarding obtaining consent for modality application or participation in therapeutic exercises. Furthermore, although individuals entering sports medicine clinics sign forms giving health care providers permission to treat them, these individuals often do not provide informed consent for specific treatments.

Often a bond of trust exists between the physically active individual and the certified athletic trainer, whereby the individual believes that the athletic trainer will provide the best possible care. Additionally, the injured person may have observed treatments administered to others and may know what to expect. These two factors lead to an implied consent to receive treatment with specific modalities and to participate in specific exercises.

Failure to receive consent prior to treatment does not routinely lead to litigation against a certified athletic trainer. However, you should not ignore this issue. Make it a habit to explain any proposed treatment to the injured person and provide an opportunity for questions. This facilitates communication in the sports medicine clinic, where the injured person is encountering an unfamiliar health care facility and providers. It is also good practice in the athletic training room, where explaining the rehabilitation plan and proposed treatments engages the injured individual and allows the certified athletic trainer to review his or her responsibilities in the rehabilitation plan (figure 1.2).

The components of informed consent, as described by Scott (1990), are presented on page 6. Clearly, items 2 through 5 are directly related to the application of therapeutic modalities. This text is intended to provide the certified athletic trainer and athletic training student with the physical and physiological principles for modality application, the mechanisms by which the therapeutic benefits of modalities are achieved, and the contraindications and precautions for modality use. With this background, the certified athletic trainer can provide physically active individuals with what they need to make informed decisions about their health care.

### Liability in Tort for Negligent Treatment and Professional Negligence

A **tort** is a private, civil legal action brought by an injured party, or the party's representative, to redress an injury caused by another person. **Negligence** entails doing something that an

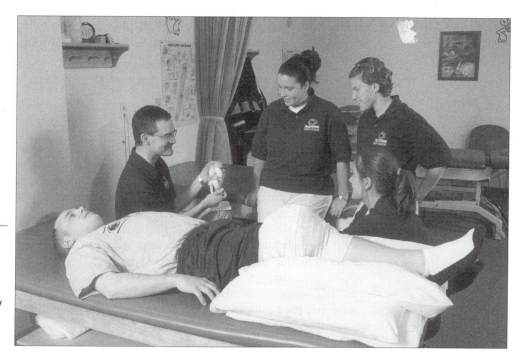

**Figure 1.2**
Explaining the rehabilitation plan and proposed treatments allows the athletic trainer to review his or her own responsibilities as well as inform the injured individual.

## Components of Informed Consent

The injured physically active person should be informed of the following:

1. The diagnosis or findings of a physical examination
2. The recommended treatment procedures and rehabilitation plan
3. The prognosis if the recommended treatment is administered or rehabilitation plan completed
4. The risks and benefits of the recommended treatment and rehabilitation plan
5. Reasonable alternatives to the proposed treatment and rehabilitation plan, with the potential risks, benefits, and prognosis
6. The prognosis if no treatment is administered or rehabilitation completed

Adapted by permission from Scott 1990.

ordinary person under like circumstances would not have done (a negligent act or an act of commission), or failing to do something that an ordinary, reasonable, prudent person would have done under similar circumstances. This general definition can be more clearly focused if *ordinary person* is replaced with *certified athletic trainer*. The professional standards established through national certification, the NATA *Code of Ethics* and Standards of Practice, and state regulation of athletic training have created a level of expectation for athletic training.

When a certified athletic trainer fails to act appropriately or acts inappropriately in providing athletic training services and injures an individual, the certified athletic trainer may be found negligent in tort. In relation to the application of therapeutic modalities, negligence in tort is likely to involve a negligent act. The certified athletic trainer is responsible for ensuring that the equipment used to apply modalities is properly maintained and calibrated and is in good working order, and that the modalities are applied in a manner that does not harm the individual. Negligent acts include burns caused by a moist heat pack with too little toweling for insulation, cold-induced nerve injury caused by inadequate instructions for applying ice packs at home, or electrical shock caused by faulty wiring on a poorly maintained transcutaneous electrical nerve stimulator. The certified athletic trainer must recognize when the application of a modality is contraindicated, must know how to apply a modality safely, and must instruct the individual properly if he or she is to self-administer a modality. Failure to do any of these things may constitute negligence if harm occurs with use of a therapeutic modality.

## THE REHABILITATION PLAN OF CARE

A team approach to treating physically active individuals is necessary because no single health care provider has all of the skills and resources needed to guide the athlete through rehabilitation. The rehabilitation plan of care is founded on the medical diagnosis provided by the physician and the physical examination of the injured athlete by the certified athletic trainer. The medical diagnosis is critical to determine whether surgery is necessary, to determine whether medications are indicated, and to estimate the rate of progression that the healing tissues will tolerate.

The physician and certified athletic trainer must also identify specific short-term goals for the injured athlete. A medical diagnosis may be a Grade II lateral ankle sprain. However, the rehabilitation plan of care addresses not the lateral ankle sprain but the pain, loss of motion, loss of strength, decreased neuromuscular control, and inability to fully bear weight, walk, run, jump, cut, or play basketball: in other words, the signs, symptoms, impairments, disabilities, and handicaps resulting from the injury. In addition, the physician and certified athletic trainer must identify factors that may limit adherence to rehabilitation, including the athlete's psychological-emotional response to the injury. Finally, the short-term goals that are established to address specific needs such as pain control or improved neuromuscular control must be tied to the individual's achievement of long-term goals. Thus, the medical diagnosis is only part of determining the best approach to rehabilitation.

Developing a rehabilitation plan of care may sound difficult; however, some basic concepts make the process much easier. First, a basic rehabilitation model should be used as the framework for the plan of care. Second, the plan of care must address the problems identified in the physical examination; thus, a plan of care is individualized. Third, the plan of care should be progressive, with clearly identified performance or time-specified criteria for progression to more complex and challenging activities.

Clinicians generally agree on the order of priorities in a progressive rehabilitation plan of care. The model presented in figure 1.3 provides a guide to progression of a rehabilitation plan of care. Following a complete clinical examination, the first priority in all health care is to do no harm. It is necessary to protect injured tissues from further damage and to allow for healing and the restoration of tissue integrity. The control of pain and swelling is also of high priority early in the rehabilitation process. Pain is one of the worst of human experiences; it makes us miserable, affects sleep, and alters neuromuscular control and function. Once a diagnosis is established, pain has served its purpose (warning the individual that something is wrong) and should be alleviated to the greatest degree possible.

Once the certified athletic trainer is assured that damaged tissues have been properly protected and pain and swelling have been addressed, attention is given to restoring range of motion about the involved joints. Injury and inflammation result in swelling, muscle guarding, and loss of motion. Functional recovery usually requires normal amounts of joint range of motion.

In addition to working to restore motion lost due to injury, the certified athletic trainer must work to restore neuromuscular control and muscular endurance (neuromuscular control is discussed in detail in chapters 6 and 15). Pain, swelling, and joint instability alter how the nervous system coordinates muscle contractions. Neuromuscular control and muscular endurance must be reestablished so the athlete can perform the low-resistance, high-repetition activities that are the foundation of strength and power training.

As the injured athlete recovers, the rehabilitation plan is progressed to address losses of strength and power and muscular endurance. *Strength* is the ability to do work, whereas *power* is a measure of the rate at which the work is done. Success in sport requires muscular strength and power. Generally, strength is addressed first with slow, controlled exercises. Power training is then added through plyometric exercises, sprinting, and other rapid movement training. In most sports, repeated or sustained muscular activity is required. Thus, *endurance*, or the ability to repeat and sustain activity, must also be retrained.

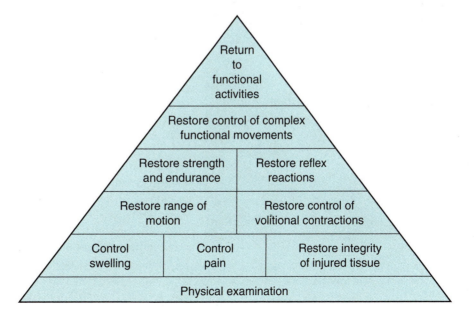

**Figure 1.3** A progressive model for rehabilitation of physically active individuals.

Reprinted by permission from Hertel and Denegar 1998.

Finally, the sport-specific needs of the athlete must be met. The functional requirements, much like the endurance requirements, differ among sports, positions, and events. A basketball player who can run, jump, and cut may not be ready to return to the game because of inability to backpedal, or a football player may not be ready to return to the offensive line because of poor footwork. Each sport and athletic activity places unique demands on the body. As a rehabilitation plan of care progresses, it should become more specific to the demands of the individual's sport and work activities.

Therapeutic modalities are primarily used to alleviate pain and allow individuals to initiate therapeutic exercises to improve range of motion and regain neuromuscular control. The certified athletic trainer should understand how the modality application affects the body and the rationale for each modality application. Modality application is not a treatment but a passive intervention that enables individuals to meet specific, short-term rehabilitation goals.

In addition to working toward specific goals related to the injury, the sports medicine team must also strive to maintain the individual's overall fitness level. Exercise to maintain cardiovascular fitness and strength should be incorporated into the rehabilitation plan as soon as it is safe to do so. Stationary cycling, stair climbing, aquatic exercising, and circuit training can be used to maintain fitness while protecting healing tissues and can provide some variety in the injured person's routine. Physically active individuals also experience a withdrawal phenomenon when their regular physical exercise routine is disrupted by injury. Including safe aerobic exercise and weight training in the rehabilitation plan helps individuals cope with this disruption. Figure 1.4 provides an example of an individualized plan of care.

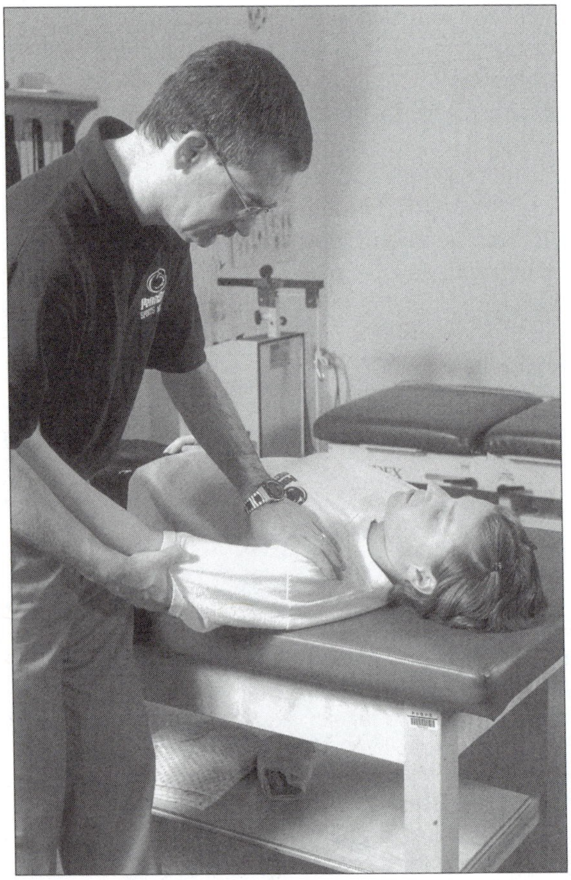

**Figure 1.4**   A plan of care is individualized with clear criteria to check progress toward more complex and challenging activities and recovery.

## *Monitoring Progress*

Progress implies change. A team physician we once worked with was fond of saying, "If things do not stay the same they will get better or worse." There are numerous potential pitfalls in evaluating and rehabilitating injured individuals. Incomplete diagnoses, poor adherence to the plan of care, and excessive activity can slow or prevent recovery from injury and return to competition. The sports medicine team must monitor an individual's progress during rehabilitation, discouraging excessive or inappropriate activities and adding challenging activities when appropriate.

Two factors guide progression. The first is tissue healing. In some circumstances, such as fractures and anterior cruciate ligament reconstruction, the time the body needs to repair the tissues is relatively well established. Although pain is often a reasonable guide for exercise progression, the team physician may specify a time frame of restricted activity.

The second factor is successful completion of short-term goals related to the earlier stages of rehabilitation. If healing tissues are adequately protected, the initial short-term goals will be based on the first three rehabilitation priorities. For example, following a lateral ankle sprain there may a considerable amount of pain. Appropriate short-term goals may include reducing pain to a rating of 2 (on a scale of 0 = *no pain*, 10 = *worst pain imaginable*) at rest in 2 days and a rating of 2 in full weight bearing in 1 week. If range of motion is lost, restoring full ankle range of motion in 10 days is a reasonable short-term goal.

Progression should be performance based. For example, a physically active person may ask how long she must remain on crutches after spraining her lateral ankle ligaments. These ligaments are not stressed by walking, only by extreme ankle inversion. Thus, a good guide for return to full weight bearing is a normal, pain-free walking gait. If walking is painful, the

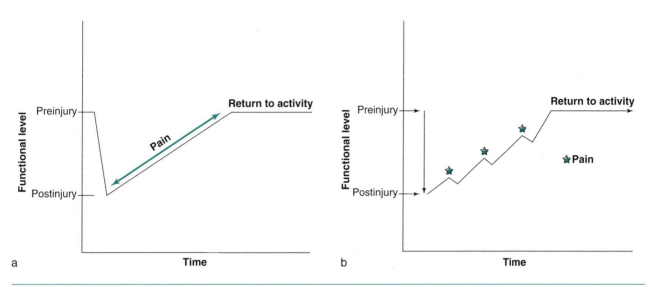

**Figure 1.5**  The return to activity is a continuum; avoiding pain with exercise as activity increases facilitates early functional recovery *(a)*. Recovery of function is delayed when the threshold of healing tissue is exceeded and pain occurs *(b)*.

Adapted by permission from Gieck and Saliba 1988.

first goal of rehabilitation has not been fully achieved. Limping is an altered neuromuscular pattern to avoid pain. Thus, to this physically active person, progression is simple and performance oriented.

Communication is essential to monitoring the injured person's progress through rehabilitation. Each individual will respond differently, and feedback from the athlete is vital. Some individuals must be cautioned repeatedly about being overly aggressive, whereas others must be encouraged to do more. Much of the individual response hinges on a person's response to pain. Some people approach therapeutic exercise with a "no pain, no gain" mentality. The sports medicine team must help such individuals interpret their pain sensation to protect healing tissues. Other people will stop exercise at the first sensation of pain, even though some discomfort is expected at various stages of most rehabilitation programs. Individuals who know what to expect will be better able to interpret their pain and make progress with their rehabilitation. Figure 1.5 shows theoretical and realistic return-to-activity models.

The final stage in recovery from injury is the return to unrestricted training, practice, and competition. Clearance to return to sport activity is a team decision. The individual must feel physically and psychologically ready. The team physician and certified athletic trainer must consider whether the injured tissues can withstand the stresses of sport and whether the individual's overall level of fitness is sufficient for him or her to play effectively without undue risk of injury. Coaches can provide valuable insight into the physical capabilities and psychological motivation of physically active individuals. Most importantly, clearance to return to play must be based on performance assessment as well as physical examination. The person evaluated solely in an office or athletic training room may appear capable of returning to sport, yet field evaluation may reveal significant losses of sport-specific agility, power, or endurance. Ideally, the certified athletic trainer and coaches should evaluate the individual's functional performance and gain physician approval before giving final clearance for unrestricted activity.

## Documenting Progress

Paperwork is the bane of health care providers. Preparing and maintaining good records is often challenging, but it is essential work. This subject is given considerable attention in the final text in the series: *Management Strategies in Athletic Training, Third Edition* (Ray 2005). However, it would be remiss not to mention documentation in this chapter.

## Patient Pain and Activity Inventory

Name _____    Date _____

1. Date of injury or date of onset of symptoms: _____
2. New injury: ☐ Yes ☐ No     Reinjury: ☐ Yes ☐ No
3. Please rate your general health (circle one):
   Excellent     Good     Fair     Poor
4. Please rate your pain with 0 being no pain and 10 being pain as bad as it can be since injury or in the last four weeks.

| | | | | | | | | | | | |
|---|---|---|---|---|---|---|---|---|---|---|---|
| Now | 0 | 1 | 2 | 3 | 4 | 5 | 6 | 7 | 8 | 9 | 10 |
| Best | 0 | 1 | 2 | 3 | 4 | 5 | 6 | 7 | 8 | 9 | 10 |
| Worst | 0 | 1 | 2 | 3 | 4 | 5 | 6 | 7 | 8 | 9 | 10 |
| With activity | 0 | 1 | 2 | 3 | 4 | 5 | 6 | 7 | 8 | 9 | 10 |

5. Please choose the best word or words that describe your pain (circle as many as apply):
   Sharp   Dull   Ache   Burning   Tingling   Numbness
6. How long does the pain last? _____ hours/day _____ days/week
7. Please mark location of your pain with an "X."

R     L     R     L

8. Please list three (3) important activities that you are unable to do or that you are having difficulty doing as a result of your problem with 0 being unable to perform the activity and 10 being able to perform activity at preinjury level.

| Activities: | | | | | | | | | | | |
|---|---|---|---|---|---|---|---|---|---|---|---|
| 1. | 0 | 1 | 2 | 3 | 4 | 5 | 6 | 7 | 8 | 9 | 10 |
| 2. | 0 | 1 | 2 | 3 | 4 | 5 | 6 | 7 | 8 | 9 | 10 |
| 3. | 0 | 1 | 2 | 3 | 4 | 5 | 6 | 7 | 8 | 9 | 10 |

**Figure 1.6**   A sample patient self-report.
Reprinted by permission from Houglum 2005.

Good records are needed to assess the benefits of treatment and rehabilitation. There is an increasingly greater demand in the managed care environment for health care providers to demonstrate that what they do makes a difference in patient care. The use of patient self-reports (figure 1.6) can facilitate communication between the athlete and the certified athletic trainer. These forms allow the athlete to document improving or worsening symptoms. Patient self-reports can also improve our understanding of which interventions are most beneficial in the treatment of the injured athlete.

Good records also are essential in a defense against a charge of negligence. Malpractice cases often take years to reach the courtroom, and a good memory will never prevail over good documentation. Figure 1.7 provides an example of an individual injury evaluation and treatment record.

Without a complete record of the case, specific details of the individual's problem and treatments will not be available. Develop good record-keeping skills and make a habit of documenting the modalities and specific parameters you select in treating each individual.

## Individual Injury Evaluation and Treatment Record

Name _____ Sport _____ Body part _____

Date injury occurred _____ Date injury reported _____ New _____ Old _____

Primary complaint _____ Secondary complaint _____

Subjective evaluation:

Objective evaluation:

Assessment:

Plan:

Evaluator's initials _____

| Date | Treatments and progress |
|------|-------------------------|
|      |                         |
|      |                         |
|      |                         |
|      |                         |
|      |                         |
|      |                         |
|      |                         |
|      |                         |
|      |                         |

**Figure 1.7**   A sample form used to record the evaluation and treatment of an injured athlete.
Reprinted by permission from Ray 1994.

## SUMMARY

1. Discuss how state regulation of athletic training may influence the use of therapeutic modalities in the care of physically active individuals.

   Athletic training is regulated in many states through state practice acts. The state practice act defines what an athletic trainer may do, whom the athletic trainer may treat, and where treatments can be administered. Although the certified athletic trainer may be educated and trained to use therapeutic modalities to treat musculoskeletal injuries, state regulations may restrict modality application depending on the setting, amateur or professional status of the individual being treated, or modality used.

2. Identify the hierarchy of components in a progressive rehabilitation plan.

   A progressive rehabilitation plan consists of six stages: (1) a complete clinical examination; (2) controlling pain and swelling and protecting damaged tissues; (3) restoring range of motion and volitional neuromuscular control; (4) restoring reflexive neuromuscular control, strength, and muscular endurance; (5) restoring power and control over complex functional movement; and (6) resuming sport-specific training.

3. Discuss guidelines for progressing an athlete through a comprehensive plan of care.

   Progression through a comprehensive rehabilitation plan of care is based on protecting healing tissues and achieving short-term goals. If healing tissues are adequately protected, pain during and following activity is the primary guide to progression. Active exercise should be pain free, and the individual should be able to do tomorrow what was done today.

## CITED SOURCES

Hertel J, Denegar CR: A rehabilitation paradigm for restoring neuromuscular control following athletic injury. *Athletic Therapy Today* 3(5/12-16, 1998).

National Athletic Trainers' Association: *Code of Ethics.* Dallas, NATA, 2005, www.nata.org//about/codeofethics.htm

National Athletic Trainers' Association: *Athletic Training Educational Competencies for the Health Care of the Physically Active.* Dallas, NATA, 1999.

Board of Certification for the Athletic Trainer: *Role Delineation Study*, 5th ed. Omaha NE, National Athletic Trainers' Association Board of Certification, Inc, 2004.

Perrin DH, Gieck JH. *Principles of Therapeutic Exercise in the Injured Athlete*, 3rd ed. Philadelphia, Lippincott-Raven, 1999.

Ray R: *Management Strategies in Athletic Training*, 3rd ed. Champaign, IL, Human Kinetics, 2005.

Sacket DL, Straus SE, Richardson WS, Rosenberg W, Haynes RB: *Evidence-Based Medicine: How to Practice and Teach EBM*, 2nd ed. Philadelphia: Churchill Livingstone, 2000.

Scott RW: *Health Care Malpractice.* Thorofare, NJ, Slack, 1990.

## ADDITIONAL READINGS

Canavan PK: *Rehabilitation in Sports Medicine.* Stamford, CT, Appleton & Lange, 1998.

Herbert DL: *Legal Aspects of Sports Medicine.* Canton, OH, Professional Reports Corp., 1990.

Worrell TW, Reynolds NL: Integrating physiologic and psychological paradigms into orthopaedic rehabilitation. *Orthop Phys Ther Clin North Am* 3:269-289, 1994.

Zachazewski JE, Magee DJ, Quillen WS: *Athletic Injuries and Rehabilitation.* Philadelphia, Saunders, 1996.

# CHAPTER 2

# Psychological Aspects of Rehabilitation

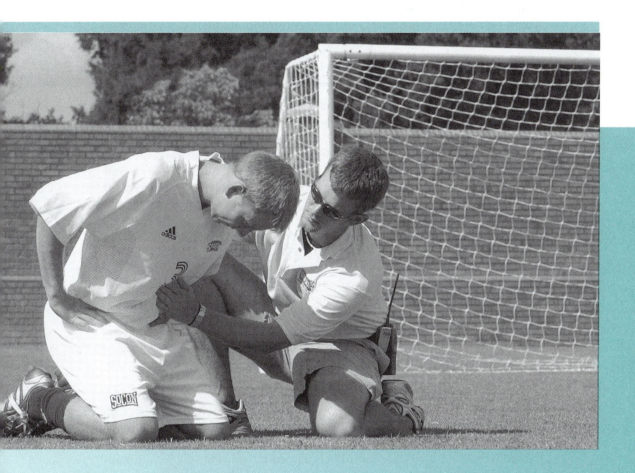

## Objectives

After reading this chapter, the student will be able to

1. compare and contrast the contemporary stage model and biopsychosocial model of psychological response to injury;

2. discuss the impact that cognitive appraisal can have on the athlete's psychological and emotional response to injury;

3. identify influences over an individual's ability to cope with an athletic injury;

4. identify factors that improve an athlete's adherence to a rehabilitation plan;

5. identify common barriers to successful completion of rehabilitation; and

6. discuss assessment of treatment outcomes in the context of natural history, placebo, and "true" treatment effect.

A retired man who is an avid golfer enters a sports medicine clinic for treatment of his shoulder, which was injured when he tripped while carrying his golf bag. He complains of stiffness and a loss of motion in the shoulder. However, his primary concern is that the injury is preventing him from playing golf and that this disability might be permanent. Physical examination reveals an extensive contusion to the right shoulder; however, the joint appears to be stable and the rotator cuff intact. He responds well to transcutaneous electrical nerve stimulation (TENS) and moist heat, prescribed to reduce pain and spasm, and active assistance and active range of motion exercise during his initial treatment. Swinging a short iron is included in the initial therapy session. The patient is far less anxious on leaving the clinic than when he entered.

He complies well with his home care program and requires just four additional treatments in the clinic. He gradually progresses his golfing activities, beginning on the driving range, then playing 9 holes, and after 4 weeks of recovery playing 18 holes.

Effective rehabilitation requires a comprehensive plan of care with specific, progressive goals. This text was written to develop your skills in applying therapeutic modalities to achieve some rehabilitation goals. Two important concepts were introduced in chapter 1: (1) A rehabilitation plan of care is based on medical diagnosis and evaluation of the injured person's needs; and (2) each individual will respond uniquely to injury, requiring you to individualize the plan of care to treat the person, not just the injury.

Perhaps the most important concept in treating individuals with musculoskeletal injuries is that the mind and body are connected. In the situation described at the beginning of this chapter, the patient's program included swinging a golf club, a sport-specific exercise that alleviated much of the individual's anxiety about playing golf again. The anatomical connection is obvious and not a new concept. The relationships between physical injury and psychological response, and between psychological dysfunction and somatic pain, are complex. This chapter is about those relationships. Before applying a therapeutic modality, you will need to appreciate the psychological aspects of rehabilitation, just as you understand the physical aspects of injury.

This chapter is based on the clinical skill and the wisdom of mental health professionals, physicians, certified athletic trainers, and physical therapists who have shared their knowledge and experience. Certified athletic trainers work closely with individuals before and after injury; and the understanding, personal attention, and caring attitude that athletic trainers can provide significantly influence a person's psychological and physical recovery. This chapter presents several issues related to the mind–body connection including the psychological response to injury, compliance with a treatment plan, barriers to success in rehabilitation, and placebo effects.

Each of these issues relates to an individual's response to treatment with therapeutic modalities. Furthermore, the complex interrelationships among psychological, physical, and social factors present the greatest obstacle in evaluating the efficacy of therapeutic interventions. Treatment outcomes studies will indicate which therapeutic interventions are most effective. Until more is known, the optimal treatment plan for each individual will result from a holistic approach to evaluation and treatment. Rather than present only the physical aspects of rehabilitation (treatment outcomes), this book takes a more holistic approach, which is why this chapter precedes discussion of the physiology of injury, modality application, and therapeutic exercise.

# PSYCHOLOGICAL RESPONSE TO INJURY

Many athletic trainers were introduced to the concept of psychological response to injury by way of Kubler-Ross's writings about death and dying. Kubler-Ross (1969) described a five-stage psychological response to terminal illness, which included stages of denial and isolation, anger, bargaining, depression, and acceptance. Early scholars applied this paradigm to injury, suggesting that the injured person first denies the severity of the injury and then expresses anger. A bargaining stage might include statements such as "If the ligament isn't torn I will train in the weight room every day." Unrealistic bargaining was thought to give way to depression, followed by acceptance of the injury and the consequences. More recent work has emphasized that physically active individuals may experience some of these responses following injury, but they are not dying. Furthermore, these individuals do not progress through stages. These people may express anger at the time of the injury, or not until they become bored with the routine and slow progression of rehabilitation. Most injured athletes do not experience depression. Thus, the paradigm described by Kubler-Ross does not adequately describe the typical psychological response to athletic injury.

This death-and-dying model of psychological response to athletic injury has been challenged and over time replaced. More recent models are predicated on the uniqueness of the individual response to an injury and the recognition that many factors influence how people cope and how well they adhere to a plan of care following injury.

## Biopsychosocial Models of Disease and Injury

Several biopsychosocial models are used to describe psychological response to athletic injury. Nagi (1965) described a model with four components of injury and response: disease, **impairment,** functional limitation, and **disability.** If *musculoskeletal injury* replaces *disease*, this model is easily applied to injured physically active people (figure 2.1).

For example, consider a volleyball player who injured her knee. The injury was diagnosed as a Grade II tibial collateral ligament sprain. The sprain to the ligament was the musculoskeletal injury. The player experienced pain, loss of motion, and loss of strength following the injury. These impairments resulted in **functional limitations,** among them the inability to walk without assistance or perform physical tasks including sport-specific activities such as running and jumping. This volleyball player could not play her sport, work part-time as a waitress on the weekends, participate in physical education, or go hiking with her family. These limitations on performance in sport, school, employment, and family activities represent her disabilities.

In this model, injury is more than tissue damage; attention is focused on the individual's entire response to the injury. This model presents an enlightening concept: To understand the physically active person's psychological response to an injury, one needs to appreciate the impact of the injury on the athlete's life, not just the pathology.

## Cognitive Appraisal Models

In response to the inadequacies of stage models such as the death-and-dying paradigm, cognitive-based appraisal models have been developed. The common feature in these models is that an individual's psychological and emotional response to injury depends on his or her appraisal or understanding of the injury and the stressors present in the context of the injury and rehabilitation. Recall the case study of the golfer presented at the beginning of the chapter.

**Figure 2.1** Nagi model of the process of disablement in the context of musculoskeletal injury in physically active people.

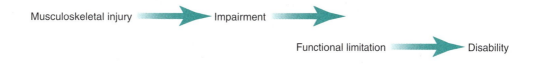

Musculoskeletal injury → Impairment → Functional limitation → Disability

His response to injury changed dramatically after he understood the nature of his injury and the limitations it was likely to place on his life. He did not work through stages of response to injury; rather, his psychological and emotional response was altered by his cognitive appraisal of his injury, impairments, functional limitations, and disabilities.

The cognitive appraisal models are distinguished from the stage models in three important ways. The first distinction is that some or most of the labeled stages may be absent in the cognitive appraisal models. For example, as already mentioned, most injured athletes do not become depressed (Wegener 1999). Depression can be a significant barrier to recovery and must be recognized and treated when it occurs, but its occurrence is the exception rather than the rule.

The second distinction is that the psychological and emotional response to injury does not progress in a structured order in the cognitive appraisal models (Wegener 1999; Yukelson and Heil 1998). Injured individuals may express little anger and frustration following an injury, accept their situation and cope, and then become angry and confrontational following a setback in rehabilitation. Such a response may also be associated with individuals' perceptions that their progress is slower than expected. This response seems to be associated with programs that vary little from day to day and week to week.

The third distinction is that cognitive appraisal models imply that the individual's psychological and emotional response to injury is affected by his or her understanding of the injury and the psychosocial environment (figure 2.2). Thus, whether a physically active person adapts and copes effectively following injury or demonstrates **maladaptive behaviors** can be influenced by members of the sports medicine team as well as the athlete's peers, friends, family, and coaches.

Again, recall the golfer described at the beginning of this chapter. Understanding the physically active person's perception of the injury and our natural fear of the unknown is crucial. Had attention been focused solely on the injured shoulder and not the person, the golfer's primary concern and goal may have been overlooked. More important, however, the certified athletic trainer would have lost the opportunity to affect the psychological response to the injury. Swinging a golf club is not standard in shoulder rehabilitation programs. However, including this activity assured the athlete that his season was not over.

Knowledge and understanding (cognition) alter the psychological-emotional response to injury (Wegener 1999). Providing the type and amount of information that injured people need takes experience and practice. Some individuals ask a lot of questions and want detailed information. For others, the information needs to be more general and less detailed. Finding the right level is important and quite subjective. Don't be overly simplistic and "talk down," but don't try to impress someone with your knowledge. If an injured person wants more information than is provided, he or she often has less confidence in the care providers and is less compliant with a plan of care. However, an individual who feels overwhelmed by information will be confused and anxious. You must listen and observe; the initial evaluation is a critical time to promote effective coping following injury.

## Personality and Environmental Influences

An individual's ability to cope following injury is influenced by many factors. Some people are natural worriers, tending to overreact to life's frustrations, whereas others seem to manage the ups and downs effectively. Someone's ability to cope also

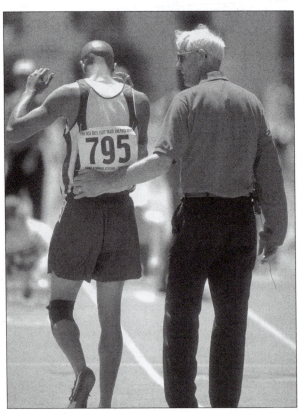

**Figure 2.2** An athlete's peers, friends, family, and coaches can influence how an athlete adapts and copes with an injury.

depends on his or her current situation and life stressors. An athlete who coped effectively with an off-season injury in high school may maladapt to a similar in-season injury in college, because the college environment, the pressure to return to competition, and decreased daily support from family, teammates, and coaches alter the individual's stressors and coping resources (Wegener 1999).

The sports medicine team cannot influence all of the factors that promote a maladaptive response. However, a holistic approach to care of the physically active individual will improve understanding of the individual's situation. An athletic training room and clinical environment that promote attention to the individual's needs are essential. Crowded, noisy facilities can leave the injured person asking, "Does anybody care?" Such an environment also diminishes the likelihood of identifying maladaptive behaviors, intervening within the limits of one's training and ability, and making appropriate referrals (Fisher and Hoisington 1998; Fisher et al. 1993).

An injury will force the athlete to adapt. Whether that adaptation is functional or dysfunctional depends on many factors. Certainly the severity of the injury, timing of the injury, and coping resources available to the athlete strongly influence the individual's response. The psychological and emotional response does not proceed through a series of stages, and the response can differ significantly from person to person and within the same individual under different circumstances. The sports medicine team must create an atmosphere conducive to compliance with rehabilitation, must respect the unique nature of each person's response, and must identify barriers to treatment compliance and recovery.

# MAXIMIZING COMPLIANCE WITH A REHABILITATION PLAN OF CARE

Perhaps the greatest influence on adherence to rehabilitation and a positive psychological and emotional adaptation following injury is the rapport established with the injured athlete's caregivers. Certified athletic trainers are often in a unique position among health care professionals in that a working relationship with the physically active individual is established before an injury occurs. Additionally, high school and college athletes are usually familiar with the athletic training room environment and have confidence in the ability of the sports medicine staff to provide a high standard of care.

One major difference between working in a high school, college, or professional setting and working in a sports medicine clinic is the nature of the initial encounter with the injured person. Because a preestablished rapport between the injured individual and the certified athletic trainer, present when the certified athletic trainer works with a team on a daily basis, is usually absent in the clinical setting, individuals are uncertain and anxious about what they will experience. Many general orthopedic patients enter the sports medicine clinic believing that therapy and rehabilitation are unlikely to relieve their condition or will be a painful experience. Thus, there is a premium placed on the initial encounter. A caring, empathetic demeanor is essential. The certified athletic trainer must learn about the problem in terms of the injury, impairment, disability, and handicap. The injured individual should leave with an understanding of these issues, the program that will be used to address rehabilitation goals, and his or her responsibilities in resolving the problem. Conducting a successful initial evaluation in a sports medicine clinic requires practice, refined attention to verbal and nonverbal communication, and portrayal of oneself as a competent, caring health care provider.

## Set Goals

The importance of setting obtainable yet challenging short- and long-term rehabilitation goals has been noted by sport psychologists and sport rehabilitation specialists (Gieck 1990; Locke and Latham 1985; Worrell and Reynolds 1994). Often these goals seem obvious to the certified athletic trainer; however, the establishment and achievement of rehabilitation goals are novel to the injured individual. Figure 2.3 shows short- and long-term rehabilitation goals for the senior golfer with the sore shoulder described earlier.

**Short-term goals**

• Pain relief at rest and early motion exercises within 5 days

• Independent in-home exercise program within 5 days

• Pain-free golf swing with short irons and putting within 10 days

**Long-term goals**

• Pain-free golf swing with woods and long irons and putting within 3 weeks

• Return to golf within 4 weeks

**Figure 2.3**   Short- and long-term goals for an injured golfer.

The injured individual and the certified athletic trainer must agree on rehabilitation goals. Often clinicians establish treatment goals without listening to what the patient views as important. On the other hand, the athletic trainer cannot adopt unrealistic goals expressed by the injured person to guide rehabilitation. Individuals with injuries tend to look only at the ultimate goal: return to competition. Often the time frame for achieving the ultimate goal is unrealistic, and important steps in a progressive plan of care are ignored. By incorporating the individual's ultimate goal into the plan of care, you can educate athletes on the need to achieve simpler, short-term goals (e.g., achieve full knee range of motion) as part of the comprehensive plan to achieve the ultimate goal (e.g., return to playing varsity soccer following anterior cruciate ligament [ACL] reconstruction).

The injured person may not value the short-term goal until it is placed in the context of achieving the ultimate goal. Adherence to a plan of care and achievement of short-term goals are improved when the goals and values are addressed as the plan of care is formulated.

Establishing short-term goals that are integral to returning to sport has an additional positive influence, especially when the recovery period is lengthy. The person recovering from a surgery such as ACL reconstruction can become frustrated by the perception that day-to-day progress is too slow. This can be countered by the positive reinforcement provided when short-term goals are achieved. Short-term goals that can be realistically accomplished in 1 to 3 weeks yet are challenging seem to work best. The individual who is reminded of the short-term goals accomplished can better cope with the frustrations inherent in a long course of rehabilitation.

## Share Responsibility

Treatment and rehabilitation of the injured individual are not *done to* the individual but are *done by* the individual. Through active involvement in establishing goals, the individual learns what responsibilities he or she has if rehabilitation is to be successful (figure 2.4). You must remember that the injury is not your problem. Often young clinicians can become overly possessive of the patient and the patient's problem. The duty of the certified athletic trainer, as for all other care professionals, is to provide a high standard of care, not to accept all of the responsibility for achieving goals.

Physically active individuals like supervision by a certified athletic trainer during their rehabilitation (Fisher and Hoisington 1998; Fisher et al. 1993). The presence of a certified athletic trainer during rehabilitation encourages individuals to do what is expected of them. In a busy athletic training room, however, daily supervision is not always possible. Furthermore, in the current managed care environment, most people treated in a sports medicine clinic must be willing to comply with a program of independent or home-based exercises due to limitations on the number of covered treatment sessions. Thus, you must effectively teach and convey the importance of the exercise program.

To increase adherence to a home exercise program, you can (1) have the individual perform each exercise before leaving the sports medicine clinic, (2) provide written instructions as well as illustrations, (3) provide an exercise log to record performance, and (4) have the

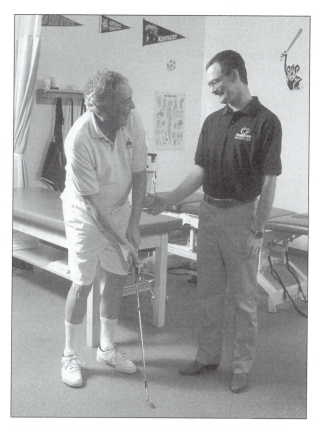

**Figure 2.4** The injured individual should be actively involved in establishing goals if the rehabilitation plan of care is to be successful.

individual demonstrate the exercise program at the beginning of the next treatment session. Proper performance of the exercise program should be positively reinforced. If an injured person is unable to complete the exercise program, he or she has not complied with the plan of care. In this situation you must first reconsider the appropriateness of the program. If some exercises increased pain or were beyond the individual's capacity, the exercise program must be modified. However, if the individual has no specific complaints about the exercise program, a nonjudgmental review of the exercise should dominate the treatment session. Failure to have successfully completed the exercise program on the next return visit is strong evidence that the person is unwilling or unable to accept responsibility for getting better. Although this type of person is frustrating to work with, remember that it is the individual's problem, not yours.

## Focus on Today

The longer time a rehabilitation plan will require to complete, the more imposing the task appears. Individuals can get lost in the big picture of their rehabilitation and lose focus and motivation. Thoughts can become irrational and catastrophic in nature. "I will never be able to play again" is sometimes heard from the individual who is frustrated by the pace of recovery and anxious about the future. You can help such patients work through these problems by focusing on what can be accomplished today. Successful rehabilitation requires a lot of small accomplishments, not a miracle cure. Focus the injured person on the short-term goals to be achieved today or this week. Be patient and empathetic. Use thought stopping and positive imagery, as well as examples of successful outcomes, to combat irrational thinking and assist the individual during periods of frustration and doubt. For example, following a lateral ankle sprain, a soccer player becomes frustrated by his slow return to full weight bearing. His thought, "I will never be able to play again," is "stopped" and replaced with "Rehabilitation takes time; Bobby hurt his knee badly last year but is now playing better than ever." The soccer player is encouraged to stop negative thinking, replace negative thoughts with positive ones, and envision his return to top-level play.

## Minimize Suffering

Pain is a universal human experience and a signal that something is wrong. Pain is usually what causes people to seek medical care. Although nearly all humans experience pain, the psychological and emotional response is very individual. One of the challenges in health care is understanding each individual's response in relation to the severity of the injury or illness.

Pain control is almost always the first goal in a comprehensive rehabilitation plan. Many of the therapeutic modalities discussed in this book have analgesic (pain relieving) effects. Through a professional and empathetic demeanor and effective initial treatment (including pain control), the certified athletic trainer can build a bond of trust with the injured individual. If the athletic trainer fails to decrease the person's pain during the first one to two treatments, adherence with the rehabilitation program may decline or the individual may seek care elsewhere.

Physically active people often have a different perspective on pain than nonactive people, which has important implications for the certified athletic trainer. Physically active people view the pain experienced in training and conditioning as a challenge to be overcome. Thus, during rehabilitation, these people may have difficulty differentiating pain due to irritation of healing tissues (bad pain) from the pain of strenuous effort (good pain) and may be overly aggressive in rehabilitation. You must help physically active individuals interpret whether the pain they are experiencing during and after rehabilitation indicates further tissue injury, which will ultimately slow their recovery.

Physically active people are very attuned to their bodies. The self-inflicted pain of conditioning is expected and tolerated. However, the same is not true of the pain associated with medical procedures and rehabilitation. Byerly et al. (1994) reported that the more pain athletes experienced during their rehabilitation, the less they adhered to their plan of care. Athletes, however, reported that pain during therapeutic exercise was less of a deterrent to rehabilitation adherence than athletic trainers perceived it to be (Fisher and Hoisington 1998). Thus, you must monitor the rehabilitation plan closely and make modifications when self-reported pain affects compliance. Athletes and athletic trainers agree that an accurate appraisal of the pain to be experienced is important to adherence with a plan of care. Discuss issues related to pain with your athletes honestly and with empathy. Individuals who feel they are suffering unnecessarily will not comply with a plan of care and will often seek treatment elsewhere.

Finally, although each individual responds differently to pain and injury and these individual differences should be respected, physically active people are generally more willing to begin and progress through a rehabilitation plan. This is important for the certified athletic trainer used to working with highly competitive athletes; he or she may encounter relatively less active people in a clinical environment. Physically active people like to exercise, want to exercise, and feel comfortable with exercise. The differences between physically active and sedentary individuals are great. The sedentary person often struggles to learn therapeutic exercises, views exercise as a chore rather than a means of recovery, and stops at the slightest discomfort or exertion. These patients require greater instruction and supervision as well as patience on the part of the health care provider. You must be sensitive to the lower tolerance to pain and effort as well as the greater need for positive reinforcement and encouragement in less active people.

# BARRIERS TO SUCCESSFUL REHABILITATION

Injured physically active and relatively nonactive individuals present to the certified athletic trainer with personal and psychological issues that can affect their successful completion of rehabilitation. Sometimes you can help physically active individuals overcome these barriers by building a bond of trust and simply caring and listening. Sometimes you can identify someone who would benefit from psychological or psychiatric care. Unfortunately, there are some barriers to successful rehabilitation that you cannot change. It is important to remember that the patient has the problem and not to become physically and emotionally exhausted trying to change what you cannot. This section identifies some of the barriers to successful rehabilitation that are common to physically active as well as nonactive people.

## Secondary Gain

A physically active individual whose performance has not lived up to expectations may find solace in the fact that he or she tried to play while hurt but could not. Another individual may avoid the wrath of coaches or the media through a slow recovery. Others may use an injury to gain freedom from a sport in which they no longer wish to participate. In some cases, the individual may perceive that there is more to be gained by not getting better.

Secondary gain relates to tangible and intangible rewards received following injury. The notion of secondary gain is more associated with automobile accident victims with pending civil litigation or injured workers receiving nearly full salary while away from a job they dislike. However, there are many forms of secondary gain. Illness and injury can alter how others interact with a person. The injured person may gain additional attention from parents and others; may be relieved of some responsibilities at home, work, or school; or may experience other "positive" responses to injury. In some situations, the rewards of being ill or injured outweigh the rewards of returning to health.

The pursuit of secondary gain may be a poorly disguised conscious effort or a more subtle behavioral pattern. There is no single solution to treating the individual who can gain from slow progress or failure. Most work their way "through the system." You must not label someone as a malingerer without thoroughly reviewing the case (see chapter 5) yet you must also guard against self-doubt and a sense of failure when those with more to gain by being injured do not respond to appropriate care.

## Substance Use and Abuse

Alcohol and drug abuse continues to be a significant problem in our society. The media have reported on numerous athletes facing substance abuse problems. Collegiate athletes also tend to consume more alcohol than the average nonathletic student. Substance abuse decreases adherence to rehabilitation in general and especially affects performance of self-care and home exercise programs. Substance abuse is a sensitive issue, and few certified athletic trainers receive adequate training in the recognition, not to mention treatment, of this problem. It is a problem most certified athletic trainers do not want to confront. Drug and alcohol use increases the risks of, and impairs recovery from, injury. Thus, members of the sports medicine team should be trained to identify substance abuse, and a plan for physician involvement and appropriate treatment referral should be implemented to assist those with substance abuse problems.

## Social and Environmental Barriers

Injuries require adjustments in daily routine. Rehabilitation based in both the athletic training room and the sports medicine clinic utilizes special equipment and requires a time commitment from the physically active individual. Some people will find it difficult to adhere to a rehabilitation plan because of personal commitments, time demands, and lack of access to equipment and facilities. Certified athletic trainers in college and high school settings may be less affected by these barriers to successful rehabilitation than clinic-based trainers, but all athletes present with unique circumstances that favor or deter successful rehabilitation.

Many physically active individuals live in rural areas without a convenient sports medicine clinic. Their local schools have very limited training facilities, and the nearest fitness club is usually many miles away. Because they have to travel considerable distances to the sports medicine clinic, they may be unable to attend formal therapy sessions as often as they and their physicians would like. Creative home exercise programs must be developed for these people to overcome the lack of equipment, facilities, and hands-on care (figure 2.5).

Similarly, individuals with family and work responsibilities may be less compliant with rehabilitation because they lack support from others who can assume some of their responsibilities. You must account for these limitations as you develop a plan of care. Sometimes you will have to modify a program to meet the individual's needs and accept that the rate of progress may be slower. The injured individual must believe that she or he will be able to complete the rehabilitation program. If the plan of care conflicts with the time and energy available, the person probably will not adhere to the rehabilitation plan.

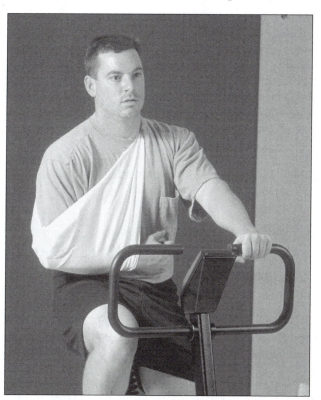

**Figure 2.5** Some physically active individuals find it difficult to adhere to a rehabilitation plan of care. Creative plans must be developed to fit the individual's needs, such as prescribing exercises that can be done at home or with limited equipment.

In the traditional setting, injury often also results in separation from a team and the loss of social support. The certified athletic trainer and the injured athlete's coach should explore ways to keep the athlete involved with the team, which will maximize support from peers and minimize disruption of the athlete's daily routine.

## Depression, Anxiety, and Sleep Disturbances

People who suffer serious injuries may develop concomitant problems related to depression and anxiety. These problems and persistent pain alter sleep patterns, which further depletes the individual's energy and coping resources.

**Depression** affects many people at some time in their lives. It is estimated that 9.5% of those over 18 years will suffer from depression in a given year, with 5% of the general population suffering a major depressive disorder (National Institute of Mental Health 2001). This rate is increased in injured persons and in patients following spinal cord injury, stroke, and heart attack. Depression is not a normal stage in the psychological response to injury but can be a significant barrier to successful rehabilitation (Wegener 1999).

Signs and symptoms of depression are discussed in more detail in chapter 5 in relation to persistent pain and somatization. The certified athletic trainer usually interacts with the injured individual more than do other members of the sports medicine team and is, therefore, in a position to recognize these signs. Depression is a treatable psychological illness that deserves medical attention. However, there is a stigma in our society regarding psychological conditions. When depression affects an individual's rehabilitation efforts, the sports medicine team must strive to provide the psychological care needed. Failure to recognize and treat depression will delay or prevent successful recovery from injury and a return to sport participation.

Anxiety disorders are characterized by excessive worry. The incidence of anxiety disorders is believed to be less than that of depression, and the effect of injury on the incidence of anxiety disorders is unknown. It is normal for an injured person to be anxious about the impact of the injury on her or his ability to participate, advancement on a team, or potential for scholarship or professional opportunities. However, extreme and unfounded worry can lead to sleep disturbances and adversely affect rehabilitation adherence. Informal counseling and relaxation techniques can be very effective in controlling anxiety. However, if someone continues to struggle, referral for psychological care is essential.

Depression, anxiety, and pain affect sleep. Anxiety is most associated with sleep onset problems, pain with midsleep awakening, and depression with early awakening (Wegener 1999). Regardless of the cause, a sleep disturbance affects a person's mood and general vitality.

## Case Study

A physically active man in his mid-50s was diagnosed with shoulder impingement syndrome and sought care at a sports medicine center. He was always attentive and complied with his rehabilitation plan of care but often seemed impatient and easily agitated. His primary complaint upon initial evaluation was that his shoulder pain awakened him several times each night. In fact, the effect of the pain on his sleeping over the previous 2 months had caused him to seek care from an orthopedic surgeon. The rehabilitation plan of care did not relieve the shoulder pain. A magnetic resonance image (MRI) revealed a tear of the rotator cuff. Surgery performed to repair the damaged rotator cuff resulted in near-complete relief of pain within a week. He was pleased because he could now get a full night's sleep. The difference in his mood was dramatic. He was far more pleasant and easy-going, and his wife commented that he was "his old self." This physically active man was not, in the opinion of the medical staff, depressed or overly anxious. However, the sleep disturbance resulting from the persistent shoulder pain was a significant issue. Sleep disturbances due to persistent pain can increase the risk for clinical depression. You should inquire about the impact of injury and persistent pain on sleep and recognize long-term sleep disturbance as a barrier to successful rehabilitation as well as a risk factor for depression.

# CLINICAL OUTCOMES AND EFFICACY OF THERAPEUTIC MODALITIES

Clinical outcomes data related to the efficacy of therapeutic modalities and other interventions used in athletic training or physical therapy are increasingly being entered into databases and systematically reviewed. At present, there are relatively few data related specifically to the impact of therapeutic modalities on the recovery of injured athletes. Much can be learned, however, from published clinical trials and systematic reviews. Historically, athletic trainers have used treatment strategies that "appear to work." As athletic trainers have shared their experiences with one another, new approaches to injury management have evolved. The treatments administered by athletic trainers have received less scrutiny than other areas of health care. There can be four reasons for this phenomenon.

The first is simply cost and complexity. Good outcomes studies are difficult to conduct, largely due to the difficulties of controlling for the psychosocial issues discussed previously.

Second is the natural history of most musculoskeletal injuries. The vast majority of musculoskeletal injuries sustained by physically active individuals will resolve over time without treatment. Intervention by the sports medicine team provides the individual with information about the nature of the injury, symptomatic relief, and guidance regarding activity restriction. Additionally, the sports medicine team can often safely return the physically active person to sport while tissues heal. The sports medicine team cannot, however, speed tissue repair and maturation.

The third reason for the lack of study of therapeutic interventions is that the treatments administered by certified athletic trainers are administered safely. Greater investigation into the use of therapeutic modalities by certified athletic trainers has not been triggered, because there are few reports of injury during treatment by certified athletic trainers. The education of certified athletic trainers has resulted in well-prepared health care providers who practice safe treatment techniques.

The fourth reason for the lack of inquiry into the treatments administered by athletic trainers is that in traditional settings, care is free to the athlete. Thus, there is no scrutiny from third-party payers asking for evidence of effective treatment.

This situation is changing. Because we better understand the pathophysiology of musculoskeletal injury and the physiology of tissue repair, some long-held beliefs about the ability of modalities to facilitate healing have been challenged. Judgments about the efficacy of individual modality applications, therapeutic exercises, or rehabilitation plans of care are increasingly based on studies that control for no treatment or studies that control for crossover effects of other treatments or modalities. Questions are being raised about the use of some therapeutic modalities (Denegar et al. 1992; Penderghest, Kimura, and Gulick 1998) and the need for extensive, supervised rehabilitation (Cherkin et al. 1998; Decarlo and Sell 1997). Researchers are studying which modalities promote the achievement of therapeutic goals, which conditions treatments are most effective for, and when and how frequently treatments should be applied. These investigations are complex; it is difficult to find a necessary number of similar patients to test treatment efficacy, and it is difficult to separate the effects of various components of a treatment plan. However, evidence is emerging that some modalities do not have the effects that they were once believed to have.

Because of these efforts, certified athletic trainers will be able to use their time and resources more effectively to provide optimal care in terms of cost and benefit. These efforts may also identify overworked athletic training staffs and overcrowded athletic training facilities. However, much of the research has focused on return to activities of daily living or work. The demands of sport are different from those of daily life, and athletes are motivated by the desire to compete. To examine the impact of athletic training services on return to sport, certified athletic trainers must assess outcomes. If we fail to do so, research involving the return of nonactive individuals to daily activities and work will be generalized to treatment of the physically active and will decrease the effectiveness of sports medicine care for this population.

# A WORD ABOUT PLACEBO

The vast majority of people treated by certified athletic trainers and physical therapists believe that treatments with therapeutic modalities and other interventions enhanced their recovery from injury. This observation can be explained by the natural history of most musculoskeletal injuries and the known benefits of treatment with therapeutic modalities and exercise. There is, however, another influence that the certified athletic trainer can use to help the injured athlete: placebo. The term *placebo*, derived from the Latin "I will please" (*Miller-Keane Encyclopedia* 1992), refers to a powerful influence on therapeutic interventions that is difficult to measure. Placebo is often thought of as a positive response to an inactive intervention such as providing a sugar pill in lieu of a real medication. However, bona fide interventions have a **placebo effect.** Believing that a medication or treatment will help can benefit the individual.

Placebo is not a treatment effect on gullible or unstable patients. It is a very real, positive mind–body response. The certified athletic trainer who can alleviate the injured person's anxiety by accurately assessing the nature and severity of an injury and establishing a plan for recovery builds a bond of trust. When the certified athletic trainer and the individual believe in the chosen treatment course, there is a high probability of success. How much of an individual response is due to treatment and how much to placebo? We do not know and can only say that a placebo effect is surely at work to some degree. Is a placebo effect bad? Absolutely not; the placebo effect helps people feel better and recover. In fact, today's managed care system, with its lack of personal touch and empathy, suffers from the loss of placebo.

Certainly, certified athletic trainers should continue to study the effects of treatments and rehabilitation programs. However, we should also remember the power of placebo and view it as a positive influence on recovery.

The mind–body relationship is complex and strongly influences response to injury as well as recovery, and a single chapter is not sufficient to cover all related issues. This chapter discussed the psychological and emotional response to injury. This response is individual and does not proceed through a series of stages as was once believed. The certified athletic trainer can facilitate adherence to rehabilitation and should attempt to identify and address barriers to successful rehabilitation. Certainly not all of an individual's problems lie within the certified athletic trainer's expertise and scope of practice. The sports medicine team should be prepared to use teamwork and appropriate referral to provide injured individuals with the care they need. Finally, the chapter addressed the placebo response, a poorly understood but positive influence on recovery that the athletic trainer should use to the injured individual's benefit.

## SUMMARY

1. Compare and contrast the contemporary stage model and the biopsychosocial model of psychological response to injury.

   The psychological response to injury has been described as occurring in stages, based on Kubler-Ross's work on death and dying. More recent literature suggests that the psychological response to injury is highly individual. Individuals do not experience all of the psychological responses described by Kubler-Ross, and the characteristics of the psychological response do not progress in ordered stages.

2. Discuss the impact that cognitive appraisal can have upon the athlete's psychological and emotional response to injury.

   The biopsychosocial model of psychological response to injury holds that an individual's understanding of the nature of the injury, its severity, and the prognosis, as well as other factors, alters the psychological response. Thus, cognition, or knowing about and understanding the injury, modifies the psychological response following that injury.

3. Identify influences over an individual's ability to cope with an athletic injury.

Multiple factors influence an individual's ability to cope with an athletic injury. Some, such as the tendency to worry and overreact, are intrinsic. Others, such as stresses from school, family, and athletic responsibilities and support from friends, family, teammates, and caregivers, are extrinsic. The sports medicine team cannot control all of these influences but can help individuals cope more effectively by identifying those who are struggling and the factors contributing to their stress.

4. Identify factors that improve an athlete's adherence to a rehabilitation plan.

Adherence to a rehabilitation plan can be enhanced by building rapport with the injured person, setting appropriate short- and long-term goals, establishing the injured person's responsibility to the rehabilitation program, focusing on the task at hand rather than the long haul, and minimizing the individual's suffering.

5. Identify common barriers to successful completion of rehabilitation.

Multiple factors are barriers to successful rehabilitation. Secondary gain, in terms of money or avoidance of situations or responsibilities, affects the rehabilitation process. Substance abuse, depression, anxiety, and sleep disturbances also impede rehabilitation. Family and work responsibilities and inconvenience of location or timing of appointments deter the progress of many individuals, especially those outside of high school and university settings.

6. Discuss assessment of treatment outcomes in the context of natural history, placebo, and "true" treatment effect.

It is very difficult to determine the true effects of treatments with therapeutic modalities. Most musculoskeletal injuries sustained by physically active people heal with time, allowing return to full athletic participation. In addition, a placebo response is common following treatment by medical and allied medical professionals. Extensive investigation is needed to identify which therapeutic modalities facilitate achievement of treatment goals and speed the rehabilitation process.

## CITED SOURCES

Byerly PN, Worrell T, Gahimer J, Domholdt E: Rehabilitation compliance in an athletic training environment. *J Athl Train* 29:352-355, 1994.

Cherkin DC, Deyo RA, Battie M, Street J, Barlow W: A comparison of physical therapy, chiropractic manipulation, and provision of an educational booklet for treatment of patients with low back pain. *New Engl J Med* 339:1021-1029, 1998.

DeCarlo MS, Sell KE: The effects of number and frequency of physical therapy treatments on selected outcomes of treatment in patients with anterior cruciate ligament reconstruction. *J Orthop Sports Phys Ther* 26:332-339, 1997.

Denegar CR, Yoho AP, Borowicz AJ, Bifulco N: The effects of low-volt microamperage stimulation of delayed onset muscle soreness. *J Sport Rehab* 1:95-102, 1992.

Fisher AC, Hoisington LL: Injured athletes' attitudes and judgments toward rehabilitation adherence. *J Athl Train* 28:43-47, 1998.

Fisher AC, Scriber KC, Matheny ML, Alderman MH, Bitting LA: Enhancing athletic injury rehabilitation adherence. *J Athl Train* 28:312-318, 1993.

Gieck J: Psychological considerations in rehabilitation. In Prentice WE (Ed), *Rehabilitation Techniques in Sports Medicine*. St. Louis, Mosby, 1990, 107-121.

Kubler-Ross E: *On Death and Dying*. New York, Macmillan, 1969.

Locke E, Latham GP: The application of goal setting in sports. *J Sport Psychol* 7:205-211, 1985.

*Miller-Keane Encyclopedia & Dictionary of Medicine, Nursing, & Allied Health*, 5th ed. Philadelphia, Saunders, 1992.

Nagi SZ: Some conceptual issues in disability and rehabilitation. In Sussman MB (Ed), *Sociology and Rehabilitation*. Washington, DC, American Sociological Association, 100-113, 1965.

National Institute of Mental Health. 2001. The numbers count: Mental disorders in America. www.nimh.nih.gov/publicat/numbers.cfm. Accessed 10/20/04.

Penderghest CE, Kimura IF, Gulick DT: Double-blind clinical efficacy study of pulsed phonophoresis on perceived pain associated with traumatic tendinitis. *J Sport Rehab* 7:9-19, 1998.

Wegener ST: *Current Concepts and Clinical Approaches in Psychology of Rehabilitation.* Paper presented at the National Athletic Trainers' Association 49th Annual Meeting and Clinical Symposia, Baltimore, MD, June 17, 1998, and the 50th Eastern Athletic Trainers' Association Annual Meeting, January 11, 1999.

Worrell TW, Reynolds NL: Integrating physiologic and psychological paradigms into orthopaedic rehabilitation. *Orthop Phys Ther Clin North Am* 3:269-289, 1994.

Yukelson D, Heil J: Psychological considerations in working with injured athletes. In Canavan PK (Ed), *Rehabilitation in Sports Medicine.* Stamford, CT, Appleton & Lange, 1998, 61-70.

## ADDITIONAL READINGS

Davis CM: *Patient Practitioner Interaction.* Thorofare, NJ, Slack, 1989.

Heil J: *Psychology of Sport Injury.* Champaign, IL, Human Kinetics, 1996.

Porter K, Foster J: *The Mental Athlete.* New York, Ballantine Books, 1986.

Purtillo R: *Health Professional and Patient Interaction,* 4th ed. Philadelphia, Saunders, 1990.

# CHAPTER 3

# Tissue Injury, Inflammation, and Repair

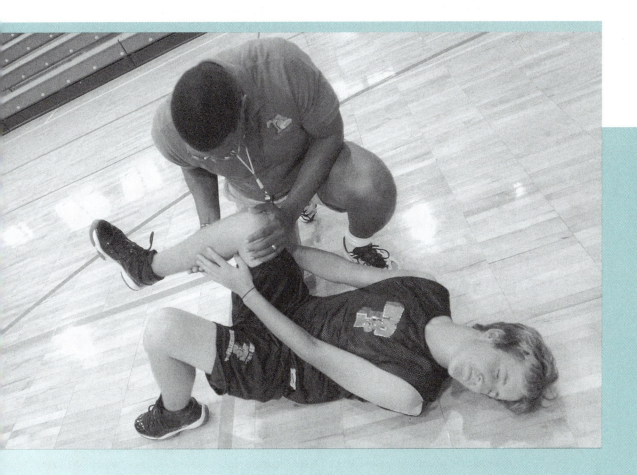

## Objectives

After reading this chapter, the student will be able to

1. describe the role of the inflammatory response in tissue healing;
2. identify key events in the acute inflammatory, repair, and remodeling phases of tissue healing;
3. identify the causes of chronic inflammation;
4. describe the events and controlling chemical mediators of the acute inflammatory response;

5. discuss the relationship between the signs and symptoms and the physiological events characteristic of the acute inflammatory response; and
6. discuss the physiological events responsible for swelling associated with tissue injury, as well as treatment strategies for swelling.

A soccer player is assisted into the athletic training room. You and the team physician examine the player, finding that she has a Grade II sprain of the tibial collateral ligament. The physician believes that the athlete can return to soccer participation in about 6 weeks. Initially the athlete is placed in a knee immobilizer and instructed to partially bear weight using crutches. She is advised to use ice several times each day to control pain. After a few days the knee is much less painful, and gentle active range of motion exercises and quadriceps setting with straight leg raises are initiated. Biofeedback with electromyography (EMG) is used to improve neuromuscular control of the quadriceps. Once active, pain-free range of motion is restored, open and closed chain resistance exercises are added to the program. After 4 1/2 weeks the athlete has full motion and strength, and stress testing of the injured ligament reveals no pain or laxity. The athlete is cleared to begin an aggressive, sport-specific program of exercises in preparation for return to top competition. What physiological events take place over these 6 weeks as the injury is repaired? Can treatment interventions speed tissue healing? When does the tensile strength of the injured ligament return to normal?

As illustrated in the soccer player's case, understanding the physiology of inflammation and applying therapeutic modalities accordingly will best meet the needs of physically active individuals and facilitate their return to activity. Tissue injury triggers an elaborate response by the body to remove injured tissue and repair the damage. Inappropriate treatment can delay or even halt repair. This chapter provides an overview of events from the time of tissue damage until tissue repair and maturation are completed.

## HEALING TISSUES AND INFLAMMATION: AN OVERVIEW

Damage to the body's tissues initiates a series of events that remove damaged tissue, provide the necessary materials for repair, and result in the maturation of new tissue. This process can take days, weeks, or many months. The specific tissue damaged, the severity of the damage, and the overall health of the individual determine the length of time required for healing. Regardless of the time frame, the events that result in tissue healing occur in order and are mediated by the same controlling factors.

**Inflammation** is the body's mechanism to remove damaged tissue, which is essential for tissue healing. Pain, loss of function, heat, redness, and swelling are the cardinal signs of inflammation, indicating that an injury has occurred and the body has begun healing.

Inflammation occurs in **vascularized** tissue in response to tissue injury; **avascular** or poorly vascularized tissue will not heal. Injury to the inner margins of the menisci is a good example. These tissues will not heal and must be resected from the knee if joint dysfunction occurs. The inflammatory response is nonspecific to cause, tissue type, or location; the same events occur under the influence of the same mediators during inflammation. This is in contrast to the body's immune response, which is highly specialized. Inflammatory and immune responses work together to defend the body against diseases and promote recovery after injury. The inflammatory response is also responsible for the symptoms that cause the athlete to seek medical attention. These symptoms also cause the athlete to refrain from painful activities and protect the injured tissues.

The inflammatory response described in this chapter is based on a model of musculoskeletal injury. Inflammation occurs in response to other conditions, including infections, autoimmune diseases, illnesses, and exposure to chemical and particulate irritants. Some of these causes are discussed later in this chapter in the section "Chronic Inflammation."

The healing process (or inflammatory response) can be divided into three phases: acute, repair, and maturation. The three phases are not distinct, separate processes but are overlapping events. Figure 3.1 illustrates the overlap of events occurring at each phase of

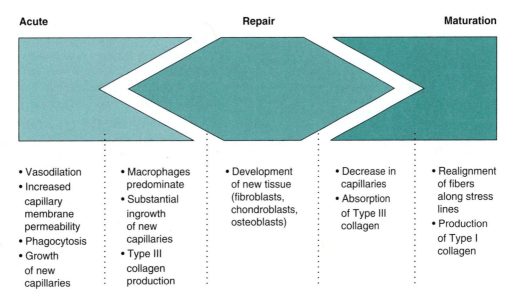

**Figure 3.1** Phases of the inflammatory response.

the inflammatory response. Because the phases have different regulatory mechanisms and purposes, we will explore each phase individually.

# ACUTE PHASE OF THE INFLAMMATORY RESPONSE

Immediately following injury, the body mounts an acute response to limit blood loss and then remove debris and allow growth of new capillaries that will transport the materials needed for tissue repair. The acute inflammatory response begins within seconds of the injury and may last up to several days depending on the severity of tissue damage.

The acute inflammatory response is initiated and controlled by more than 180 chemical mediators released from cells or activated plasma proteins (Merrick 2003). Some of the chemical mediators of the acute inflammatory response stimulate free nerve endings and cause pain, which results in muscle spasm and triggers the body's protective mechanisms. Muscle spasm can cause more pain, resulting in a cycle of pain and spasm and a loss of function, which affects the individual's ability to be physically active. Modalities are generally applied during the acute response to injury or in the treatment of persistent pain. If healing tissues can be protected, the certified athletic trainer can speed the individual's recovery by interrupting the pain–spasm cycle and restoring functional ability.

Other chemical mediators cause an opening of the capillary beds, called **vasodilation.** The increase in blood in the area results in redness and warmth over the inflamed tissue. Vasodilation also slows the rate at which the blood flows, resulting in **hemoconcentration.** Hemoconcentration allows for **leukocytes** (white blood cells) to fall out of circulation and migrate to the capillary walls. Along with vasodilation, the walls of the capillary become more permeable, allowing leukocytes and plasma proteins to leak out. These proteins, along with proteins from the walls of the cells damaged in the injury, attract water. Thus, there is more water in the space between the cells, which causes swelling.

The acute inflammatory response lasts until the damaged tissue has been removed and a new capillary network has been formed to support tissue repair. The acute response overlaps with the repair phase but must resolve before the symptoms associated with injury and inflammation fully resolve.

## Limiting Blood Loss

When injury occurs, small-diameter vascular structures (capillaries, arterioles, and venules) are damaged. Larger vascular structures (arteries and veins) may also be injured, which results in a loss of blood volume and can be life threatening. Fortunately, most athletic injuries do not

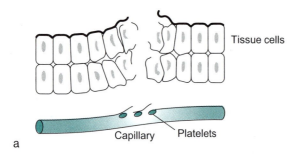

Tissue cells

Capillary   Platelets

a

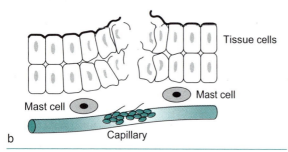

Tissue cells

Mast cell   Mast cell

b   Capillary

**Figure 3.2**   Early response to tissue damage. Tissue injury and damage to capillaries and tissue cells (a). Platelet and fibrin repair of capillary damage (b).

damage the large vessels. Within seconds after injury to soft tissues (ligaments, tendons, muscle) or bone, platelets adhere to the site of damage in the small blood vessels and pile up (figure 3.2a). When blood contacts damaged tissues, a complex series of events converts plasma protein fibrinogen to fibrin. **Fibrin** forms a meshlike network of a clot, which prevents the further loss of red blood cells into the space between cells **(interstitium)**. Epinephrine and substances released from platelets, especially thromboxane A2, result in vasoconstriction. Thus, immediately following tissue damage, the body's defense mechanisms are at work to repair damage to blood vessels and prevent further blood loss (figure 3.2b).

When large blood vessels are injured and the athlete is bleeding externally, the athletic trainer must control bleeding. Compression and elevation can help control external bleeding provided that these actions do not cause further injury. If large vessels are damaged and the bleeding is internal, the injured athlete will go into **hypovolemic** shock. The certified athletic trainer must recognize the signs of shock and immediately stabilize the individual and activate an emergency response plan.

Most musculoskeletal injuries sustained by physically active individuals do not damage large blood vessels. Damage to the small vessels is plugged very rapidly. Athletic trainers used to be taught to immediately apply ice to an injury to control bleeding and thus prevent swelling. Although the application of cold has a place in the management of acute musculoskeletal injuries, cold has little effect on the loss of blood. The body's own mechanisms control blood loss. It is more important to carefully examine the injury than to rapidly apply cold.

The events that limit the loss of blood from small vessels begin within seconds and end in minutes. Once damage to the blood vessels has been plugged, the events of the remainder of the acute response begin.

The events that occur in acute inflammation are complex. Substances released by mast cells, the activation of various plasma proteins, and substances released by leukocytes as well as substances formed by the breakdown of phospholipids contribute to the events that characterize acute inflammation. In a single chapter it is not possible to fully detail all of the events and mediators associated with acute inflammation. Key mediating factors and the responses they trigger are described. Specific events are presented separately in this text. It is important, however, to appreciate that the actions caused by various mediators occur simultaneously. There are also multiple triggers for inflammation. For example, mast cell degranulation initiates the inflammatory response following musculoskeletal injury, whereas a bacterial infection will activate the complement cascade of plasma proteins, which in turn activate mast cell degranulation.

## Signs of Shock

- Rapid, weak pulse
- Low blood pressure
- Rapid, shallow breathing
- Cool, clammy skin
- Lethargy

## Mast Cell-Mediated Events

**Mast cells** are found in the connective tissues adjacent to many of the capillaries. These cells have within them large basophilic granules that contain histamine, neutrophil chemotactic factor, serotonin, and heparin. Like most cells in the body, mast cells also release prostaglandins and leukotrienes. When surrounding tissue is damaged, the body mounts an immune response. The mast cells are exposed to toxins or chemical stimulants causing the mast cells to release the contents of the granules and synthesize prostaglandins and leukotrienes. These chemicals stimulate an inflammatory response.

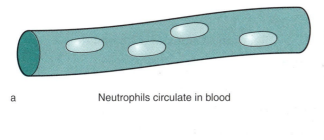

a          Neutrophils circulate in blood

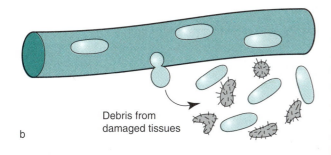

Debris from
damaged tissues

b

**Figure 3.3**  Neutrophils circulate in the blood *(a)* and emigrate through pores in the capillary membrane to phagocytize debris *(b)*.

Histamine is a potent vasodilator and also increases the permeability of the capillary membrane. Neutrophil chemotactic factor attracts neutrophils (a type of white blood cell) to the area of tissue damage. Neutrophils are **phagocytes** that have a primary role in the body's defense against bacteria. These two chemical mediators increase local blood flow and bring more neutrophils to the area, allow for them to move from the circulation into the interstitium (space between the cells), and attract them to the site of tissue damage (figure 3.3). Large numbers of neutrophils arrive in the area of tissue damage and perpetuate the inflammatory response.

Serotonin also increases capillary membrane permeability. The increase in capillary membrane permeability is essential to the inflammatory process. Normally the pores in the capillary wall are too small to permit the passage of leukocytes (white blood cells). Thus, the increase in capillary membrane permeability permits leukocytes (especially neutrophils and monocytes) to move into the area of tissue damage. Unfortunately, when the capillary membrane permeability increases, many plasma proteins, which are too large to slip into the interstitium under normal conditions, escape. These proteins exert an osmotic (water attracting) force. The fluid these proteins draw into the interstitium accounts for the swelling associated with tissue injury and inflammation. A more in-depth discussion of the causes and resolution of swelling is presented later in this chapter.

Heparin is a strong anticoagulant, a chemical substance that prevents clotting. It is released in small quantities under normal conditions to maintain blood flow into the capillaries. It performs the same function in an acute inflammatory response, ensuring that the leukocytes can reach the damaged tissues.

The chemical mediators released from mast cells are responsible for many of the events associated with the acute inflammatory response (table 3.1). The mediators attract neutrophils and ease the movement of these cells from the blood to the area of tissue damage. The removal of the damaged tissues sets the stage for tissue repair and maturation (figure 3.4).

**Table 3.1    Summary of the Mediators, Symptoms, and Purposes of the Acute Inflammatory Response**

| Mediator | Purpose | Relation to signs of inflammation |
|---|---|---|
| **Mast cells** | | |
| Histamine | Vasodilation | Heat and redness |
| Neutrophil chemotactic factor | Attract neutrophils to phagocytize necrotic tissue | Swelling, indirectly, because increased membrane permeability is required for neutrophil emigration |
| Serotonin | Increase capillary membrane permeability | Swelling |
| Heparin | Prevent occlusion of capillary blood flow | No direct relationship |
| Prostaglandin E2* | Increase capillary membrane permeability | Pain and swelling |
| Leukotrienes* | Attract neutrophils to phagocytize necrotic tissue | Swelling, indirectly, because increased membrane permeability is required for neutrophil emigration |

*(continued)*

**Table 3.1** *(continued)*

| Mediator | Purpose | Relation to signs of inflammation |
|---|---|---|
| **Plasma proteins** | | |
| Clotting cascade | Prevent loss of red blood cells | No direct relationship |
| Kinin cascade | Increase capillary membrane permeability | Pain and swelling |
| Complement cascade | Facilitate all aspects of acute inflammatory response | Increases all signs of inflammation |
| **Leukocytes** | | |
| Cationic proteins | Increase capillary membrane permeability, attract monocytes, promote phagocytosis | Swelling |
| Neutral proteases | Facilitate all aspects of acute inflammatory response | Increase all signs of inflammation |

* Products of the breakdown of phospholipids released from damaged cells in addition to synthesis in mast cells.

**Figure 3.4**
Neutrophils and macrophages remove necrotic tissue from wound areas by surrounding and engulfing the dead and damaged material.

Neutrophil

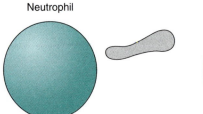 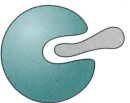 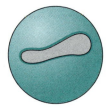

# Phospholipid Breakdown

Prostaglandins and leukotrienes also have a regulatory influence over the inflammatory process, as well as a number of other bodily functions including gastric acid output and renal activity. Prostaglandins and leukotrienes are derived from arachidonic acid, which is produced from phospholipids (figure 3.5). In addition to prostaglandin and leukotriene production by cells, including mast cells, these substances can be derived from the breakdown of damaged cells. When cells are damaged, as occurs in acute musculoskeletal injury, the phospholipids liberated are acted upon by enzymes (phospholipase) forming arachidonic acid that is then transformed into prostaglandins and leukotrienes.

Prostaglandin E2 (PGE2) is one of many prostaglandins that regulate a variety of physiological functions. Prostaglandin E2 interacts with histamine to increase capillary membrane permeability. Along with the plasma protein bradykinin, PGE2 stimulates free nerve endings, resulting in the sensation of pain. Evidence of the role PGE2 plays in the sensation of pain is found in the effects of nonsteroidal anti-inflammatory drugs (NSAIDs). All drugs in this class of medications affect the synthesis of PGE2, which is responsible for their analgesic effects.

Leukotrienes are chemicals that attract leukocytes. They are similar to neutrophil chemotactic factor, described earlier. However, leukotrienes are chemotactic to other white blood cells in addition to neutrophils. Basophils, eosinophils, lymphocytes, and macrophages are also leukocytes. Macrophages, which mature from monocytes, are very active in the later stages of an acute inflammatory response. Basophils, eosinophils, and lymphocytes are involved with the inflammatory responses to invading organisms and toxins. These leukocytes have a more limited role following musculoskeletal injury.

The actions of cyclooxygenase (see figure 3.5) on arachidonic acid are not limited to prostaglandin synthesis. During the transformation from arachidonic acid to stable prostaglandins, **free radicals** are released (Kerr, Bender, and Monti 1996; Ward, Till, and Johnson 1990).

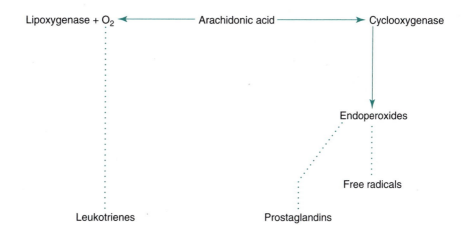

**Figure 3.5** Synthesis of leukotrienes and prostaglandins from arachidonic acid.

These free radicals activate proteases such as collagenase, which break down adjacent cell membranes (Kerr, Bender, and Monti 1996; Ward, Till, and Johnson 1990). The purpose of the proteases is to break down the membranes of damaged cells; however, some surrounding healthy cells may be damaged by this process, resulting in secondary cell death or a secondary zone of injury. The issue of secondary tissue injury is discussed further in chapter 8. A more detailed discussion of secondary tissue injury is provided by Merrick (2002) and is highly recommended reading for the student and certified athletic trainer alike.

## Plasma Protein-Mediated Events

Many proteins are found in the plasma, many in inactive states. They may be activated by antigen–antibody responses, bacteria, and chemicals released from damaged cells. The activation of some plasma proteins sets off a chain reaction that activates other plasma proteins. These chain reactions are called protein cascades.

### Antigen–Antibody Responses

Antibodies, also referred to as immune bodies, are formed when B-lymphocytes respond to an antigen. An antigen is a substance that triggers an immune response. Antigens include toxins and bacteria as well as foreign proteins contained within viruses. When the body detects an antigen for which an antibody has been developed, an immune response is triggered. Such a response will include activation of plasma protein cascades and ultimately inflammation.

Three protein cascades are associated with the acute inflammatory response. The clotting cascade results in a fibrous framework for tissue repair (figure 3.6). The kinin cascade results in the formation of bradykinin. The complement cascade affects all aspects of the acute inflammatory response. These protein cascades interact and occur simultaneously with other events of the acute inflammatory response.

The clotting cascade converts the plasma protein fibrinogen to fibrin. Fibrin forms a mesh-like web with platelets to temporarily repair damaged vascularized tissues. The first protein in the clotting cascade, Factor XII, or the Hageman factor, also activates the kinin cascade (figure 3.7), first converting the plasma protein prekallikrein to kallikrein, which then activates the conversion of kininogen to bradykinin. Bradykinin increases capillary membrane permeability and interacts with prostaglandins to stimulate free nerve endings, causing pain.

The complement cascade is a family of plasma proteins that participate in virtually every aspect of the inflammatory response including lysis (breakdown) of membranes of dead

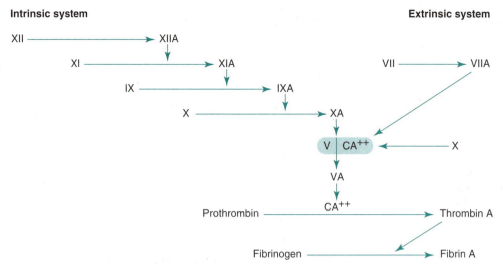

**Figure 3.6** Clotting cascade theory. Activation of the Hageman factor in response to tissue injury initiates a cascade of events culminating with formation of fibrin.

Adapted from Langley 1974.

"A" indicates active form of plasma protein.

cells, chemical attraction of leukocytes, and increased capillary membrane permeability. The complement cascade also stimulates mast cell degranulation. The complement can be activated by antigen–antibody reactions (such as those occurring in rheumatoid arthritis), proteins of the clotting cascade, and toxins released by bacteria.

The protein cascades function with the chemical mediators released from the mast cells. It should be apparent that these cascades interact. An injury or illness activates one or more cascades. If mast cell degranulation occurs first, it will trigger the plasma protein cascades. If the plasma protein system is activated first, other plasma protein systems will be activated and will stimulate mast cell degranulation. Thus, the inflammatory response is said to be nonspecific. The same events occur regardless of the precipitating stimulus.

## Leukocyte-Mediated Events

The leukocytes are drawn to the area of inflammation by chemical attraction. Following a musculoskeletal injury, neutrophils are the predominant leukocytes in the area of tissue damage. The principal role of neutrophils is to fight infection by attacking bacteria. Neutrophils are relatively short-lived. When neutrophils die, chemical mediators are released from the lysosomes. Two groups of lysosomal enzymes perpetuate the inflammatory response: cationic proteins and neutral proteases.

Cationic proteins, released from the lysosomes, increase the permeability of capillary membranes and are **chemotactic** to monocytes. Monocytes mature into large leukocytes

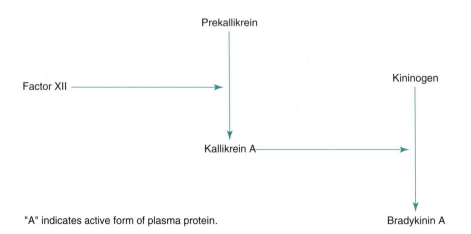

**Figure 3.7** Conversion of kininogen to bradykinin.

"A" indicates active form of plasma protein.

(macrophages) that are capable of phagocytizing the debris from damaged tissue. Thus, since neutrophils cannot remove damaged tissue, the body has a mechanism to attract larger phagocytic cells. Late in the acute inflammatory response, macrophages are the predominant leukocyte in the area of tissue damage. The large leukocytes are also found in high concentrations in the inflamed joints of people with rheumatoid arthritis; these cells attack the articular cartilage of the joints, resulting in the joint dysfunction associated with this disease.

The other group of lysosomal enzymes released from neutrophils is composed of neutral proteases. These chemical mediators stimulate the complement cascade and the kinin system. Through the lysosomal enzymes, the inflammatory response is perpetuated until the damaged tissues are removed.

Oxygen free radicals are also produced by neutrophils (Kerr, Bender, and Monti 1996; Leadbetter 1995; Ward, Till, and Johnson 1990). As noted previously, free radicals activate proteases, such as collagenase, which break down adjacent cell membranes and are believed to contribute to secondary tissue injury.

# REPAIR PHASE OF THE INFLAMMATORY RESPONSE

Repair implies the growth of new tissue. Once injury debris is removed and the vascular network to support tissue growth is in place, repair is well under way. The rate of repair and the type of tissue generated are influenced by several factors. The cell type of the tissue determines the course of the repair process.

Tissues are classified according to the proportion of cells in mitosis (actively dividing) normally present (Martininez-Hernandez and Amenta 1990). Tissues such as the epidermis contain cells that are continuously being replaced, classified as labile cells. Bone marrow and the cells lining the respiratory, gastrointestinal, and genitourinary tracts are also labile cells. Tissues made of labile cells have excellent regenerative capacity.

Stable cells have less regenerative capacity. Cells that make up the tissues of the liver, pancreas, and kidneys, as well as fibroblasts, osteocytes, endothelial cells, and chondrocytes, are classified as stable cells. Fibroblasts synthesize collagen and elastin, which are the major components of ligaments and tendon. Osteoblasts, which mature into osteocytes, form bone; and chondroblasts, which mature into chondrocytes, form cartilage. Thus bone and cartilage can regenerate but do so more slowly than tissues made up of labile cells.

Cells that have no regenerative capacity in adults are classified as permanent cells. The nerves of the central nervous system, the lenses of the eyes, and cardiac muscle have no regenerative capacity. Advances have been made in understanding why some tissues lose regenerative capacity after birth—work that has special application in the treatment of spinal cord injuries.

Skeletal muscle has limited regenerative capacity. As with other permanent tissue, large areas of muscle tissue damage are repaired by the laying down of scar tissue. Scar is made up primarily of collagen formed by fibroblasts. When injury is more limited, such as that associated with delayed soreness, satellite cells mature into myofibrils, restoring functional muscle tissues.

Because excessive stress to healing tissues disrupts repair and slows recovery, you must understand how damaged tissues are repaired and the time frame over which repair occurs. In the second chapter of *Therapeutic Exercise for Musculoskeletal Injuries, Second Edition* (Houglum 2005), the repair of musculoskeletal tissues is covered in depth to provide a foundation for safe, progressive programs of therapeutic exercise.

# MATURATION PHASE OF THE INFLAMMATORY RESPONSE

As the repair process progresses, healing tissues are able to withstand greater stresses. As ligaments and tendons heal, Type III collagen is replaced with stronger Type I collagen (Andriacchi et al. 1988). Fiber alignment improves, and the links between fibers become stronger. In bone, new tissue matures and the mineral content increases. The rate at which tissues heal varies, and the skilled athletic trainer progresses each athlete's rehabilitation at a rate that allows healing tissue to adapt. If too much stress is applied too soon, the tissue fails and reinjury occurs. Applying too little stress does not fully prepare the tissues to withstand the demands of sports, and reinjury occurs when the individual returns to activity. In this phase, rehabilitation should advance the physically active individual through a course of functional activity and return him or her to sport participation. The rate of progress will depend on the nature and extent of the injury, the athlete's overall fitness, and the demands of the particular sport.

# CHRONIC INFLAMMATION

Normally the symptoms of acute inflammatory response resolve within 3 to 10 days, indicating that repair is well under way. However, in some circumstances the symptoms of acute inflammation persist. The causes of chronic inflammation can be divided into four categories.

1. Contamination by a foreign body or bacteria
2. Invasion of microorganisms that are able to survive within large phagocytes (macrophages) such as the microorganisms responsible for tuberculosis and syphilis
3. Antigen–antibody reactions such as those that occur in rheumatic diseases like rheumatoid arthritis
4. Constant irritation by mechanical stress or chemical and particulate matter

It is unlikely that a certified athletic trainer will treat patients with tuberculosis. However, when inflammation persists, the certified athletic trainer must explore the reason. Excessive mechanical stress due to an overly aggressive treatment plan or the individual's failure to comply with instructions to rest the injured area is a common cause of chronic inflammation in athletes. Infection must also be ruled out as a cause of chronic inflammation, even when the skin has not been disrupted. In the sports medicine clinic, the certified athletic trainer may encounter athletes with rheumatoid arthritis, a disabling autoimmune disease resulting in destruction of the articular cartilage.

Chronic inflammation can result in chronic pain. The causes and treatments of persistent pain are discussed in chapter 5.

## Reviewing the Signs and Symptoms of Inflammation

At this point it may be helpful to review the **signs** (responses that you must look or test for, such as heat) and **symptoms** (responses that the athlete must tell you about, such as pain) of acute inflammation and identify why they occur. Heat and redness result from the vasodilation triggered by plasma proteins of the complement cascade and histamine released from mast cells. Pain results from the synthesis of PGE2 and the formation of bradykinin, which in turn stimulate free nerve endings. Other chemical mediators including **substance P,** which is released from free nerve endings, also cause pain. Finally, mechanical stress due to pressure and swelling contributes to pain. Loss of function is the body's natural response to pain. Muscles contract involuntarily (spasm) to splint and protect the injured area. Thus, the chemical mediators described cause the events that allow the body to clear away damaged tissues and result in the heat, redness, pain, and loss of function associated with inflammation.

# SWELLING

Prevention and elimination of swelling used to be dominant themes in the education of athletic trainers. Athletic trainers would apply ice as soon as possible to slow the bleeding that would result in swelling following musculoskeletal injury. Students were also instructed in treatment strategies that supposedly would increase blood flow and reduce the swelling around injured tissues. Over the years, the validity of these treatments has been questioned.

Swelling, a key sign of inflammation, occurs following injury to the bones, ligaments, tendons, and muscles. However, in the absence of injury to large vessels, very few red blood cells are found in the fluid responsible for the increase in tissue volume or swelling. Because of the very rapid vasoconstriction around the tissue damage, the immediate attraction of platelets to the damaged area, and the formation of fibrin, little bleeding into the tissues occurs after the first moments following injury. Thus, applying ice immediately to prevent bleeding has little impact, because the body's natural reactions have bleeding well under control.

However, if the loss of whole blood does not cause swelling, what does? Earlier, the impact of increased capillary membrane permeability was introduced. When capillary membrane permeability increases, leukocytes can enter the area of damaged tissue because these cells are small enough to fit through the pores in the capillary walls. Red blood cells are too large to leak out. However, large numbers of plasma proteins do leak out. Proteins exert an osmotic pressure; that is, the proteins attract water. Thus, the increase in proteins in the interstitium and the osmotic pressure the proteins exert are responsible for swelling. Osmotic pressure is caused not only by the proteins that leak from capillaries. The cells of the damaged tissues also have a protein component; and when dead cells are broken down, proteins that helped form the cell walls add to the accumulation of free proteins in the interstitium and increase the osmotic pressure.

The increase in free proteins in the interstitium disrupts normal capillary filtration balance, and swelling occurs (figure 3.8). The osmotic force exerted by plasma proteins is essential to the function of the cardiovascular system. Dissolved nutrients and gases are delivered to the tissues by fluid forced into the interstitium by the pressure that plasma exerts against the capillary wall (hydrostatic pressure). However, fluid that is forced from the capillaries must be absorbed, or the body would literally burst due to fluid accumulation. Because plasma proteins are large, few pass through the capillary wall. The concentration of protein increases at the venule end of the capillary. These proteins exert an osmotic pressure that pulls fluid and dissolved waste products back into the capillary. This system prevents fluid accumulation while providing a mechanism to deliver nutrients and remove waste from the tissue.

In the normal balance, plasma is forced into the interstitium under hydrostatic pressure. Nutrients are delivered to the cells and waste products removed. Plasma is reabsorbed into capillaries and venules due to osmotic pressure exerted by plasma proteins. In a disrupted process, neutrophils and plasma proteins migrate through capillary membrane pores expanded under the influence of histamine, serotonin, and other chemical mediators. The increased number of free proteins to the interstitium limits absorption of plasma from the interstitium.

A few plasma proteins do leak from the capillaries under normal conditions. These proteins cannot be absorbed into the capillary or postcapillary venule. If they were to accumulate, the osmotic pressure exerted would disrupt normal capillary filtration balance and there would be persistent swelling. However, the lymphatic system parallels the capillary system and absorbs free protein from the interstitium, thus preventing the accumulation of free proteins and chronic swelling.

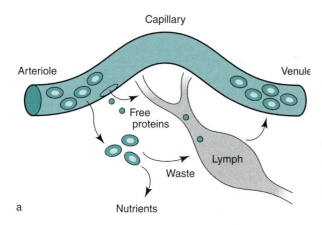

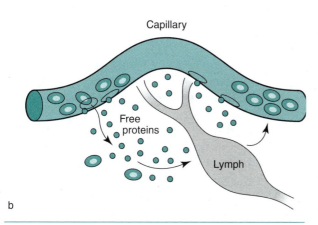

**Figure 3.8**   Normal capillary filtration pressure balance (a) and an increase of free proteins, which disrupts normal capillary filtration pressure balance (b).

How does the capillary filtration system relate to the swelling associated with inflammation? As noted previously, several chemical mediators increase the permeability of the capillary membrane. The increased size of pores in the capillary walls allows plasma proteins to leak into the interstitium in large quantities. The proteins left from the lysis of cell membranes add to the protein concentration. The osmotic force exerted by these proteins alters normal capillary filtration pressure balance and results in the retention of interstitial fluid, or swelling.

Can the certified athletic trainer influence how much swelling occurs following injury? By understanding capillary filtration pressure and the function of the lymphatic system, you can identify strategies to minimize swelling. Elevation reduces hydrostatic pressure, so less fluid is forced into the interstitium. External pressure may minimize the osmotic pressure exerted by the free proteins in the interstitium. These strategies should be incorporated into treatment following injury or surgery.

Can the application of therapeutic modalities affect the development of swelling? The effects of ice on the development of swelling have not been fully investigated. Although ice has been used for many years to treat musculoskeletal injuries, its impact on the development of swelling in humans remains speculative. This question is addressed in greater depth in chapter 8. Recent studies have suggested that electrical currents may alter capillary membrane permeability, as discussed further in chapter 9.

Despite efforts to minimize swelling, some fluid will accumulate in the tissues. To eliminate the fluid, the free proteins that are attracting the fluid must be removed. As noted previously, these free proteins are not absorbed back into the capillary or postcapillary venule but must be absorbed by the lymphatic system. Lymph is pumped through lymphatic vessels by the contraction of surrounding muscles. Thus, movement is the best means of pumping lymph from the area surrounding the damaged tissue and stimulating the absorption of free proteins and fluid. However, the activity used to increase lymphatic drainage must not perpetuate the inflammatory process, or more protein will leak from the capillaries.

Do modalities help resolve swelling? Muscle contraction facilitates lymphatic drainage, but muscle spasm limits lymph flow. Thus, modality applications that decrease muscle spasm will promote lymphatic drainage (figure 3.9). However, modalities to increase local blood flow do little to resolve swelling, because the lymphatic, rather than vascular, capillaries absorb the free proteins. Thus, an understanding of capillary filtration pressure tells you why swelling is associated with inflammation, how to speed the resolution of swelling, and what limits prevention strategies.

## Joint Effusion

The model described in the previous section explains why swelling occurs in interstitial space following tissue damage. However, sometimes a fluid increase within a joint capsule is unrelated to alterations in capillary filtration pressure balance. Synovial joints are lined by a synovial membrane that produces fluid to lubricate and nourish joint surfaces (Tsang 2001). When the synovial membrane is irritated by a loose body or torn meniscus, protein leaks out from capillaries supplying the synovial membrane and an excessive amount of fluid accumulates. Joint effusion impairs the function and normal mechanics of a joint.

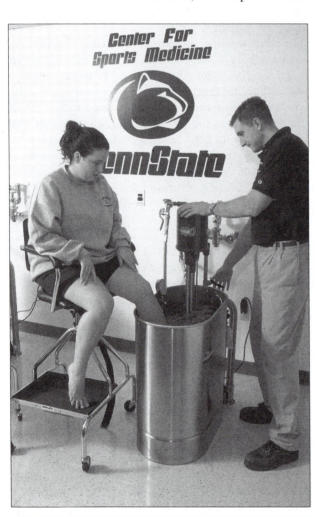

**Figure 3.9**  Modality applications that decrease muscle spasm will promote lymphatic drainage and thereby reduce swelling.

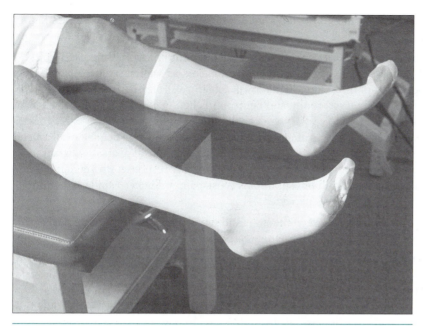

**Figure 3.10** The accumulation of fluid in some individuals is caused by failure of the valves in the leg veins. Compressive stockings can help control this swelling.

## Swelling in the Lower Extremity Due to Venous Insufficiency

Some individuals may experience chronic swelling in their feet and ankles but have no history of recent trauma. This fluid accumulation is caused by failure of the valves in the leg veins. With age, the one-way valves in the veins fail. Thus, blood in the veins that is normally pumped toward the heart backwashes. This blood exerts a hydrostatic pressure at the postcapillary venule that opposes the absorption of fluid from the interstitium. Thus, fluid accumulates in the tissues, and swelling is observed. Because the concentration of free proteins in the interstitium does not increase, this swelling is more easily resolved. Elevating the feet allows gravity to pull venous blood toward the heart, decreases hydrostatic pressure at the venule, and promotes interstitial drainage. The use of a compressive stocking increases the interstitial resistance to fluid loss and can help control edema in the feet and ankles (figure 3.10).

## SUMMARY

1. Describe the role of the inflammatory response in tissue healing.

   Inflammation is the process by which the body removes damaged tissues and establishes a blood supply to support repair. Once damaged tissues have been removed by the phagocytic cells, damaged tissues regenerate or are repaired with scar tissues.

2. Identify key events in the acute inflammatory, repair, and remodeling phases of tissue healing.

   The acute inflammatory response begins with vasoconstriction and clotting. Vasoconstriction results from the actions of epinephrine and thromboxane. The clotting cascade is activated to minimize hemorrhage. This is a rapid and relatively short process. Once further blood loss is prevented, vasodilation and increased capillary membrane permeability allow for the invasion of neutrophils and later macrophages. The cells attack bacteria and phagocytize damaged tissue. As phagocytosis occurs, a new network of capillaries is formed to support the repair phase. During repair, new tissue is formed by fibroblasts, osteoblasts, or chondroblasts, depending on which tissues have been damaged. Over time, stress to new tissues increases tensile strength as remodeling occurs.

3. Identify the causes of chronic inflammation.

   Sometimes inflammation does not proceed to repair and maturation, and the body remains in a chronic inflammatory state. There are four general causes of chronic inflammation: contamination by a foreign body or bacteria, invasion of microorganisms, antigen–antibody reactions, and constant irritation by mechanical stress or chemical and particulate matter.

4. Describe the events and controlling chemical mediators of the acute inflammatory response.

The acute inflammatory response can be divided into mast cell-mediated, plasma protein-mediated, and leukocyte-mediated events as well as events mediated by the products of phospholipid breakdown. Chemicals released from the mast cells, including histamine, serotonin, and neutrophil chemotaxic factor, collectively promote vasodilation and capillary endothelial permeability and cause pain. Plasma proteins from the clotting, kinen, and complement cascades participate in all aspects of the inflammatory response. Cationic proteins and neutral proteases attract macrophages to the area and perpetuate the inflammatory response. Prostaglandins and leukotrienes formed from phospholipids cause pain, influence capillary membrane permeability, and attract leukocytes.

5. Discuss the relationship between the signs and symptoms and the physiological events characteristic of the acute inflammatory response.

The signs and symptoms of acute inflammation include heat, redness, pain, loss of function, and swelling. Heat and redness occur with vasodilation, which is caused by histamine and complement cascade proteins. Pain is caused by irritation of free nerve endings by PGE2, bradykinin, and pressure created by swelling. Loss of function stems from pain. Swelling results from the attraction of water to free proteins accumulating in the interstitium. Normally, very few plasma proteins pass through the capillary membrane. However, several chemical mediators of inflammation increase the permeability of the capillary membrane, allowing plasma protein to escape. In addition, the breakdown of the cell membranes of damaged tissue contributes to the pool of free protein in the interstitium. In short, injury and acute inflammation disrupt normal capillary filtration pressure balance. Interstitial fluid will accumulate until a new pressure balance is reached. Swelling will resolve when free proteins are removed from the interstitium by lymphatic drainage.

6. Discuss the physiological events responsible for swelling associated with tissue injury, as well as treatment strategies for swelling.

Swelling results from a disruption of normal capillary filtration pressure balance. Swelling can be minimized through elevation, which decreases capillary hydrostatic pressure, and external compression, which introduces a counterforce to increased interstitial osmotic pressure. Cold application may also limit swelling through vasoconstriction but should be used in combination with compression and elevation for maximum benefit.

## CITED SOURCES

Andriacchi T, Sabiston P, DeHaven K, Dahners L, Woo S, Frank C, Oakes B, Brankd R, Lewis J: Ligament: Injury and healing. In Woo S, Buckwalter JA (Eds), *Injury and Repair of the Musculoskeletal Soft Tissues*. Park Ridge, IL, American Academy of Orthopaedic Surgeons, 1988, 103-128.

Houglum PA: *Therapeutic Exercise for Musculoskeletal Injuries*, 2nd ed. Champaign, IL, Human Kinetics, 2005.

Kerr MA, Bender CM, Monti EJ: An introduction to oxygen free radicals. *Heart Lung* 25:200-209, 1996.

Langley L: *Dynamic Anatomy and Physiology*, 4th ed. New York, McGraw-Hill, 1974.

Leadbetter WB: Anti-inflammatory therapy in sports injury. *Clin Sports Med* 14:353-410, 1995.

Martinez-Hernandez A, Amenta PS: Basic concepts in wound healing. In Leadbetter WB, Buckwalter JA, Gorden SL (Eds), *Sports-Induced Inflammation*. Park Ridge, IL, American Academy of Orthopaedic Surgeons, 1990, 25-54.

Merrick MA: Secondary injury after musculoskeletal trauma: A review and update. *J Athl Train* 37: 209-217, 2002.

Merrick MA: *Inflammation and Secondary Injury*. Paper presented at the Penn State Athletic Training Conference, March 28, 2003.

Tsang KKW: The Effects of Induced Effusion of the Ankle on Neuromuscular Control. Doctoral dissertation, Penn State University, 2001.

Ward PA, Till GO, Johnson KJ: Oxygen-derived free radicals and inflammation. In Leadbetter WB, Buckwalter JA, Gorden SL (Eds), *Sports-Induced Inflammation*. Park Ridge, IL, American Academy of Orthopaedic Surgeons, 1990, 315-324.

## ADDITIONAL READINGS

Berne R, Levy M: *Physiology*. St. Louis, Mosby, 1988.

Leadbetter WB, Buckwalter JA, Gorden SL (Eds): *Sports-Induced Inflammation*. Park Ridge, IL, American Academy of Orthopaedic Surgeons, 1990.

Woo SLY, Buckwalter JA: *Injury and Repair of Musculoskeletal Soft Tissues*. Park Ridge, IL, American Academy of Orthopaedic Surgeons, 1988.

# Pain and Pain Relief

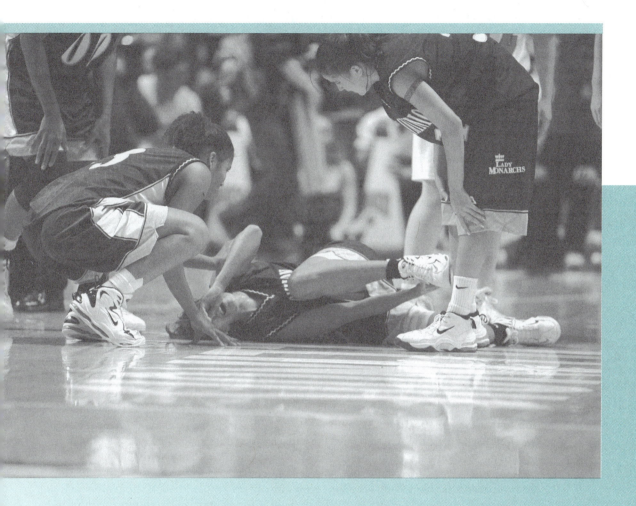

## *Objectives*

After reading this chapter, the student will be able to

1. describe the multidimensional nature of pain;
2. explain the role of pain in preserving health and well-being;
3. discuss how the pain response can assist in evaluating an injured athlete;
4. describe how pain is sensed and how the "pain message" is transmitted to the central nervous system; and
5. discuss contemporary theories on modulating the pain message in the central nervous system.

A tennis player presents to the athletic training room complaining of severe, well-localized back pain. What questions should you ask to determine the nature of the injury?

After evaluating this tennis player, you conclude that the pain and muscle spasm are resulting from **hypomobility** at one or more lumbar facets. In a subsequent evaluation, a team physician agrees with this assessment. How does the dysfunction at the facet result in pain? The perception of pain is a complex neurophysiological phenomenon and will be a focus of this chapter. The tennis player is upset because the physician tells her that her back will take a few days to respond to treatment and she is unlikely to play in a match this weekend. Is there an emotional response to injury, pain, and dysfunction?

You treat this athlete with transcutaneous electrical nerve stimulation (TENS) and ice before performing joint mobilization. The tennis player reports much less pain after treatment with TENS and ice. What mechanisms would explain such a response? Understanding pain and ways to manage pain are important when you are using modalities.

Pain is critical to human survival. Pain causes the injured person to seek medical attention. However, pain is misery, and it limits function. The certified athletic trainer must thoroughly understand pain and the psychological response to pain and loss of function. In the case study at the beginning of this chapter, the tennis player's pain brings attention to her injury. Clinical experience and findings of the physical examination guide the physician's prognosis concerning return to competition. Your knowledge of injury, pain, and associated muscle spasm allows for appropriate treatments to minimize suffering and, in this case, speed return to sport. Pain is also used as a guide for therapeutic exercise. If an overzealous athlete pushes him- or herself too hard during rehabilitation and exercises to the point of pain, progress is slowed while the injury calms back down.

The application of modalities can modulate pain during the rehabilitation process, allowing controlled exercise that further perpetuates pain resolution. Relieving pain is often a focus of therapeutic modalities. Pain during rest or beyond what is necessary to protect the athlete should be treated with medication, modalities, and activity modification. The goal is to reduce pain so that therapeutic exercise can be performed. Heat, ice, ultrasound, electrical stimulation, and mechanical therapies all have the capacity to reduce pain. Therapeutic modalities including TENS and ice are intended to *reduce* pain, but they do not eliminate pain.

In the previous chapter, pain was identified as one of the cardinal signs of inflammation. However, pain is far more complex than a symptom caused by the chemical stimulation of free nerve endings. As suggested in the case study, pain is a warning sign that limits function and affects an individual psychologically and emotionally. This chapter addresses the questions that arise from the case study and provides an in-depth review of the anatomy and physiology of pain and the body's pain-relieving mechanisms. The chapter defines pain; addresses the function, multidimensionality, and physiology of pain; and identifies nervous system structures that carry and receive sensory input. The clinical evaluation and interpretation of pain are reviewed. Finally, contemporary theories of pain control are described.

## WHAT IS PAIN?

Pain is defined by the International Association for the Study of Pain (IASP) as "an unpleasant physical and emotional experience which signifies tissue damage or the potential for such damage" (IASP 1979, p. 249). This definition points to the complexities of the pain experience. Pain is not simply a physical experience. Pain affects the entire organism, altering physical and psychological processes. The certified athletic trainer must appreciate the impact of injury and pain on the athlete and treat from a holistic perspective. Failure to understand the emotional component of pain can affect the relationship between the health care provider and the injured individual and can slow recovery.

Much of the early intervention following injury involves relieving pain. However, despite the unpleasantness associated with pain, it is essential for human survival. Pain can protect the body by warning of impending injury. Pain also signifies that something is wrong. Most people who seek the services of a certified athletic trainer do so because of pain. Inflammation, pain, and loss of function are interrelated. Using therapeutic modalities to decrease pain allows the injured person to perform therapeutic exercise that will then facilitate the return of normal movement and function.

The skillful athletic trainer incorporates questions regarding pain into the interview portion of the physical exam. The answers provided by the athlete narrow the diagnostic possibilities and focus the remainder of the physical exam. Thus, although pain relief is usually the first priority of treatment, the pain experience motivates the injured athlete to seek care and helps the sports medicine team make an assessment.

## PAIN AND THE PHYSICAL EXAM

Although the physical examination process is discussed in great detail in *Examination of Musculoskeletal Injuries, Second Edition* (Shultz, Houglum, and Perrin 2005), the interpretation of pain warrants review in this chapter. When evaluating an injured person, you should ask numerous questions to narrow the diagnostic possibilities. The interview should result in a working diagnosis that is then confirmed or refuted by the physical exam. Questions regarding when and how the injury occurred are obvious. However, you may need to ask follow-up questions to fully interpret the answers and develop a clinical diagnosis.

### P-Q-R-S-T

One approach for asking questions about pain follows a **P-Q-R-S-T** format. This is easy to remember, because **P, Q, R, S,** and **T** are the waves of an electrocardiogram.

**P** is for provocation. Ask how the injury occurred and what activities increase or decrease the pain.

**Q** is for quality, or characteristics of pain. For example, does the individual experience aching shoulder pain, suggesting impingement syndrome; burning pain, suggesting nerve irritation; or sharp pains, suggesting acute injury?

**R** is for referral or radiation. Referred pain occurs at a site distant to damaged tissue that does not follow the course of a peripheral nerve. Pain in the jaw and left shoulder is a common referral pattern during a heart attack. Radiating or radicular pain follows the course of a peripheral nerve. Pressure on a nerve due to a herniated intervertebral disc will result in radiating pain.

**S** is for severity. Judging the severity of pain is subjective, but sometimes one knows that the problem is serious just from the severity of pain.

**T** is for timing. When does pain occur? Night pain may indicate cancer or another nonmusculoskeletal problem since provocative activity is minimized during rest. Pain in the sole of the foot with the first steps in the morning is consistent with plantar fasciitis.

Certainly an acute injury with a well-described mechanism of injury will point to a working diagnosis. Trauma leads to fractures, strains, and sprains. The injured physically active person can often describe the instant and mechanism of these injuries. When the athlete cannot identify the moment of injury or a specific mechanism, the athletic trainer needs to use deductive reasoning and be more discerning of the **etiological factors** leading to the pain.

For example, a baseball pitcher complained of shoulder pain but was unable to identify a specific injury or onset of pain. Further questioning revealed that this athlete's shoulder pain had started following a tournament in which he pitched three times in four days. Injuries with an insidious onset and a poorly defined mechanism broaden the diagnostic possibilities and should not be ignored. This baseball pitcher developed impingement syndrome due to overuse of the throwing muscles. Repetitive microtrauma can injure tendons, cause stress fractures, and lead to conditions such as plantar fasciitis, medial tibial stress syndrome, patellofemoral pain, and, as in this case, glenohumeral impingement syndrome. Thus, understanding the onset of symptoms focuses the injury evaluation and the physical exam.

Other aspects of the pain experience also will help establish the diagnosis. The quality of pain can be difficult to assess, but with experience you will appreciate the difference between the sharp, well-localized pain of a fracture and the diffuse pain associated with myofascial pain syndrome. Pain that radiates within a dermatome indicates pressure on a nerve and is often caused by injury to an intervertebral disc or a vertebral fracture.

Referred pain is another type of pain that occurs when there is pain in another area separate from the pathology. Referred pain can be mysterious yet have predictable patterns. Pain in the left shoulder and jaw during a heart attack and left shoulder pain with a spleen injury are two examples of referred pain. Table 4.1 identifies several medical problems with well-established patterns of referred pain. Unlike the skin and soft tissue, the **viscera** have very few sensory organs. When the sensory information synapses at the spinal cord, an activation of interneurons at that level takes place. The interneurons converge on the neurons that localize pain to the dermatome or myotome at the same spinal cord level. The brain interprets the pain as arising from the soft tissues rather than the involved organ. A thorough evaluation of the injury should identify the area of pathology so that the injury is treated rather than the pain site. The severity of pain indicates severity of the problem. If you have a close working relationship with the athlete, it is easier to interpret his or her reaction to pain and injury.

## Table 4.1 Common Referred Pain Patterns

| Problem | Location of pain |
| --- | --- |
| Myocardial infarction | Neck, jaw, and left shoulder |
| Spleen injury | Left shoulder |
| Appendicitis | Lower abdomen and right groin |
| Pancreatic injury or pancreatitis | Left shoulder, low back, and middle left abdomen |
| Cholecystitis (gallbladder) | Right shoulder and midscapular region |
| Renal (kidney) disorder | Low back and left shoulder |
| Stomach and upper small intestine (duodenum) disorder | Left shoulder |

Finally, the timing of the pain can yield clues about the problem. The fact that pain occurs with specific movements or at certain times of the day may be significant. For example, a person suffering from iliotibial band friction syndrome usually complains of pain while climbing stairs or running up and down hills. Plantar fasciitis is almost always very painful upon arising in the morning and with weight bearing on the injured foot. Questioning the individual about these issues usually provides a working diagnosis, allowing you to focus and organize the physical exam rather than randomly conduct a series of tests. Furthermore, finding out what activities cause more pain helps to determine what activity modifications are necessary. If stairs cause pain, then step-ups should not be included in the rehabilitation plan until changes are made in strength, flexibility, and biomechanics. If possible, the injured athlete should avoid provocative activities.

## PAIN ASSESSMENT

Pain is difficult to assess because it is a symptom rather than a sign. Quantification of pain is very subjective since it is a sensory phenomenon with an affective-motivational dimension (Melzack 1983).

### The Sensory Component of Pain

The sensory component relates to what the individual feels. In order to determine whether your treatments are helping the injured athlete, an attempt to quantify the pain is necessary.

Dull ache — Discomfort during activity

Slight pain — Awareness of pain without distress

More than slight pain — Pain that distracts attention during physical exertion

Painful — Pain that distracts attention from routine occupations such as writing and reading

Very painful — Pain that fills the field of consciousness to the exclusion of other events

Unbearable pain — Comparable to the worst pain you can imagine

**Figure 4.1** Visual analog scale.

Reprinted by permission from Denegar and Perrin 1992.

No pain ———————————————————————————— Unbearable pain

| Dull ache | Slight pain | More than slight pain | Painful | Very painful |

Pain measurement should be reliable and valid. To assess the **intensity** of pain, you can use a simple pain scale, for instance by asking the individual to rate the pain from 0 = *no pain* to 10 = *worst pain ever*. This type of pain assessment is quick and simple but becomes less effective when the athlete is asked for a score several times throughout the evaluation and treatment. For example, the athlete will remember reporting a "5" before the treatment and subconsciously use that figure as a reference for reporting his or her score after the treatment is over.

A visual analog scale (VAS) (figure 4.1) has no demarcations, so the patient cannot use a previous score as a reference point. The VAS uses a 10-cm-length line with the words "no pain" on one end and "unbearable pain" on the other end. The upper end should imply postsurgical or excruciating pain. The clinician measures the horizontal distance from the left to the athlete's mark of the extent of his or her pain in centimeters for the pain score.

More complex assessments involve pain charts (figure 4.2) or a comprehensive questionnaire such as the Pain Disability Index (figure 4.3) to assess the impact of pain on function (Pollard 1984). The more simple scales can be used to quickly assess recovery from injury. The more comprehensive evaluations are more time-consuming but yield valuable insight about persistent and chronic pain. These instruments can also be used to study the effects of therapeutic interventions.

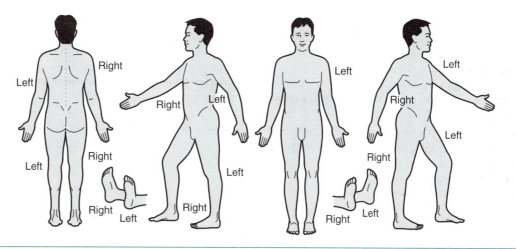

**Figure 4.2** Pain chart. The injured individual uses the figures to show exactly where his or her pain is and where it radiates. As precisely and with as much detail as possible, the individual uses a blue marker to indicate painful areas, a yellow marker for numbness and tingling, a red marker for burning or hot areas, and a green marker for cramping.

Reprinted by permission from Margolis 1983.

**1** Family/home responsibilities. This category includes chores and duties performed around the house (e.g., yard work) and errands or favors for other family members (e.g., driving the children to school).

| 0 | 1 | 2 | 3 | 4 | 5 | 6 | 7 | 8 | 9 | 10 |
|---|---|---|---|---|---|---|---|---|---|----|

No disability                Total disability

**2** Recreation. This category includes hobbies, sports, and other leisure activities.

| 0 | 1 | 2 | 3 | 4 | 5 | 6 | 7 | 8 | 9 | 10 |
|---|---|---|---|---|---|---|---|---|---|----|

No disability                Total disability

**3** Social activity. This category refers to activities involving friends and acquaintances other than family members. It includes parties, theater, concerts, dining out, and other social functions.

| 0 | 1 | 2 | 3 | 4 | 5 | 6 | 7 | 8 | 9 | 10 |
|---|---|---|---|---|---|---|---|---|---|----|

No disability                Total disability

**4** Occupation. This category refers to job-related activities, including nonpaying jobs, such as housework or volunteer work.

| 0 | 1 | 2 | 3 | 4 | 5 | 6 | 7 | 8 | 9 | 10 |
|---|---|---|---|---|---|---|---|---|---|----|

No disability                Total disability

**5** Sexual behavior. This category refers to the frequency and quality of sex.

| 0 | 1 | 2 | 3 | 4 | 5 | 6 | 7 | 8 | 9 | 10 |
|---|---|---|---|---|---|---|---|---|---|----|

No disability                Total disability

**Figure 4.3** Pain Disability Index. For each category, the injured individual circles the number on the scale that describes the level of disability she or he typically experiences. A score of 0 means no disability at all, and a score of 10 signifies that all of the person's normal activities have been totally disrupted or prevented by pain.

Reprinted by permission from Pollard 1984.

**6** Self-care. This category includes activities of personal maintenance and independent daily living (e.g., taking a shower, driving, getting dressed, etc.).

| 0 | 1 | 2 | 3 | 4 | 5 | 6 | 7 | 8 | 9 | 10 |
|---|---|---|---|---|---|---|---|---|---|----|

No disability                Total disability

**7** Life-support activity. This category refers to basic life-supporting behaviors, such as eating, sleeping, and breathing.

| 0 | 1 | 2 | 3 | 4 | 5 | 6 | 7 | 8 | 9 | 10 |
|---|---|---|---|---|---|---|---|---|---|----|

No disability                Total disability

## Sensory and Affective-Motivational Components of Pain

The affective-motivational component of pain relates to the impact of pain on the individual. For example, following injury, pain signifies that something is wrong. However, until the person understands the severity of an injury and the impact it will have on his or her ability to compete, pain may cause considerable anxiety. Persistent pain can lead to withdrawal and depression, responses that compose the affective-motivational aspect of pain.

The response to pain is highly individual and can be influenced by several factors, such as previous pain experiences, family and cultural background, and the specific situation. The certified athletic trainer must learn to accept individual differences in pain response and help the injured person cope with pain.

When pain persists or becomes chronic, the affective-motivational component of the pain experience becomes even more significant in evaluation and treatment. Lasting pain affects virtually every aspect of day-to-day life, from sleep patterns, to the ability to concentrate and study, to social and personal relationships. The causes and treatment of lasting pain are presented in depth in chapter 5.

## TRANSMISSION OF THE PAIN SENSATION

The most common use of therapeutic modalities in athletic training is to relieve pain. These modalities ultimately alter the neural input transmitted to brain centers where pain perception and response occur. Intervention can be at any anatomical level of pain transmission: periphery, spinal level, ascending pathway, supraspinal level, or descending pathway. To understand how modalities can alter a pain experience, you must understand the pathways for transmission of painful (noxious) and nonnoxious sensory information (touch, temperature, vibration, and proprioception).

## Pathways for Transmission of Pain

Acute pain travels along the neospinothalmic tract, which is a fast, three-neuron pathway from the periphery to the cortex. The paleospinathalmic tract is slower and more complex as the information travels to the cortex.

### Acute Pain Pathway

Pain is transmitted from the injured area to the brain in a systematic fashion. Acute pain is a rapid, three-neuron sequence to provide accurate information about the location of injury. The nociceptor is the sensory organ in the tissues that is sensitized to the painful stimulation. The information travels to the spinal cord via the sensory nerve. This fiber is known as the first-order neuron. All sensory nerve fibers have their cell bodies in the dorsal root ganglia and synapse in the spinal cord in the dorsal horn. The second-order neuron crosses to the opposite side of the spinal cord (decussates) and transmits the information up to the thalamus. The second-order neuron is commonly termed the "T" cell. This generic term is used since various sensory input (touch, deep pressure, vibration, temperature, proprioception, and pain) travels in organized columns of axons from the spinal level to the brain. At the thalamus, there is a synapse onto the third-order neuron that carries information to the sensory cortex of the brain where the pain is acknowledged. The three-neuron pathway describes the neospinothalamic system (figure 4.4). This pathway represents the "first pain" (Bolay and Moskowitz 2002), which is well localized, discriminative, and lasts as long as the acutely painful stimulus is applied.

The following neurological components are important in the acute pain pathway:

1. Nociceptor (in the skin, soft tissue, and periosteum).
2. Sensory nerve (cell body is in the dorsal root ganglion and synapses in the dorsal horn of the spinal cord). This is the first-order neuron.

*(continued)*

(continued)

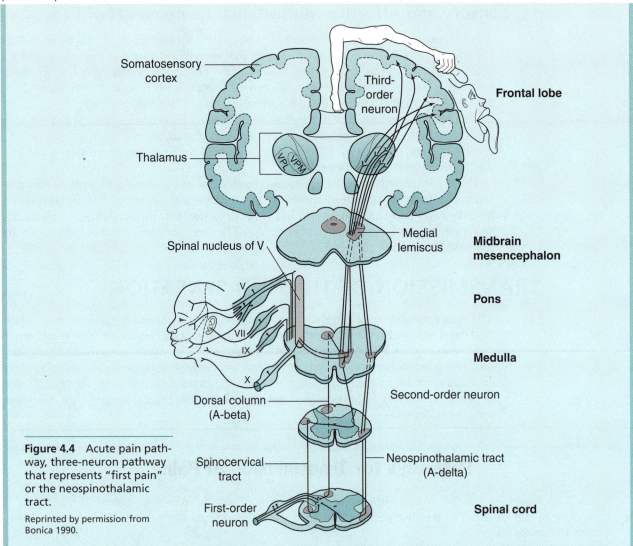

**Figure 4.4** Acute pain pathway, three-neuron pathway that represents "first pain" or the neospinothalamic tract.

Reprinted by permission from Bonica 1990.

3. T cell: Second-order neuron that "transmits" a signal to the thalamus. The name "T cell" is given to this neuron since pain, temperature, light touch, vibration, and deep touch are carried on different tracts. Therefore "T cell" is a generic name for the second-order neuron.

4. Thalamus: Cell bodies of the third-order neuron are clustered in nuclei organized according to the stimulus and its origin. This area also sends information to emotion centers of the brain that causes some of the typical responses to a pain sensation.

5. Sensory cortex: Area of the brain that identifies the location of pain.

## Paleospinothalamic Tract Pain

"Second pain" is associated with the affective-motivational aspects of the pain experience. More intense stimuli activate polymodal nociceptors and promote a diffuse, unpleasant, and persistent burning sensation that lasts beyond the acutely painful stimulus. The transmission to the spinal cord is similar; but there is more time for a vast, diffuse network of interneurons to be activated in the central nervous system. Wide dynamic range neurons that are second-order nociceptive neurons responding to both somatic and visceral stimulation are activated. These signals infiltrate many neurological centers as the input ascends to the supraspinal areas in the brain. The limbic system that is responsible for emotional responses is affected as well as the pituitary gland and hypothalamus that control vegetative and endocrine functions. Additionally, centers for attentiveness, well-being, sleep, and motor activity such as the periaqueductal gray area, the reticular formation, and the Raphe nucleus are activated. These brain centers also have a role in descending pain modulation when targeted specifically. The second pain neurological pathway is termed the paleospinothalamic system (figure 4.5).

Neurological structures associated with second pain include the following:

1. Nociceptor.

2. Sensory nerve (typically C fiber) or first-order neuron.

3. Synapses in the dorsal horn of the spinal cord and activates nociception-specific neurons in lamina I and II and becomes the second-order neuron.

4. Supraspinal networking:

   • Reticular formation: Diffuse network of neurons that mediate motor, autonomic, and sensory functions.

   • Periaqueductal gray (PAG): Directs descending inhibition.

   • Hypothalamus: Regulates vegetative and endocrine functions throughout the body.

   • Pituitary: Controlled by hormonal or neuronal signals from the hypothalamus. The pituitary is the master gland of the endocrine system.

   • Thalamus: Final gateway/relay center for all afferent input (except olfactory). Specific nuclei direct the function of the thalamus.

   • Limbic system: Role in motivational, emotional, and affective behavior. Has input from the thalamus, hypothalamus, and cortex.

5. Sensory cortex: Area of the brain that identifies the location of pain. Receives input from all sensory and associated cortical areas and projects to the reticular formation and limbic system. Central processing center.

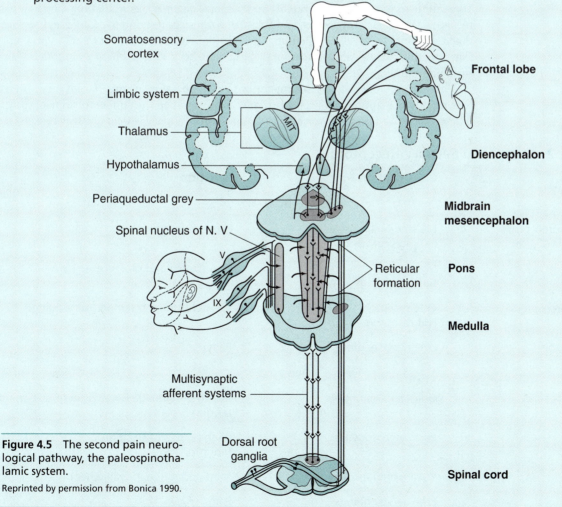

**Figure 4.5** The second pain neurological pathway, the paleospinothalamic system.

Reprinted by permission from Bonica 1990.

# Peripheral Sensory Receptors

All information related to our environment and the relationship of our bodies to the environment is transmitted to higher brain centers from peripheral sensory receptors. Sensory receptors can be classified as special, visceral, superficial, or deep. Special receptors provide the senses of sight, taste, smell, and hearing and contribute significantly to balance. Visceral receptors perceive hunger, nausea, distension, and visceral pain. These two groups of sensory receptors have little impact on the perception of, and response to, the pain of musculoskeletal injury. The peripheral sensory receptors, however, provide the central nervous system with information about pain, touch, vibration, temperature, and proprioception. These receptors are very important in transmitting information about the status of the musculoskeletal and integumentary systems.

The superficial receptors transmit sensations such as warmth, cold, touch, pressure, vibration, tickle, itch, and pain from the skin (Berne and Levy 1993). The deep receptors transmit information regarding position, kinesthesia, deep pressure, and pain from the muscles, tendons, fascia, joint capsules, and ligaments (Berne and Levy 1993). The superficial and deep peripheral receptors transmit the impulses that result in the perception of pain following injury. Table 4.2 identifies the categories and functions of peripheral sensory receptors.

## Superficial Receptors

The superficial receptors, also called cutaneous receptors, can be subdivided into three categories based on the type of stimuli to which they respond: mechanoreceptors, thermoreceptors, and nociceptors. Mechanoreceptors respond to stroking, touch, and pressure. Some of these receptors adapt rapidly and perceive changes in stimulation. The hair follicle receptors, Meissner's corpuscles, and Pacinian corpuscles respond to changes in pressure and touch. In contrast, Merkle cell endings and Ruffini endings, which respond to pressure and skin stretch, are more slowly adapting (Berne and Levy 1993). These receptors respond to sustained stimuli.

Thermoreceptors respond to temperature and temperature change. Cold and warm receptors are slowly adapting but discharge in phasic bursts when the temperature changes rapidly. These receptors respond over a large temperature range. However, warm receptors stop

## Table 4.2    Peripheral Sensory Receptors

| Receptor | Classification | Function |
| --- | --- | --- |
| **Superficial** | | |
| Mechanoreceptors | Meissner's corpuscles Pacinian corpuscles | Pressure and touch |
| | Merkle cells Ruffini endings | Skin stretch and pressure |
| Thermoreceptors | Cold receptors Hot receptors | Temperature and temperature change |
| Nociceptors | Free nerve endings | Pain |
| **Deep** | | |
| Proprioceptors | Golgi tendon organs | Changes in muscle length and muscle spindle tension |
| | Pacinian corpuscles | Change in joint position Vibration |
| | Ruffini endings | Joint end range, possible heat |
| Nociceptors | Free nerve endings | Pain |

discharging at temperatures that damage the skin. The pain of thermal burn results from the stimulation of free nerve endings and **nociceptive** afferent pathways. Cold receptors continue to discharge when tissue cooling is perceived as painful. However, cooling slows the conduction velocity of the nerves between the sensory receptor and the spinal cord (Berne and Levy 1993; Knight 1995). Thus, tissue injury due to cold (frostbite) is not particularly painful. However, when the frostbitten tissue thaws, there is considerable inflammation and pain.

Nociceptors form the third category of superficial receptor. Nociceptors, also labeled free nerve endings, are stimulated by potentially damaging mechanical, chemical, and thermal stress. These receptors are sensitized by prostaglandins, bradykinin, substance P, serotonin, and other chemical mediators of inflammation or by pressure and distension. Polymodal nociceptors contain the neurotransmitter l-glutamate and conduct painful stimuli from various noxious input.

## Deep Tissue Receptors

Ligaments and other deep tissues are supplied by mechanoreceptors (figure 4.6) and nociceptors. In muscle, specialized mechanoreceptors called Golgi tendon organs (GTO) and muscle spindles sense changes in muscle length and tension. Some muscle receptors may also be sensitive to chemical stimuli.

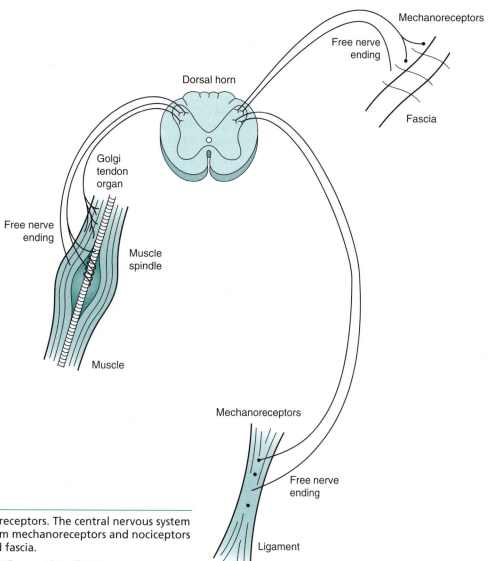

**Figure 4.6**   Deep tissue receptors. The central nervous system receives information from mechanoreceptors and nociceptors of muscle, ligament, and fascia.

Adapted by permission from Wilmore and Costill 1999.

Joint structures are supplied by rapidly and slowly adapting mechanoreceptors and nociceptors. Pacinian corpuscles adapt rapidly and respond to changes in joint position and vibration. Ruffini end organs (or Ruffini endings) are slowly adapting and are most active at the end of joint range of motion. Nociceptors or free nerve endings signify that motion has exceeded normal limits and that stabilizing structures are at risk of failing or that injury has already occurred.

The body's connective tissue or fascial network is also supplied with sensory receptors. Fascia, the "glue" that holds the body together, surrounds the muscles and organs and literally connects the body from head to toe. The innervation of fascia has not been fully explored. However, input from mechanoreceptors and nociceptors affects the resting length and tension of muscle and is likely the underlying cause of complex pain patterns labeled myofascial pain syndrome, discussed more extensively in chapters 5 and 13.

## Afferent Pathways

Impulses generated at the sensory receptors are transmitted to higher centers by afferent, or sensory nerves (figure 4.7). A first-order afferent is a nerve fiber in the periphery (outside the central nervous system), and has its cell body in the dorsal root ganglia and synapses in the spinal cord. The afferent nerves are classified according to structural and functional characteristics. Specifically, categories of sensory nerve fibers are grouped by the diameter or width of the nerve, the degree of myelination, and the nerve's function. The function of nerve fibers determines the type of sensory information carried by that nerve: light touch, pressure, pain, or temperature. The conduction velocity relates to the diameter and the degree of myelination of the nerve fiber. Larger-diameter, heavily myelinated fibers are fast-conducting nerves compared to smaller-diameter, nonmyelinated nerves. For the purposes of understanding pain and pain modulation theories, differences in the nerve fibers must be understood. The first-order neurons are classified in table 4.3. There are numerous other first-order neuron types, but these do not have a function in pain and pain modulation so they are not included.

The A-beta fibers originate from hair follicles, Meissner's corpuscles, Pacinian corpuscles, Merkle cell endings, and Ruffini endings. These fibers transmit sensory information regarding touch, vibration, and hair deflection. They are large-diameter, myelinated nerves. These characteristics make the A-beta fiber a fast-conducting nerve fiber. The A-beta fiber has a relatively low threshold, making it easily stimulated.

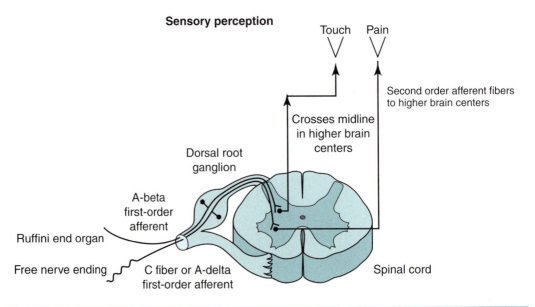

**Figure 4.7**   Primary afferents synapse with second-order afferent fibers in the dorsal horn of the spinal cord. Sensory information is perceived in the opposite sensory cortex; the pain fibers cross at the level of synapsing, but touch and vibration cross in the higher brain centers.

## Table 4.3    First-Order Afferents

| Type and group | Diameter (μm) | Conduction velocity (μs) | Location | Information transmitted |
|---|---|---|---|---|
| **Myelinated** | | | | |
| A-beta | 6-12 | 36-72 | Skin | Touch, vibration |
| A-delta | 1-6 | 6-36 | Skin | Touch, pressure, temperature, pain |
| **Unmyelinated** | | | | |
| C | <1 | 0.5-2 | Muscle Skin | Pain Touch, pressure, temperature, pain |

Adapted by permission from Denegar and Bownan 1996.

The A-delta fibers transmit information from warm and cold receptors, a few hair receptors, and free nerve endings, thus transmitting pain. The free nerve endings supplied by A-delta fibers primarily respond to noxious mechanical stimulation such as pinching, pricking, and crushing. The A-delta fibers are myelinated, but are smaller than A-beta fibers and thus have a slower conduction velocity.

The "C" fibers are the smallest afferent peripheral nerves that are associated with pain. They are unmyelinated and also include the **efferent** postganglionic fibers of the sympathetic nervous system. Those fibers that originate at deep receptors are primarily mechanoreceptors and nociceptors. A few Type C afferents are thermoreceptors. The C fibers are the slowest of the sensory nerve fibers in conduction and require a greater stimulation than the others to elicit a response.

## Ascending Pathways

Once the afferent peripheral nerve enters the spinal cord, it synapses in the **dorsal horn.** The cell body of the second-order neuron is within the dorsal horn, making this area gray. The dorsal horn is organized into laminae or layers that are numbered 1 through 10. The different fiber types synapse in specific laminae according to their function. The second-order neuron's axon makes up the ascending pathways. Axonal areas of the spinal cord have a white appearance.

Multiple pathways or tracts carry sensory input to the brain. The spinal cord is well organized into tracts that bundle types of sensory input together and transmit the information to higher centers in the brain. The tracts are further organized according to the location where the sensory input originated. For example, axons carrying information from the L5 dermatome are medial, while axons carrying information from C3 are lateral. "Sensation," meaning light touch or proprioception, is carried by A-beta fibers. The A-beta fiber synapses in the dorsal horn, and the impulse is transmitted via the dorsal columns. The dorsal columns are on the ipsilateral (same) side as the sensory receptor and do not cross the spinal cord (decussate) until the midbrain level at the medulla; then they travel upward to the thalamus (figure 4.8).

## Supraspinal Centers

The target for the second-order neuron in both pleasant and noxious sensory input is the thalamus, just above the brainstem in the diencephalon. The cell bodies of the third-order neuron are located in clusters, or nuclei of the thalamus. Here the sensory information is organized, and the thalamus becomes a relay center with facilitatory and inhibitory circuits. Figure 4.9 represents the organization of the thalamus. The ventral posterior lateral (VPL) and ventral posterior medial (VPM) nuclei are identified as the most significant for pain

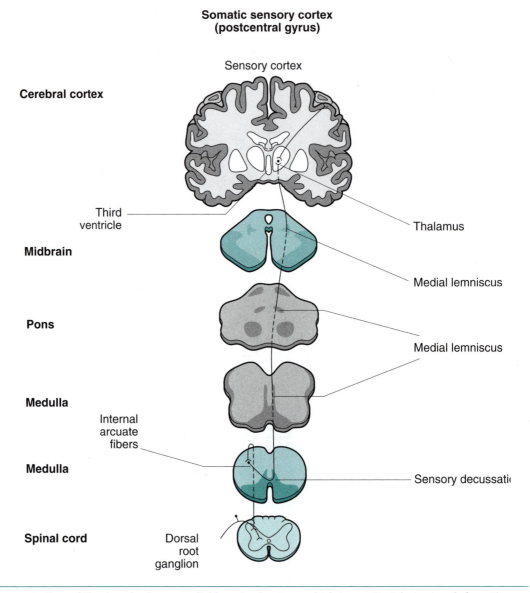

**Somatic sensory cortex
(postcentral gyrus)**

Sensory cortex

**Cerebral cortex**

Third
ventricle

Thalamus

**Midbrain**

Medial lemniscus

**Pons**

Medial lemniscus

**Medulla**

Internal
arcuate
fibers

**Medulla**

Sensory decussatio

**Spinal cord**    Dorsal
root
ganglion

**Figure 4.8**  General organization of the dorsal column-medial lemniscal system, which transmits A-beta signals from the periphery to mediate tactile sensation and limb proprioception.

Adapted by permission from Kandel, Schwartz, and Jessell 2000.

transmission and pain modulation (Berne and Levy 1993). The fibers ascending from the body synapse in the VPL, whereas the fibers from the head and face synapse in the VPM. The thalamus modulates input from the ascending nerves prior to transmitting it to the **somatosensory** cortex. Ultimately, the localization and discrimination of pain occur in the postcentral gyrus of the cortex of the brain. The thalamus also relays input to the limbic system, which regulates the emotional, autonomic, and endocrine response to pain. Thus, the thalamus relays sensory input that provides for the sensory-discriminatory and affective-motivational aspects of pain.

## Descending Pathways

The previous characterization of the three-neuron pathway describes an efficient mechanism for perceiving, locating, and discriminating both painful and nonpainful stimuli. This allows for reflex action for protection and a cognitive awareness of a potentially dangerous situation. However, we know that pain is a multifaceted experience encompassing sensory and affective behaviors. The emotional response and the physiological changes of the body due to stress and

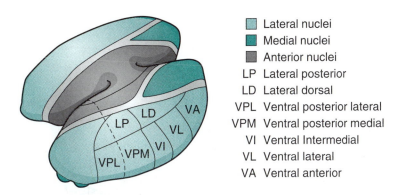

Lateral nuclei
Medial nuclei
Anterior nuclei
LP    Lateral posterior
LD    Lateral dorsal
VPL   Ventral posterior lateral
VPM   Ventral posterior medial
VI    Ventral Intermedial
VL    Ventral lateral
VA    Ventral anterior

**Figure 4.9**   The organization of the thalamus.

discomfort are the result of a complex networking of interneurons and activation of various centers in the central nervous system. Some of the centers are activated during the ascending pathway, especially with pain carried by C fibers, while some are activated after the cortex has acknowledged the painful stimulation. Any activity after the cortex has received the input describes the descending pathways. The descending tracts ultimately have an excitatory or inhibitory action on new impulses that are being transmitted in the spinal cord.

The paleospinothalamic tract describes the diffuse ascending pathways of noxious stimulation. Some of the second-order neuron afferents terminate directly in the periaqueductal gray (PAG) formation in the midbrain. The noxious stimulation causes specific neurotransmitters to activate other brain centers such as the reticular formation and the Raphe nucleus. The reticular formation is in the brainstem and helps to control autonomic functions, has some motor function, and helps to provide collateral sensory signals to higher brain centers. The Raphe nucleus is an area that controls the level of arousal and affects the individual's perception of well-being. These brain areas, the PAG, the reticular formation, and the Raphe nucleus, all have the potential to affect the perception of pain through a descending mechanism. For example, in a painful situation, continual impulses are sent from the receptor to the spinal cord and to the cortex where the pain is acknowledged consciously. Inflammation and its chemical mediators sensitize receptors increasing the pain impulse. When the PAG is activated, a network is initiated that can calm the person and help to filter out some of the pain signals by exciting the reticular formation and the Raphe nucleus. The pituitary gland also produces hormones and neuropeptides that help regulate the signals at the spinal cord level. These brain centers ideally lessen the impulses to the cortex. Evoking these descending modulation areas is the goal of pain management, through either medication, modalities, or stress relief. The neuroanatomic representation of these important relay centers is depicted in figure 4.10.

The diffuse network of messages and activation of brain centers during a painful event may exacerbate the situation. The hypothalamus, pituitary, reticular formation, and Raphe nucleus control subconscious, vegetative functions such as respiration, heart rate, attention, sleep, and general feelings of impending doom. When these areas are not inhibited, the affective-emotional response to pain is similar to shock. Painful stimulation continues to flow to the cognitive areas, and the perception of pain is increased. It becomes more difficult to concentrate on other activities, and the injured person's functional capacity is limited. These areas of the brain respond neurochemically and are strongly affected by medications. They are not controlled by consciousness, although calming, reassuring techniques are often helpful. A phenomenon known as "windup" describes how noxious stimulation can spiral out of control, resulting in a pain syndrome that exceeds its benefit of alerting the injured person of potential harm. The presence of peptide neurotransmitters such as substance P, combined with the release of the excitatory amino acid glutamate in central nociceptive nerve terminals, results in temporal summation. This alters the response characteristics of the second-order cells in the spinal dorsal horn resulting in a sustained C fiber input. The sensitization of the postsynaptic nerves to such sustained input results in a state of hyperstimulation.

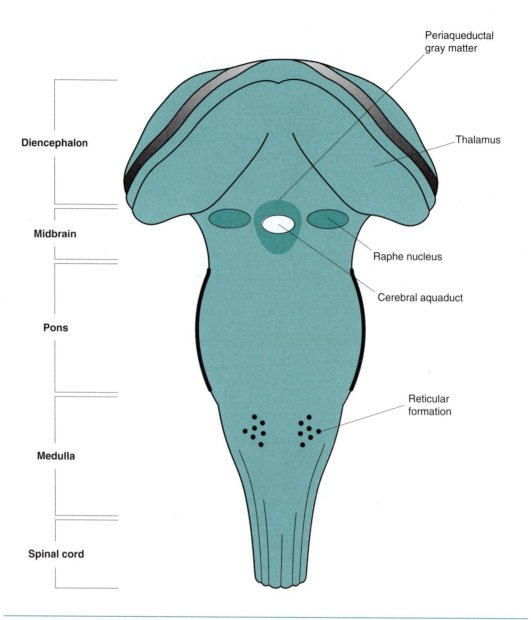

**Figure 4.10**    Brainstem structures involved in pain perception and modulation.

Efforts should be made to control pain with activity modification (rest, splinting), pharmacological agents if needed, stress reduction to prevent neurogenic shock, and therapeutic modalities. Proper treatment usually prevents the hyperstimulated state in an acute injury. However, windup may occur insidiously with persistent pain syndromes. Persistent pain is discussed further in chapter 5.

## Synaptic Transmission and Transmitter Substances

Communication from one nerve fiber to the next takes place at the **synapse** between the two nerves. Impulses from a presynaptic nerve may stimulate depolarization of the postsynaptic nerve by releasing a **transmitter substance.** When this occurs, the transmitter substance is facilitatory. However, not all substances released from presynaptic nerves stimulate depolarization from postsynaptic nerves. Some transmitter substances are inhibitory and block the depolarization of the postsynaptic nerve.

Neuroscience has significantly advanced the understanding of transmitter substances. More than 30 biogenic amine transmitters, amino acid transmitters, and neuroactive peptides have been found to influence synaptic transmission somewhere in the nervous system. Discussion of each of these neuroactive substances is beyond the scope of this text but can be found in the neuroscience texts listed in the reference section. However, a few substances, like glutamate and substance P, play a significant role in nociception and are discussed next.

Glutamate, an amino acid, and substance P, a neuroactive peptide, are believed to facilitate synaptic transmission in the nociceptive pathways (Jessell and Kelly 1991), which intensifies the pain perception. **Beta endorphin,** dynorphin, methionine enkephalin, and leucine enkephalin are classified as opioid peptides because they bind to the same sites as the opiate drugs. Because these neurochemicals are produced by the body, they are considered endogenous opioids and inhibit the transmission of pain impulses. Beta endorphin is a large peptide chain found in distinct locations within the central nervous system (Jessell and Kelly 1991). Beta endorphin has a half-life of about 4 h, so it can produce long-lasting pain modulation. Dynorphin and the enkephalins are smaller amino acid chains and are more widespread. They have a much shorter half-life, ranging between 45 sec and 20 min. Endogenous opioids compete for the same receptor sites as narcotic drugs. When an individual is prescribed pain medication, pain modulation through endogenous opioids becomes less effective.

It is believed that enkephalins and perhaps other opioid peptides inhibit the action of glutamate and substance P. Contemporary pain theories suggest that the body has opioid pain control systems that can be stimulated through external stimuli.

## PAIN CONTROL THEORIES

Understanding how pain is perceived is a prerequisite to studying the body's analgesic mechanisms. The pain-relieving effects of touch, acupuncture, and other treatments have been recorded since ancient times. How these treatments altered pain was unknown because of inadequate information regarding the human nervous system. As recently as the 1960s, pain and pain control theory revolved around the pattern theory and the specificity theory.

The pattern theory denied the existence of pain receptors and suggested that pain occurred when the rate and pattern of sensory input exceeded a threshold. Different sensations were thought to be represented by the pattern of action potentials within the nerve, much like Morse code. The specificity theory suggested that pain was perceived when pain receptors in the periphery were stimulated and that these pain receptors were connected directly to sensory areas in the brain. All sensory input was thought to be directly communicated by a specific receptor, to a specific nerve, and to a localized area of the brain. Neither theory plausibly explained the pain-relieving effects of treatments long recognized as effective.

In 1965, Melzack and Wall published proposals concerning their gate control theory of pain relief. This theory plausibly explained why therapeutic modalities controlled pain, and it initiated the development of new treatment approaches including TENS. Since 1965, more has been learned about the anatomy and physiology of the nervous system, and the theoretical base has expanded. Positron emission tomography (PET scan) and functional magnetic resonance imaging (MRI) are used to visualize working areas of the brain, and the understanding of neurochemical function is constantly expanding. The theories presented here reflect these advances. However, as our knowledge base continues to grow, the validity of these theories will be challenged and the scientific basis for clinical application of modalities will continue to evolve.

The scientific basis of athletic training has advanced considerably in the past few decades; however, it remains incomplete. Although athletic trainers have always applied therapeutic modalities, the rationale behind these treatments was often based on observations handed down from athletic trainers to students. As the profession has grown, some of the assumptions made regarding therapeutic modalities have been discovered to be unfounded. Thus, the scientific and theoretical basis of athletic training has evolved.

As more has been learned about the neuroanatomy and neurophysiology of the human body, new theories have emerged and have been modified, and this information is essential in the application of therapeutic modalities. Research is vital to explain why modalities are applied and why they produce desired clinical outcomes.

In much the same way pain transmission is organized, pain modulation models reflect the point of intervention: at the periphery, spinal level, supraspinal level, and descending pathway. One other theorized technique that a sports medicine clinician can use for the modulation of pain is to evoke an action potential failure. This technique is nerve block pain modulation. You should know where the pain modulation takes place. The pain modulation techniques used in therapeutic modalities are named for the type of stimulation used to evoke the analgesia. For example, in the gate theory, "sensory" stimulation presynaptically inhibits the pain transmission to the lateral spinothalamic tract. In contemporary physical medicine terminology, subsensory, sensory, motor, noxious, and action potential failure are mechanisms to modulate pain with electrical stimulation. Pain modulation with electrical stimulation, or electroanalgesia, is covered in chapter 9.

## Peripheral Pain Modulation

Pain modulation techniques can target the desensitization of peripheral nociceptors. If the receptor has a higher threshold, or is more difficult to stimulate, then fewer pain impulses are propagated to the spinal cord. Basically, the athletic trainer attempts to counteract the effects of acute inflammation that sensitizes free nerve endings and peripheral nociceptors. Bradykinin, prostaglandin E2, and serotonin in the periphery facilitate nociceptor sensitivity. These chemical mediators are released at the site of inflammation and alter the voltage threshold of ion channels to encourage action potentials (Cesare and McNaughton 1997).

How can the athletic trainer desensitize the peripheral nociceptors? We know that cryotherapy lessens the effects of the chemical mediators and slows conduction velocity of all sensory input. Applying ice to a painful area eventually leads to superficial anesthesia or numbness, thus minimizing the pain transmission to the spinal level.

Research on the inflammatory process and peripheral level of pain modulation demonstrates a complex matrix of chemotactic agents, immune cells, and endogenous opioids at the receptor sites. In attempts to discover new medications that act at the pain site rather than at the central nervous system, researchers are gathering new information about these mechanisms and the balance of pain and pain control. Although it has been documented that naturally occurring opioids such as beta endorphin modulate pain in the central nervous system, recent research has shown that intrinsic modulation of nociception can occur at the peripheral terminals of afferent nerves. Specifically, these studies indicate that the immune system can interact with peripheral sensory nerve endings to inhibit pain (Stein 1995).

Peripheral opioid receptors were identified when exogenously applied opioids were applied to mediate analgesia locally. The analgesic effect was most pronounced during painful inflammatory conditions when the resident immune cells in inflamed peripheral tissue secreted endogenous ligands or opioid peptides (Machelska et al. 1998). When the immune system was suppressed, the peripheral effect of beta endorphin was abolished. Environmental stimuli and endogenous substances, such as corticotropin-releasing hormone and cytokines, can stimulate the release of these opioid peptides. Means of eliciting pain relief with this method are still being explored. The potential exists for an intervention at this level by therapeutic modalities, but the mechanisms are currently unknown.

Subsensory-level electrical stimulation such as with microcurrent application has been proposed to affect pain modulation at the peripheral level. Microcurrent stimulation empirically reduces pain, but the explanation for the pain reduction is perplexing. Microcurrent application has been shown to improve healing in pressure sores (Carley and Wainapel 1985) which may be caused by an increased chemotactic effect of immune cells. This subsensory application of electrical stimulation may also be affecting the peripheral mediators of pain. Likewise, nonthermal ultrasound empirically reduces pain when applied over inflammatory conditions. The energy absorbed in the cells may lessen the sensitivity of the pain receptors. Further study is needed with both electrical stimulation and nonthermal ultrasound for pain modulation.

## Spinal Level Pain Modulation: The Gate Control Theory

Melzack and Wall proposed the gate control theory in 1965. This point is reiterated because this proposal gave credence to some of the methods used in physical medicine and redirected the research on pain modulation to facilitating the endogenous inhibitory control of pain. According to this theory, a neural mechanism in the dorsal horn of the spinal cord acts as a gate; this gate increases or decreases the flow of nerve impulses from the peripheral fibers to the central nervous system. The extent to which the gate enhances or reduces sensory transmission is determined by the relative activity of the large-diameter (A-beta) and small-diameter (A-delta and C) fibers. When the amount of information passing through the gate exceeds a critical level, it activates the neural areas responsible for pain sensation. The most likely site where spinal gating occurs is the substantia gelatinosa, an area within the dorsal horn of the spinal cord.

The model of Melzack and Wall was criticized because it emphasized presynaptic control and failed to predict the complex pattern of facilitation and inhibition observed in dorsal horn cells. In the revised model of Melzack and Wall, substantia gelatinosa contains both excitatory and inhibitory cells that project to the transmission cells. Central control mechanisms in the brain also modulate pain, via descending signals from the brain to the gate in the spinal cord, so that nociception is inhibited. The classic gate theory (figure 4.11) is presented along with a more contemporary model (figure 4.12) showing the impact of enkephalin interneurons that inhibit the transmission of pain.

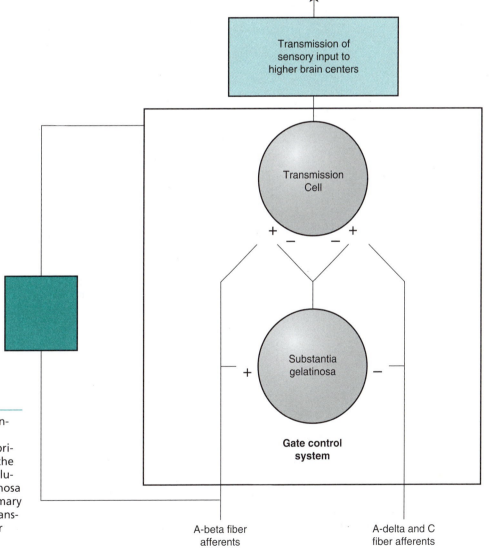

**Figure 4.11**   The gate control theory. Input along large-diameter (A-beta) primary afferents activates the presynaptic inhibitory influence of substantia gelatinosa on transmission from primary to afferent nerves to a transmission cell (second-order afferent).

The substantia gelatinosa acts as a presynaptic inhibitor that modulates pain by terminating presynaptically upon the large and small fibers just prior to their termination on the T cells. When the substantia gelatinosa is active, from neuronal input from the A-beta fibers, there is an increase in the presynaptic inhibition (gate is closed). The synapse does not produce an action potential, and the stimulation is not propagated. Ultimately, less sensory stimulation is perceived by the T cell. The idea that A-beta fibers could "close the gate" resulted in the development of TENS units to modulate pain perception.

In 1975 when endogenous opioids were identified, the gate theory was revised. It was proposed that an interneuron that utilized **enkephalin** (a naturally occurring opioid) was present in the area known as the substantia gelatinosa. The enkephalin interneuron inhibited the pain transmission within the dorsal horn (figure 4.12).

What is one of the first things you do after you bump your head? You probably rub it, and it feels better. This illustrates gate control theory. Rubbing your head activates non-nocicep-

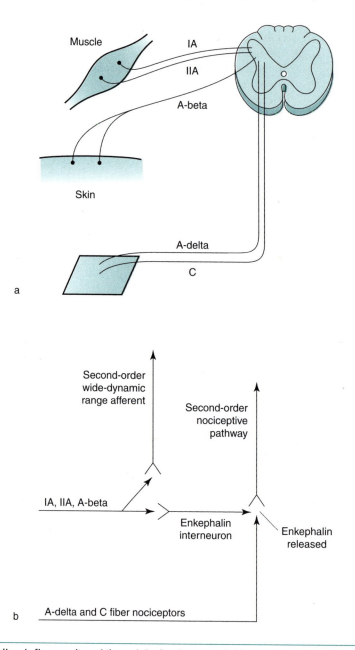

**Figure 4.12**    Ascending influence (Level I) model of pain control *(a)*. IA, IIA, and A-beta afferent nerves synapse with interneurons, which release enkephalins *(b)*.

tive touch signals carried into the spinal cord by large nerve fibers (A-beta). The inhibitory interneurons are activated by the rubbing, which then blocks the pain transmission. This explains why "counterstimulation" techniques are sometimes effective at relieving pain. One can evoke gate control by rubbing the skin (massage) or by using an electrical stimulator to excite the nerves in the skin. The electrical stimulator (TENS) stimulates the large (A-beta) sensory fibers in peripheral nerves to activate the inhibitory neurons of the dorsal horn and block pain transmission. Importantly, these devices work best when placed on or near the skin of the injured or painful region. The electrical stimulation should be strong and comfortable to maximize A-beta firing while avoiding A-delta stimulation. (More information on this technique is presented in chapter 10.)

# Supraspinal and Descending Pain Modulation

Pain transmission occurs through a complicated network of interneurons that activates numerous brain or supraspinal structures. These areas are in an intricate balance between alerting the individual that something is dreadfully wrong and calming the individual so that attention can be directed to solving the problem. As discussed previously, the descending mechanisms of pain modulation cause inhibitory signals to decrease the continued propagation of the pain message back at the spinal cord level. Descending pain modulation uses feedback loops that involve several different nuclei in the brainstem reticular formation; specifically, the PAG and the Raphe nucleus are important in controlling pain.

The PAG contains enkephalin-rich neurons that excite the Raphe nucleus, which in turn project down to the spinal cord to block pain transmission by dorsal horn cells. The descending modulation can be either direct, using an enkephalin interneuron, or by presynaptic inhibition. Presynaptic inhibition is caused by neurotransmitter release that blocks postsynaptic terminals.

A second descending system of serotonin-containing neurons exists. The cell bodies of these neurons are located in the Raphe nucleus of the medulla and, as with the noradrenaline-containing neurons, the axons synapse on cells in lamina II and III of the dorsal horn. Stimulation of the Raphe nucleus produces a powerful analgesia, and it is thought that the serotonin released by this stimulation activates inhibitory interneurons and thus blocks pain transmission. Serotonin neurons appear to inhibit somatosensory transmission and may have a function in the initiation of sleep. A complicating factor is that serotonin receptors are found in many places in the dorsal horn, including on primary afferents from C fibers. Serotonin may act to presynaptically inhibit pain by blocking the C fiber terminals for substance P and glutamate.

Additionally, the hypothalamus and pituitary gland are stimulated by the pain impulses. These centers base their function on a biofeedback loop to determine the need for neurochemical or neuroendocrine intervention. The pituitary can release precursors to powerful analgesic and anti-inflammatory agents.

The descending pain modulation mechanisms are evoked by pharmacological agents and stimulation. For research purposes and for chronic, intractable pain, electrical stimulation can be directly applied to the PAG for analgesia. This technique, because it involves applying the stimulation directly to the brain, is obviously beyond the scope of the athletic trainer's expertise. However, two different techniques of externally applied electrical stimulation have been shown to recruit descending pain modulation. These techniques use (1) a strong, pulsed motor stimulation and (2) a noxious stimulation. The following sections describe the schematic representation of the pain modulation theories, while chapter 10 describes the specific parameters necessary.

## *Motor Pain Modulation*

Endorphins are part of a complex neurophysiological system that decreases pain. They are opioids that are naturally produced (endogenous) in various locations in the body, including the central nervous system. The goal of motor pain modulation is to enhance the production of endorphins. No TENS treatment can eliminate pain, but if the pain is decreased, even temporarily, then therapeutic exercise can be initiated. The exercise along with other pain-relieving therapies such as joint mobilization and passive range of motion can contribute to the resolution of the pain–spasm–pain cycle.

Endorphins are primarily produced in the anterior pituitary through the breakdown of a large molecular complex known as beta lipotropin (figure 4.13). The beta lipotropin molecule is broken down to produce beta endorphin and certain types of enkephalins that have strong analgesic qualities. Adrenocorticotropic hormone (ACTH) is also produced in the pituitary gland and may affect cortisol production from the adrenal glands, which lie superior to the kidneys. Variations in cortisol production are normal, and subtle changes in ACTH levels are difficult to measure.

It is theorized that the endogenous opioid production is enhanced by low-frequency, high-intensity stimulation of peripheral nerve fibers. The frequency of stimulation must be in the 2 to 7 cycle per second range at intensities sufficient to evoke muscular contraction. Furthermore, endorphin has also been shown to exert a powerful influence on the Raphe nucleus and PAG that activate the descending control system. Therefore, when motor pain modulation is elicited with the rhythmical muscle contractions, along with A-delta fibers, there is an enhancement of the noxious pain modulation (descending tract) as well.

Low-frequency stimulation of trigger and acupuncture points is very valuable in the treatment of chronic and acute pain and injury. Increased corticosteroid levels from the enhanced ACTH production provide analgesic effects as well. Enhancement of pituitary production of hormonal and analgesic factors may also account for the high success rate of low-frequency TENS.

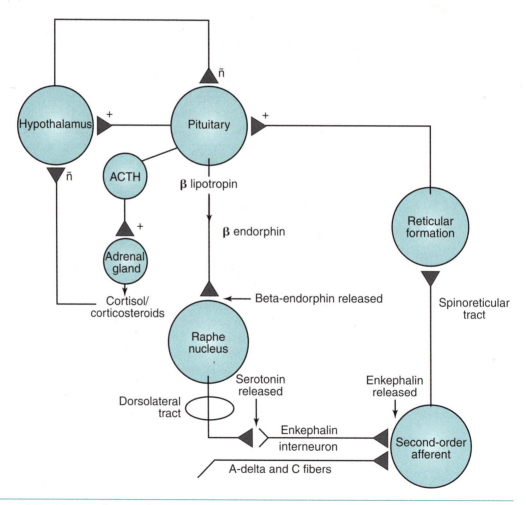

**Figure 4.13** Motor pain control. Neuroanatomic structures are stimulated by pulsed motor stimulation to elicit A-delta fiber excitation. Motor pain modulation requires strong but tolerable muscle contractions at 2 to 7 pulses per second.

## Noxious Pain Modulation

It has been shown that electrical stimulation of the PAG matter of the rat brain and human brain results in profound analgesia (figure 4.14). The Raphe nucleus, which is located in the pons and rostral medulla, receives projections from the PAG. A high density of projections from the Raphe nucleus to the substantia gelatinosa has been observed. These projections descend through the dorsolateral funiculus of the spinal cord. The analgesia evoked by the stimulation of PAG is dependent on this raphae-spinal pathway.

This type of pain modulation has been examined since the 1970s, when a researcher noted that stimulation of the PAG produced analgesia in unanesthetized rats (Mayer et al. 1971).

The Raphe nucleus tends to preferentially inhibit A-delta (over A-beta) fibers and contains serotonin-carrying neurons. Serotonergic neurons are heavily concentrated in lamina I of the dorsal horn of the spinal cord and are presumed to have a direct monosynaptic inhibitory effect on the second-order neuron, also known as the T cell.

A second system that originates in the pons also produces dorsal horn inhibition and analgesia. The descending inhibitory system may terminate directly on second-order neurons (T cells) or indirectly via an enkephalinergic interneuron.

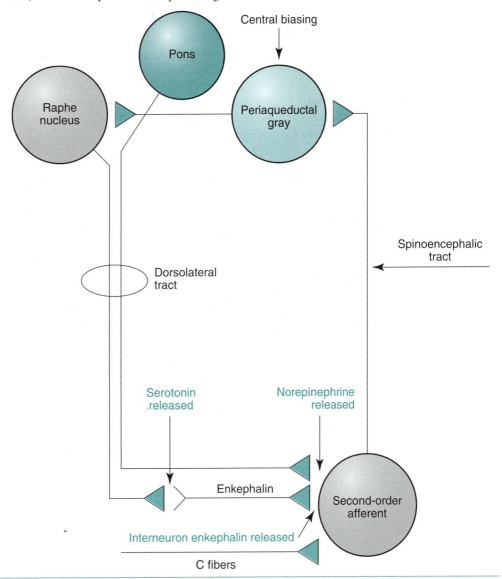

**Figure 4.14**   Noxious pain control is elicited by very painful stimulation of C fibers, usually using electrical stimulation. This causes an increase in the activity of the PAG and Raphe nucleus, producing inhibitory action on the transmission of pain at the spinal level.

This conceptual model is "turned on" by elicitation of pain (C fibers) in the affected region. The clinician can utilize certain types of electrical stimulation to excite C fibers, but a long phase duration is required (see chapter 10 for more information on electrical stimulation). Cryotherapy can also cause C fiber stimulation. When an ice pack is applied, the injured person will experience sensations of cold, burning, aching, and then numbness. The burning and aching sensations are caused by C fibers and may evoke descending pain modulation. This may explain the powerful analgesic property of ice treatment.

### Nerve Block Pain Modulation

The final technique that therapeutic modalities use to decrease pain is nerve block pain modulation or creation of an action potential failure. The application of electrical stimulation creates an "all-or-nothing" response in the nervous tissue on which it is applied. If the electrical stimulation exceeds the threshold of the resting membrane, if it is applied long enough to overcome the capacitance of the tissue, and if it is applied rapidly enough to prevent accommodation to the stimulation, an action potential will occur. This is the law of Dubois Reymond, discussed further in chapter 10. Once depolarization occurs, the nerve must "reset" itself with the sodium-potassium pump. This causes a refractory period during which the threshold is increased. If continual impulses are applied to the nerve at a fast pace (over 1,000 pulses per second), the membrane cannot continually fire because of the refractory period. Subsequent stimulation actually hyperpolarizes the membrane further, creating an inhibitory effect. The membrane is unable to keep up, and an action potential failure occurs. This is termed Wedenski's inhibition and is seen with the application of medium-frequency currents such as Russian stimulation or interferential stimulation. The area between the electrodes becomes temporarily anesthetic. This mechanism of pain control may be useful for superficial areas for a brief time period, but the analgesia lasts only as long as the stimulation.

There are still gaps in our understanding of the body's pain control systems. Melzack and Wall's notion of a central control of pain continues to intrigue researchers and clinicians. As noted at the beginning of this chapter, there are many influences on the perception of and reaction to noxious stimuli. We all have observed individuals who can block out pain or alter their pain experience. Relaxation and imagery are but two techniques to facilitate conscious, "central" control of pain.

Placebo responses to treatments are also poorly understood and are discussed in chapter 2. However, a belief that a treatment will relieve suffering may become a self-fulfilling prophecy. The placebo response confounds the investigation of therapeutic modalities used in athletic training and must be addressed by researchers in this area. However, another aspect of the placebo response is often overlooked by certified athletic trainers. Stated simply, a treatment is more likely to be effective if the individual and the athletic trainer believe it will be effective. Do not neglect the power of positive thinking in treating an injured athlete, whether you are applying a therapeutic modality or planning a rehabilitation program.

The mechanisms by which we can control our pain experience through conscious effort and subconscious processes are not fully understood. However, it is clear that the pain control systems described in this chapter are connected to a more complex process of neuromodulation that defines the pain experience.

## SUMMARY

1. Describe the multidimensional nature of pain.

   Pain can be conceptualized as having two dimensions: intensity and affective-motivational. The intensity component is pain sensation. Where does it hurt and how badly? The affective-motivational component relates to how an individual responds to pain. For example, is the person angry or withdrawn? Providing care involves more than asking about the intensity of the pain. The athletic trainer must respect each person's response to pain.

2. Explain the role of pain in preserving health and well-being.

   Pain signals that something is wrong with the body and is usually the motivation to seek medical care. Without pain, diseases and injuries (could) go undetected and therefore untreated.

3. Discuss how the pain response can assist in evaluating the injured athlete.

   Understanding the pain response following injury can help you make an accurate diagnosis. The causes, timing, locations, and severity of pain often narrow the possibilities and allow the sports medicine team to focus on special tests and examination procedures that lead to a rapid and accurate diagnosis.

4. Describe how pain is sensed and how the "pain message" is transmitted to the central nervous system.

   Free nerve endings are the body's pain receptors or nociceptors. When free nerve endings are stimulated, impulses are transmitted to the brain by specific nerves and neural pathways. Impulses are transmitted from the free nerve endings to the spinal cord by A-delta and C fiber primary or first-order afferent nerves. A-delta fibers more rapidly conduct pain, but C fibers cause a diffuse, noxious ache. The pain message is carried from the primary afferents up the spinal cord by second-order afferent nerves. The pain message can be carried on wide dynamic range, second-order nerves or on nociceptive-specific nerves. The nociceptive-specific nerves carry only pain information, whereas the wide dynamic range fibers carry all types of neural input. The second-order afferent fibers terminate at multiple brain centers. The thalamus, PAG region, and reticular formation all play important roles in accurate assessment of the pain message and in mediating the individual's response to pain.

5. Discuss contemporary theories on modulating the pain message in the central nervous system.

   In 1965, Melzack and Wall published the gate control theory of pain, which proposed that the pain message could be blocked at the spinal cord with appropriate external stimuli. With advances in neuroanatomy and neurophysiology, the basic concept of pain modulation has been refined. Descending modulation of pain is important for pain relief by the application of modalities. The noxious pain modulation model proposes that nerves descending from the Raphe nucleus can trigger the release of enkephalin and modulate pain, and that this descending pathway is stimulated by noxious input transmitted in the spinal-encephalic pathway to the PAG. This model offers a plausible explanation for pain relief induced by painful procedures such as acupressure. The motor pain modulation model proposes that pulsed, rhythmic stimulation of small-diameter afferent nerves can trigger the release of beta endorphin by connections between the hypothalamus and the Raphe nucleus. Because beta endorphin has a long half-life, this transmitter substance can stimulate the descending pathway for long periods. This model may explain how acupuncture and perhaps superficial heat relieve pain.

## CITED SOURCES

Berne RM, Levy MN: *Physiology*, 3rd ed. St. Louis, Mosby, 1993.

Bolay H, Moskowitz MA: Mechanisms of pain modulation in chronic syndromes. *Neurology* Sep 10;59(5 Suppl 2):S2-7, 2002.

Carley PJ, Wainapel S: Electrotherapy for acceleration of wound healing: Low intensity direct current. *Arch Phys Med Rehabil* 66:443-446, 1985.

Cesare P, McNaughton P: Peripheral pain mechanisms. *Curr Opin Neurobiol* Aug; 7(4): 493-499, 1997.

Denegar, CR, Perrin, D.H.: Effect of transcuteneious electrical nerve stimulation, cold, and a combination treatment on pain, decreased range of motion, and strength loss associated with delayed onset muscle soreness. *Journal of Athletic Training* 21: 200-206, 1992.

IASP: Pain terms: A list with definitions and notes on usage recommended by the IASP subcommittee on taxonomy. *Pain* 6:249-252, 1979.

Jessell TM, Kelly DD: Pain and analgesia. In Kandel ER, Schwartz JH, Jessell TM (Eds), *Principles of Neural Science*. Norwalk, CT, Appleton & Lange, 1991.

Knight KL: *Cryotherapy in Sports Injury Management*. Champaign, IL, Human Kinetics, 1995.

Machelska H, Cabot PJ, Mousa SA, Zhang Q, Stein C: Pain control in inflammation governed by selections. *Nat Med* Dec; 4(12): 1425-1428, 1998.

Margolis RB, Tait RC, Krause SJ. A rating system for use with patient pain drawings. *Pain* 24:57-65, 1986.

Mayer DJ, Wolfle TL, Akil H, Carder B, Liebeskind JC: Analgesia from electrical stimulation in the brainstem of the rat. *Science* 174:1351-1354, 1971.

Melzack R: *Pain Measurement and Assessment*. New York, Raven Press, 1983.

Melzack R, Wall P: Pain mechanisms: A new theory. *Science* 150:971-979, 1965.

Pollard CA: Preliminary validity study of the pain disability index. *Percept Mot Skills* 59:974, 1984.

Shultz SA, Houglum PA, Perrin DH: *Examination of Musculoskeletal Injuries*, 2nd ed. Champaign, IL, Human Kinetics, 2005.

Stein C: The control of pain in peripheral tissue by opioids. *N Engl J Med* 5 Jun 22;332(25):1685-1690, 1995.

## ADDITIONAL READINGS

Bonica JJ: *The Management of Pain*. Philadelphia, Lea & Febiger, 1990.

Calliet R: *Soft Tissue Pain and Disability*, 2nd ed. Philadelphia, Davis, 1988.

Calliet R: *Pain Mechanisms and Management*. Philadelphia, Davis, 1993.

Castel JC: *Pain Management: Acupuncture, and Transcutaneous Electrical Nerve Stimulation Techniques*. Lake Bluff, IL, Pain Control Services, 1979.

Kendell E, Schwartz J, Jessell T: *Principles of Neuroscience*. Norwalk, CT, Appleton & Lange, 1991.

Mannheimer JS, Lampe GN: *Clinical Transcutaneous Electrical Nerve Stimulation*. Philadelphia, Davis, 1984.

Porreca F, Lai J, Malan JT: Can inflammation relieve pain? *Nature Medicine* Dec;4(12):1359-1360, 1998.

# CHAPTER 5

# Persistent Pain and Chronic Pain

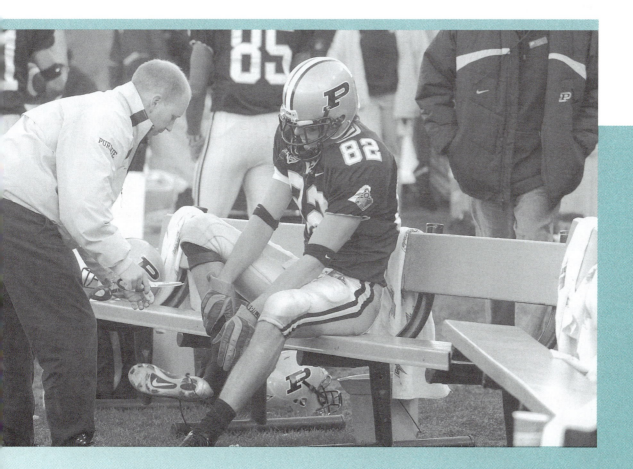

## *Objectives*

After reading this chapter, the student will be able to

1. describe the differences between acute and lasting pain;

2. identify common causes for persistent pain in active individuals, including diagnostic errors, faulty plans of rehabilitation, rest–reinjury cycle, complex regional pain syndrome, myofascial pain, and depression and somatization; and

3. define the differences between chronic and persistent pain and discuss how chronic pain may occur.

**A** 15-year-old basketball player developed patellofemoral pain during preseason. She was evaluated by the team physician and treated by the school's certified athletic trainer. She completed a rehabilitation program and returned to competition within 3 weeks. She subsequently developed a rotator cuff strain, was evaluated by an orthopedic surgeon, and again received treatment by the certified athletic trainer. She decreased her activity during Christmas break and recovered. One month later she developed low back pain. She was evaluated by the team physician and treated by the certified athletic trainer. She failed to improve and received additional treatment in a local sports medicine center. A modified plan of therapeutic exercises failed to resolve her low back pain, and she was reevaluated by an orthopedic surgeon. Reevaluation again suggested that she was suffering from mechanical low back pain. Her treatment was modified but the pain did not improve.

The athletic trainer was becoming frustrated about this athlete's situation. She always arrived in the training room on time and always complied with her rehabilitation. Finally, the athletic trainer discussed the situation with the basketball coach, learning that the athlete had moved into the school district the previous year with her mother. Her parents had recently divorced and her father now lived far away. Her older sister had earned a basketball scholarship to a major university. The coach believed that the family expected this athlete to follow her sister and attend college on an athletic scholarship. The coach also noted that the injured athlete did not really fit in with her teammates socially but often attended games with a small group of friends who were active in the school's band and chorus programs.

The athletic trainer consulted with the team physician, and they subsequently sought the advice of the school psychologist. The team physician arranged a meeting with the athlete's mother, the athlete, the physician, and the school psychologist. The meeting confirmed the circumstances relayed by the basketball coach, revealing that the athlete felt so pressured to perform well in basketball that she felt guilty about exploring her interest in singing. Her mother stated her support for her daughter and indicated that although an athletic scholarship would be nice, it was not necessary in order for her daughter to attend college. Both mother and daughter were open about the difficult adjustments they were trying to make following the divorce and move to a new area.

The mother and daughter agreed that family counseling might help them, and they were referred to a local family counselor and psychologist. The athlete decided to continue to play basketball but also became more active in the school's fine arts programs. Under the guidance of the team physician and certified athletic trainer, she continued to be treated for mechanical low back pain. She was independent in her back care within 3 weeks.

The case study presents a situation in which an athlete sought medical care because of pain that affected performance. The certified athletic trainer and team physician used pain to diagnose the injuries and plan treatments. However, psychological factors can also produce pain (Heil 1993; Peppard and Denegar 1999). The appropriate treatment of some physically active individuals requires the recognition of psychological factors, intervention, and, when necessary, referral for definitive psychological care. Somatization and depression are common psychological problems that can result in unexplained somatic pain.

In the previous chapter, pain was identified as a cardinal sign of inflammation and a warning that something is wrong with the body, and the relationship between inflammation and tissue healing was described. Logic suggests that when the inflammatory response subsides and tissues heal, pain should disappear. However, sometimes pain lasts beyond, or occurs in absence of, inflammation.

Chronic pain has been defined as pain that lasts beyond the normal time frame for healing. Some have suggested a specific length of time, 6 months, for example (Donley and Denegar 1994; Stone 1987), before lasting pain is labeled as chronic. It may be more appropriate to divide lasting pain into the categories of persistent and chronic pain. Because the term *chronic pain* implies that the pain is mysterious and untreatable, the term *persistent pain* is more appropriate in many cases.

Persistent pain is often treatable through activity modification, appropriate modality application, therapeutic exercise, and sometimes counseling. What is chronic pain? The International Society for the Study of Pain task force suggested that chronic pain is "persistent pain that is not amenable, as a rule, to treatments based upon specific remedies, or to the routine methods of pain control such as non-narcotic analgesics" (Merskey and Bogduk 1994, p. XII). Chronic pain likely involves changes in how the nervous system operates. If this definition is applied, those suffering from true chronic pain will not improve through the administration of therapeutic modalities. The sports medicine team should carefully evaluate a physically active person who has been experiencing pain lasting weeks, months, or even longer. In most cases the source of pain can be identified and effectively treated. When treatments are not effective despite reevaluation and revisions of the treatment plan, a diagnosis of chronic pain must be considered. Hopefully, advances in the understanding and treatment of chronic pain will improve pain management and the quality of life for those afflicted by this condition.

Persistent pain is a significant challenge to the sports medicine team, and it is frustrating to the physically active individual as well. Therapeutic modalities are very useful in some, but not all, cases of persistent pain. Chronic pain, by definition, fails to respond to modality application.

This chapter introduces the problem of persistent pain, identifying sources of persistent pain in the context of clinical exam findings, and touches on the treatment of persistent pain. However, uses of specific modalities to treat persistent pain are discussed in chapter 16, after each modality is introduced in intervening chapters. A brief review of central sources of chronic pain is also included here to introduce the reader to potential sources of this disabling condition.

## SOURCES OF PERSISTENT PAIN

Most injured individuals treated by a certified athletic trainer respond well to treatment and return to competition within a predictable time frame. However, some fail to respond to treatment, and their symptoms persist beyond the normal time required for tissue repair and maturation. Others present with complaints of pain without an identifiable pathology. Are these problems due to a failure to heal? Does pain linger even though tissue has healed? Is the injury imaginary? The certified athletic trainer must try to answer these questions, being ever mindful that pain is a symptom that something is wrong (figure 5.1).

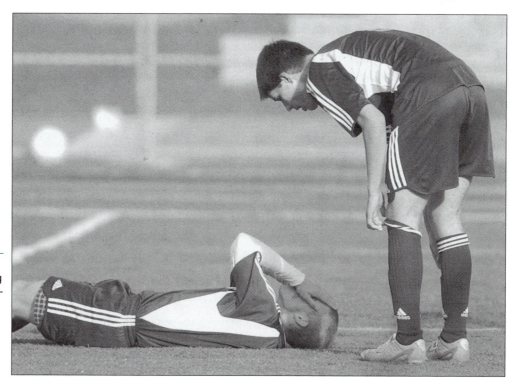

**Figure 5.1** Pain is a symptom that something is wrong. When pain persists even after an injury has been treated, the certified athletic trainer must work with the athlete to determine the underlying cause.

The causes of persistent pain span a spectrum from physical to principally psychological (figure 5.2). The physical causes involve a diagnostic error, a failure to correct faulty biomechanics, an inappropriate treatment plan, or a rest–reinjury cycle. However, physical pain may also be a symptom of somatization and depression. The causes of complex regional pain syndrome and myofascial pain syndrome are multifaceted and not fully understood. However, psychological stress appears to contribute to or exacerbate these conditions.

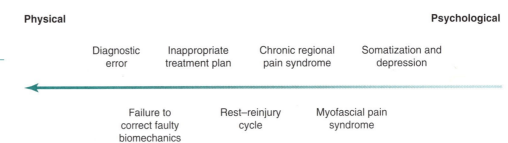

**Figure 5.2** Persistent pain spans a spectrum from physical to principally psychological.

Adapted by permission from Denegar and Peppard 1997.

## The Diagnosis

When pain persists, the certified athletic trainer should reevaluate the injury and complaint of pain as though it were a new problem. Sometimes persistent pain stems from a problem that was not recognized on initial examination. Thus, the first step in reevaluation is to reconsider the original diagnosis.

In the following case, the new diagnosis required a much different plan of care. Appropriate treatment of this runner's stress fractures resulted in complete resolution of the persistent foot pain. Although she presented with many signs and symptoms consistent with plantar fasciitis, the persistence of the problem led to a complete review of her case and, ultimately, a correct diagnosis.

## Case Study

A women's cross country runner was diagnosed by a team physician as having bilateral plantar fasciitis. She received daily treatments with ultrasound followed by massage and stretching before training, and ice massage after workouts. Because her foot pain did not improve, she was referred to an athletic trainer, who found that some of her symptoms were not consistent with plantar fasciitis. The athletic trainer discussed the athlete's situation with the team physician and an orthopedic surgeon; the orthopedic surgeon requested additional diagnostic imaging, which revealed bilateral navicular stress fractures (Denegar and Siple 1996).

This case illustrates two very important lessons. First, the application of therapeutic modalities is part of a comprehensive plan of care. Failures can occur in evaluation, treatments, or rehabilitation. When the physically active do not respond to treatment, you must explore the reasons.

Second, persistent pain problems are often complex. Modalities can mask symptoms and delay definitive care, but they can also allow pain-free therapeutic exercise. You must be capable of evaluating and treating persistent pain problems as well as symptoms of acute inflammation. This chapter provides a hierarchy of persistent pain problems that is a model for evaluation of physically active individuals.

## Biomechanics and Somatic Dysfunction

Evaluating the injured person's movement mechanics is also an essential part of a comprehensive physical exam. Failure to identify biomechanical flaws may leave the major cause of persistent pain untreated. Certified athletic trainers commonly encounter individuals who are suffering from medial tibial stress syndrome or shinsplints. Modalities may help reduce pain, but modality application does not cure the injury. Often the cause of the problem is excessive subtalar pronation, and recognizing and controlling excessive subtalar pronation may alleviate persistent shin pain with running. Thus, the solution to the problem lies in identifying and correcting the underlying cause of pain, rather than simply treating the pain.

Many other repetitive microtrauma injuries are related to movement mechanics, such as patellofemoral pain, iliotibial band (ITB) friction syndrome, and Achilles tendinopathy. In the upper extremity, improving scapular stabilization may be the key to relieving persistent shoulder pain.

Somatic dysfunction is a term that we define as a circumstance in which dysfunction or malalignment in one area is resulting in tissue overload and pain at a distant site. Stated differently, the biomechanics of a kinetic chain are being altered by a state of dysfunction or malalignment. For example, an athlete presenting with ITB friction syndrome may in fact have hypertonus in the tensor fascia lata muscle caused by pelvic rotation. The tension in the muscle tightens the ITB, causing it to rub over the lateral femoral condyle. Thus, the athlete presents complaining of lateral knee pain, but the underlying cause is pelvic malalignment. The clinician must address the underlying causes of the kinetic chain dysfunction to successfully treat the athlete-patient.

## Plan of Care

Persistent pain after injury or surgery can sometimes be attributed to an incomplete or inappropriate treatment plan. Failure to address scapular stabilization in individuals with shoulder instability and impingement is one example. Another example is an aggressive postoperative regimen of therapeutic exercises following patellar bone-tendon-bone anterior cruciate ligament reconstruction that results in patellar tendinopathy. In the second case, the exercise regimen must be modified to prevent persistent anterior knee pain.

Many treatment and rehabilitation programs for specific musculoskeletal injuries are discussed in another of the books in this series: *Therapeutic Exercise for Musculoskeletal Injuries, Second Edition* (Houglum 2005). However, because therapeutic modalities are used to treat persistent pain, this chapter discusses the plan of care as a source of persistent pain.

## Rest–Reinjury Cycle

Athletic excellence requires individuals to put forth maximum effort and push through pain in their training. When injured, physically active individuals generally will accept a period of rest until the pain is relieved. The absence of pain, however, is often interpreted as a sign that the tissue is healed and that the athlete is ready to return to unrestricted practice and competition. If the tissue is not ready, reinjury occurs and the rest–reinjury cycle begins (Peppard and Denegar 1994). Rehabilitation extends beyond specific treatments and therapeutic exercises and must include a gradual return to functional exercises.

Recognizing persistent pain involving a rest–reinjury cycle will allow the certified athletic trainer to educate the injured individual about the differences between conditioning and reconditioning after injury. Reconditioning requires careful control of exercise intensity, frequency, and duration. The exercise program must allow the person to stay within the exercise tolerance window. Exercise that results in pain severe enough to alter movement patterns must be avoided, and intensity and duration must be limited to avoid postexercise pain.

A good rule is that the injured individual should be able to do tomorrow what was done today. In other words, if someone is too sore to repeat yesterday's therapeutic and functional exercises, the exercise tolerance limit was exceeded and the rehabilitation process slowed. As a well-structured rehabilitation program progresses, the exercise tolerance window widens and the individual becomes more tolerant of exercise-induced pain. Training should be specific, structured, and, when possible, supervised. Coaches and strength and conditioning specialists can help the injured athlete progress in gradually more demanding sport-specific exercises and general reconditioning.

The certified athletic trainer should carefully evaluate the use of therapeutic modalities in all cases of persistent pain. This is especially important when a rest–reinjury cycle is involved.

Physically active individuals frequently respond well to modality application for pain control, but they may continue to seek the treatments that allowed them to return to practice and competition following the initial injury. The certified athletic trainer can perpetuate the rest–reinjury cycle by continuing **palliative care** without educating the injured individual and his or her coaches about the problem and restricting the athlete's exercise program.

## Complex Regional Pain Syndrome

**Complex regional pain syndrome (CRPS),** also commonly labeled reflex sympathetic dystrophy (RSD), is a symptom complex characterized by pain that is disproportional to the injury. The syndrome involves hypersensitivity to touch and movement, joint stiffness and muscle guarding, edema, erythema, hyperhydrosis, and osteopenia (Gieck and Burton 1986). The etiology of this condition is not fully understood, making treatment a challenge. Complex regional pain syndrome may occur after even minor injury or following surgery; it can occur immediately or may be delayed. The individual may experience a normal postinjury or postoperative course for several days before the early signs of CRPS appear. In some cases, the onset of CRPS may not appear until symptoms are nearly resolved.

Ladd et al. (1989) introduced the term *reflex sympathetic imbalance (RSI)*, a related disorder involving pain that is out of proportion to the injury. Although disproportional pain is the hallmark symptom of CRPS, other signs and symptoms may not be present initially. These authors suggested that RSI can be diagnosed solely based on the presence of disproportional pain, thus expediting recognition of many causes of CRPS. Early recognition increases the likelihood of successful treatment. If disproportional pain is present, the sports medicine team should not wait until other symptoms are present before considering a diagnosis of CRPS and initiating appropriate treatments.

CRPS progresses through three stages over several months. When it is recognized and treated early, the prognosis for recovery is good. However, CRPS can become a permanent, disabling condition if not recognized early in its development. Treatments and exercises that exacerbate pain should be discontinued, and the individual should follow up with his or her physician as soon as possible. Because CRPS can develop into a permanent and disabling condition, all members of the sports medicine team must be able to recognize its early signs. When pain appears out of proportion to what is expected with a specific injury, or at specific point in recovery from injury or surgery, the certified athletic trainer and team physician must explore the possibility of CRPS.

Medical management of CRPS may include medications as well as injections to block sympathetic pathways. The certified athletic trainer must work with the medical team to design a comprehensive plan of care. Therapeutic modalities can be very useful in treating CRPS; however, no treatment should be administered that is painful for the injured individual. Moist heat, cold, and massage must be used with caution. Biofeedback, transcutaneous electrical nerve stimulation (TENS), gentle massage and joint mobilization, and pain-free therapeutic exercises are usually better tolerated than more vigorous treatment approaches. As the condition improves, the therapeutic exercise regimen can be progressed and more vigorous stimulation will be tolerated. The bottom line is that early recognition of CRPS is critical, and treatments that cause pain exacerbate the problem and must be avoided.

## Myofascial Pain

As previously noted, when pain persists beyond the time frame for tissue repair, the certified athletic trainer should review the situation systematically and thoroughly, looking for diagnostic and treatment errors, **rest–reinjury cycles,** and CRPS. If this review does not identify the cause of persistent pain, **myofascial pain syndrome (MFPS)** or somatization must be considered.

Myofascial pain syndrome is characterized by pain emanating from the muscles and connective soft tissues. It is commonly associated with the cervical and lumbar spine; however, persistent joint pain can result in myofascial pain patterns in the extremities as well.

## Causes of Myofascial Pain Syndrome

There is no single cause of MFPS, making the condition difficult to diagnose and treat. Several factors can contribute to its development, including trauma and repetitive microtrauma with recurrent painful episodes, posture, stress, and fatigue.

In sport, repetitive microtrauma can trigger MFPS. For example, physically active individuals with long histories of knee and shin pain such as medial tibial stress syndrome or patellofemoral pain can develop secondary, or Type II, MFPS (Denegar and Peppard 1997), challenging you to treat the primary injury as well as the secondary MFPS. These athletes generally complain of very localized tenderness over inflamed tissue and a more general aching pain in the affected limb. Further evaluation will often reveal soft tissue tightness and **trigger points** in a pattern characteristic of MFPS. With experience, you will be able to locate sensitive trigger points and identify characteristic patterns related to specific areas of the body. Trigger points manifest bilaterally, and those on the contralateral side may be the most sensitive. Figures 5.3 and 5.4 depict common trigger points associated with knee, hip, elbow, back, shoulder, foot/ankle, and forearm/upper extremity pain.

A single traumatic episode can result in MFPS. Often patients in the sports medicine center, some of whom are physically active and others not, will complain of neck pain, shoulder pain, and headaches several months following automobile accidents. Often the only injury sustained was a "minor" whiplash or low back strain. Acute pain that resolved within 3 weeks and a lingering aching pain that worsens with fatigue are common findings. Increased pain while using a keyboard, while driving, and while performing other activities that place the individual in a forward-head position and stress the paraspinal musculature is a common complaint. Neck and shoulder pain is frequently accompanied by headaches. The pain often affects the individual's ability to participate in sport. In these cases, MFPS is the primary problem.

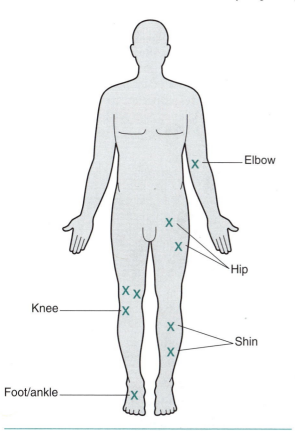

**Figure 5.3** Common trigger points associated with knee, hip, elbow, shin, and foot/ankle pain.

Reprinted by permission from Denegar and Peppard 1997.

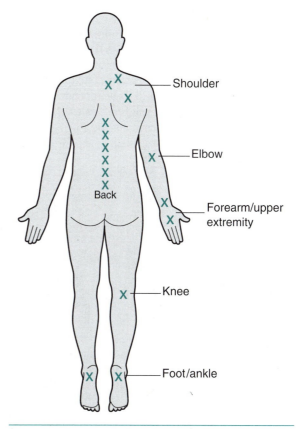

**Figure 5.4** Common trigger points associated with shoulder, elbow, back, knee, foot/ankle, and forearm/upper extremity pain.

Reprinted by permission from Denegar and Peppard 1997.

Poor posture, faulty movement mechanics, and stress play a role in the development of MFPS. A general lack of fitness and occupations that lead to postural deficits are associated with Type I MFPS affecting the trunk and neck (Denegar and Peppard 1997). Some sports such as cycling and swimming can also lead to muscle imbalances and poor posture. Often people alter movement patterns in an attempt to avoid pain, and these natural adaptations stress tissues that are not well conditioned, exacerbating the pain. Conversely, faulty movement mechanics can cause repetitive microtrauma injuries that lead to Type II MFPS. If excessive pronation is the cause of medial tibial stress syndrome or patellofemoral pain, neither the primary problem nor Type II MFPS will resolve until running mechanics are addressed, unless, of course, the individual quits running. Thus, you should assess posture and movement mechanics in all cases of MFPS.

Stress is common in our lives, and the demands of sport and pressure to succeed add to stress. Student-athletes strive to balance schoolwork, social life, family commitments, and the demands of sports. Other physically active people often squeeze training and competition in between job and family commitments. Individuals respond to the stresses of daily life differently. However, many people treated for MFPS in the back, neck, and shoulders "hold" their stress in the affected area. Many do not appreciate how much tension resides in these areas until it is relieved through treatment. Some learn to manage pain when they appreciate how their response to life events affects them. Some clinicians are very effective at helping individuals understand their response to stress and assisting with stress management. All members of the sports medicine team must be able to recognize when physical responses to stress contribute to persistent pain and must be able to assist individuals with stress management (figure 5.5).

## Recognizing Myofascial Pain Syndrome

The individual with myofascial pain will complain of pain that has persisted for several months or recurrent painful episodes. Myofascial pain is generally localized to a region but is not focal. Myofascial pain syndrome is characterized by tension in the muscles and fascia with exquisitely tender trigger points. The person usually complains of an aching, burning sensation that is worse with overuse and fatigue. Symptoms often radiate from the neck and shoulder to an upper extremity and from the low back and sacroiliac region to a lower extremity. The radiating symptoms do not usually follow a dermatomal distribution and can usually be reproduced by stimulating the most sensitive trigger points. If you suspect MFPS, explore for contributing factors previously discussed. Myofascial pain syndrome is a diagnosis of exclusion. Each case must be systematically reviewed to rule out other causes of persistent pain before the individual is treated for MFPS.

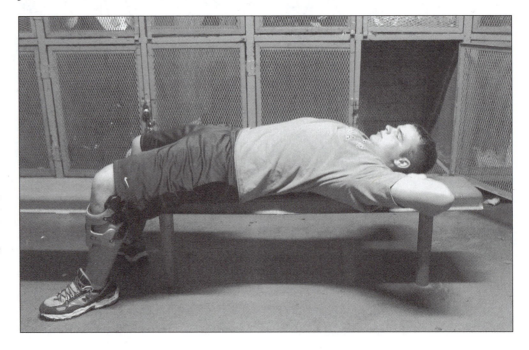

**Figure 5.5** Some physically active individuals may need help understanding their response to stress. All members of the sports medicine team should recognize when a stress response contributes to persistent pain.

### Modality Application and Myofascial Pain Syndrome

There is not a single cause of MFPS, and therefore there is not a single remedy. Orthotics to correct faulty biomechanics, therapeutic exercise and postural retraining, stress management, manual therapy, and therapeutic modalities can be used to treat MFPS.

The physical principles and the physiological responses to contemporary therapeutic modalities are presented later in this book. Touch is important in the evaluation of MFPS (figure 5.6), and chapter 13 includes an extensive introduction to manual therapies. Manual therapy, superficial heat, cold, ultrasound, and TENS may be combined to treat MFPS. Development of a plan of care for the individual with MFPS is presented in chapter 16.

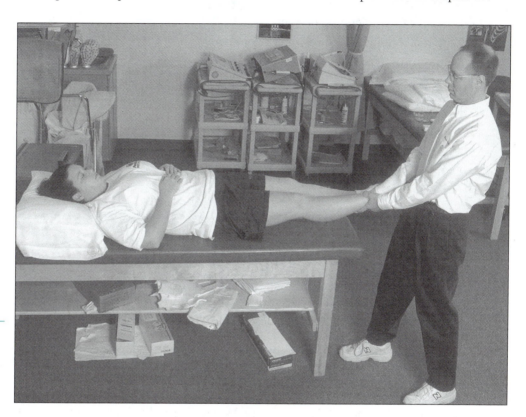

**Figure 5.6**  Touch is important in the evaluation of myofascial pain syndrome, and manual therapies can be effective in its treatment.

## Depression and Somatization

When pain fails to resolve despite additional diagnostic testing, the individual should be reexamined and multiple treatment approaches explored. The pain of a knee sprain signals the need for medical attention and treatment, but pain in the absence of physical injury also signals a need for treatment. The experienced sports medicine team must be able to read the signals and provide appropriate care.

One in eight individuals will require treatment for depression. However, only one half to one third of patients with major depressive disorders are recognized by physicians (Depression Guidelines Panel 1993). Many physically active individuals with depressive disorder are referred to certified athletic trainers and physical therapists for treatment of their somatic complaints. The close working relationship between the certified athletic trainer and the physically active person allows the athletic trainer greater opportunity to identify pain and psychological origin.

### Major Depressive Disorder

A major depressive disorder is diagnosed by the presence of at least five of the symptoms listed on page 78 (Depression Guidelines Panel 1993; Peppard and Denegar 1999). One of the first two must be present. The symptoms must be present nearly daily, for most of each day, for 2 weeks.

# Signs and Symptoms of Major Depressive Disorder

- Depressed mood
- Markedly diminished interest in or pleasure derived from almost all activities
- Significant weight loss or weight gain
- Insomnia or hypersomnia
- Psychomotor agitation or retardation
- Fatigue or loss of energy
- Feelings of worthlessness or guilt
- Impaired concentration and indecisiveness
- Recurrent thoughts of death or suicide

Features most associated with younger individuals include the following:

- Overeating
- Oversleeping
- Mood that responds to events
- Extreme sensitivity to interpersonal rejection
- Complaints of heaviness in the arms and legs

## Somatization Disorder

**Somatization** is the presentation of somatic symptoms by someone with psychiatric illness or psychological distress (Lipowski 1988). A diagnosis of somatization disorder requires a history of many physical complaints including four pain symptoms, two gastrointestinal symptoms, one sexual symptom, and one pseudoneurological symptom that are not explained by medical conditions or intentionally caused (American Psychiatric Association 1994). Undifferentiated somatoform disorder (somatization) is defined as one or more physical complaints, without identifiable cause, that last for more than 6 months (American Psychiatric Association 1994). The region and nature of the symptoms often mimic those of musculoskeletal injury. When a rehabilitation plan of care is initiated but the individual fails to improve, and other causes of persistent pain are ruled out, a diagnosis of somatization should be considered.

# Indications of Somatization

Indications that somatization may be present include the following (American Psychiatric Association 1994; Lipowski 1988):

- Increased demand on the athletic trainer's time including lengthy visits, frequent appointments, and multiple telephone calls
- Frequent requests for treatments that require special attention
- Behaviors that demonstrate a need for special attention
- Anger when the athletic trainer indicates that the condition has improved sufficiently to warrant discontinuation of treatment and a return to sport
- An individual's history inconsistent with the physical exam

Individuals with somatization disorder can be very demanding and difficult; however, recognition and appropriate care are to everyone's benefit. In treating somatization, the care provider should (1) provide care for a bona fide injury, (2) develop a sound relationship to prevent the individual from fleeing and entering a pattern of "doctor shopping" (seeking care from one doctor after another in search of a physical cause of symptoms), and (3) avoid doing harm by dismissing the individual as a malingerer or symptom magnifier.

You should not provide psychological counseling unless qualified to do so. However, many physically active individuals have benefited from informal counseling provided by members of the sports medicine team. The young physically active person often needs to talk to someone who will listen without prejudging. Listening to young athletes and reassuring them that their fears and concerns are common can help them cope during a difficult situation.

The skilled and appropriately trained certified athletic trainer can help individuals control their stress response through such techniques as biofeedback, muscle relaxation, thought stopping, deep breathing, or imagery (Peppard and Denegar 1994, 1999). Proficiency at these techniques requires formal instruction and practice, and you should not employ techniques with which you are not proficient.

Regardless of your attempts to provide excellent care, a limitation of success must be recognized. Not all injured people get better. Physical causes of the problem should be sought; however, it is often easier to continue to search for physical causes than confront psychological ones. The search for psychological causes begins with communication. Listening and interpreting nonverbal communication require training, skill, practice, and patience.

Somatic pain of psychological origin is a symptom, a crying out. The sports medicine team is well prepared to treat the pain of physical injury and illness, but detecting emotional pain requires skill as well. Sometimes all that an individual needs is a sympathetic ear and reassurance that the stresses he or she is experiencing are normal. Sometimes the skilled athletic trainer can assist with stress management and arousal control. Definitive psychological care may ultimately be required; certainly depression and somatization warrant medical and psychological attention. The sports medicine team must develop the skills to identify these problems and refer individuals to appropriate resources.

## SOURCES OF CHRONIC PAIN

In some cases individuals report severe pain that is unresponsive to the interventions of the sports medicine team. These patients may have examination findings that are consistent with persistent pain as described earlier such as mechanical dysfunction, a pattern of trigger points consistent with myofascial pain, or signs of depression. Chronic pain may be a cause of depression. In these cases the complaint of pain may be most attributable to changes in nervous system function. This is a complex issue and not entirely understood. Wright (2002, p. 48) described mechanisms of peripheral and central sensitization of the nociceptive system. In summarizing peripheral sensitization, he wrote, "It is apparent that the sensitization process is fairly complex and that different forms of sensitization may develop depending on the nature of the injury or disease." Peripheral sensitization has been linked to alterations in ion channels in nociceptors under the influence of multiple chemical mediators, activation of silent nociceptors, and phenotype changes of some afferent nerve fibers. Neuroplasticity is not limited to peripheral sites but also plays a role in central sensitization. Alterations in ion concentrations, neuroanatomical organization, and cell function within the dorsal horn have been identified as contributors to this phenomenon.

Clearly, mechanisms of truly chronic pain are not fully understood and are beyond the scope of this text. It is important, however, to appreciate that new developments increase the likelihood of effective treatment for more sufferers of chronic pain. The clinician must also recognize that the hypersensitivity of some individuals to normally non-pain-provoking stimuli is the result of complex alterations in the function of the nervous system.

## SUMMARY

1. Describe the differences between acute and lasting pain.

   Acute pain, a warning that something is wrong and requires medical attention, is associated with musculoskeletal injury. Pain that persists beyond the normal time required for tissue repair is less well understood. Often, when an individual's pain lasts for weeks or months, it is labeled chronic pain. Because the term *chronic* implies a sense of hopelessness, the term *persistent pain* was introduced to identify situations in which lasting pain is a signal that something is wrong and will respond to appropriate treatment. Chronic pain is complex and very poorly understood; however, often the causes of the persistent pain can be identified and effectively treated.

2. Identify common causes for persistent pain in active people, including diagnostic errors, faulty plans of rehabilitation, rest–reinjury cycle, complex regional pain syndrome, myofascial pain, and depression and somatization.

   Persistent pain can result from a number of causes. This chapter begins with physical causes and progresses to psychological causes of persistent pain. Physical causes include diagnostic errors and faulty plans of care. Failure to identify the problem or effectively address identified problems can lead to persistent symptoms. Physically active individuals often associate the absence of pain with complete recovery, which can lead them to overstress healing tissues and experience reinjury. This phenomenon can repeat, setting up a rest–reinjury cycle. Complex regional pain syndrome, also labeled reflex sympathetic dystrophy, is characterized by pain out of proportion to the extent of an injury as well as hypersensitivity to touch and movement, joint stiffness and muscle guarding, edema, erythema, hyperhydrosis, and osteopenia. Complex regional pain syndrome is progressive, and the prognosis for complete recovery worsens if diagnosis and treatment are delayed. Myofascial pain, which may result from many causes, is a diagnosis of exclusion characterized by tender trigger points, increased tension in muscles, and often a pattern of referred pain. Physical symptoms can result from psychological dysfunction. The somatic pain experienced by those suffering from depression and somatization is a signal that care is needed. Unfortunately, somatic symptoms stemming from psychological dysfunction are more difficult to interpret. If other sources of persistent pain are ruled out, the sports medicine team should consider psychological causes before making the diagnosis of chronic pain.

3. Define the differences between chronic and persistent pain and discuss how chronic pain may occur.

   The principal difference between chronic and persistent pain is that chronic pain will not respond to conventional treatments such as modality application and at present is reduced only with narcotic medications. Chronic pain is the result of changes within the nervous system in the periphery, spinal cord, higher brain centers, or more than one of these. The changes have only recently been identified and have not been fully understood. Hopefully, research will lead to a better understanding and treatment of chronic pain.

## CITED SOURCES

American Psychiatric Association: *Diagnostic and Statistical Manual of Mental Disorders*, 4th ed. Washington, DC, American Psychiatric Association, 1994.

Denegar CR, Peppard A: Evaluation and treatment of persistent pain and myofascial pain syndrome. *Athl Ther Today* July:38-42, 1997.

Denegar CR, Siple BJ: Bilateral foot pain in a collegiate distance runner. *J Athl Train* 31:61-64, 1996.

Depression Guidelines Panel: *Depression in Primary Care: Vol 1. Detection and Diagnosis. Clinical Practice Guidelines, Number 5*. Rockville, MD, U.S. Department of Health and Human Services, Public Health Services, Agency for Health Care Policy and Research, 1993.

Donley PB, Denegar CR: Managing pain with therapeutic modalities. In Prentice WE (Ed), *Therapeutic Modalities in Sports Medicine*, 3rd ed. St. Louis, Mosby, 1994.

Gieck J, Buxton BP: Reflex sympathetic dystrophy. *Athl Train, JNATA* 22:120-125, 1986.

Heil J: *Psychology of Sport Injury*. Champaign, IL, Human Kinetics, 1993.

Houglum PA: *Therapeutic Exercise for Musculoskeletal Injuries*, 2nd ed. Champaign, IL, Human Kinetics, 2005.

Ladd AL, DeHaven KE, Thanik J, Patt RB, Feuerstein M: Reflex sympathetic imbalance. *Am J Sports Med* 17:660-667, 1989.

Lipowski ZJ: Somatization: The concept and its clinical application. *Am J Psychiatry* 145:1358-1368, 1988.

Merskey H, Bogduk N: Classification of chronic pain. *Definitions of Chronic Pain Syndromes and Definition of Pain Terms*, 2nd ed. Seattle, WA. International Association for the Study of Pain, 1994.

Peppard AP, Denegar CR: Pain and the rehabilitation of athletic injury. *Orthop Phys Ther Clin North Am* 3:439-462, 1994.

Peppard A, Denegar CR: Depression and somatization and persistent pain in the athletic patient. *Athl Ther Today* Nov:43-47, 1999.

Stone LA: Pain in neuromuscular disorders. In Ecternach JL (Ed), *Pain*. New York, Churchill Livingstone, 1987.

Wright A: Neurobiology of pain and pain modulation. In Strong J, Unruh AM, Wright A, Baxter GD (Eds), *Pain: A Textbook for Therapists*. Edinburgh, Churchill Livingstone, 2002.

## ADDITIONAL READINGS

Travel JG, Simons DG: *Myofascial Pain and Dysfunction: The Trigger Point Manual*. Baltimore, Williams & Wilkins, 1983.

# Impact of Injury and Pain on Neuromuscular Control

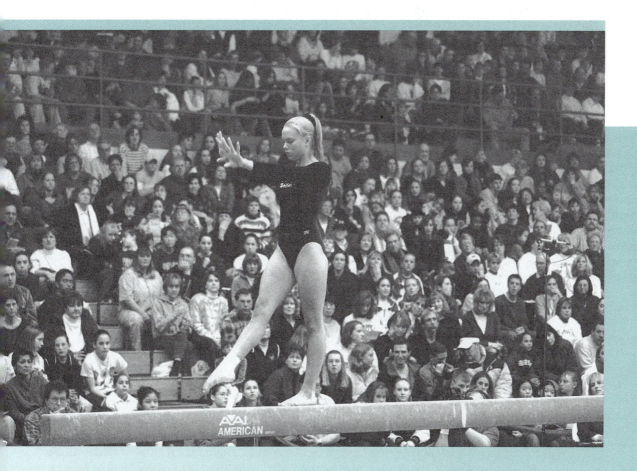

## *Objectives*

After reading this chapter, the student will be able to

1. identify the three components of neuromuscular control;

2. differentiate between neuromuscular control deficits and muscle atrophy as causes of muscular weakness; and

3. discuss the effects of swelling, pain, and altered mechanoreceptor input on neuromuscular control.

A fit, physically active 22-year-old collegiate rugby player enters the athletic training room for a preoperative consultation to review a postoperative rehabilitation plan of care. He injured his right knee 5 months ago while skiing and was diagnosed with a torn anterior cruciate ligament. He delayed surgery because of a heavy work schedule but is to undergo a patellar bone-tendon-bone allograft reconstruction in 2 days. He states he has been working out regularly to build muscle strength and maintain overall fitness. Examination of the knee reveals a positive Lachman's test, full knee range of motion, and excellent muscular development of the quadriceps and hamstrings.

On the day following surgery, he has extreme difficulty contracting his vastus medialis during a quadriceps set and is initially unable to perform a straight leg raise (figure 6.1). Why are the quadri-ceps so weak? Less than 24 h has passed since surgery, certainly too little time for muscle to atrophy. You determine that this athlete is experiencing a loss of neuromuscular control and use neuro-muscular electrical stimulation to assist in neuromuscular reeducation. Within a couple of days, you observe substantial improvement.

This case study illustrates that pain, swelling, and joint instability can impair neuromuscular control. The certified athletic trainer must be able to detect and correct deficits in neuromuscular control to progress a rehabilitation plan into strength, power, and sport-specific retraining.

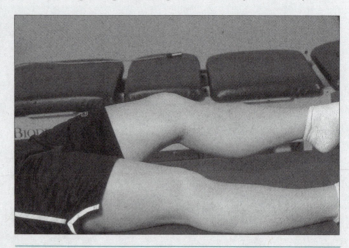

**Figure 6.1**  Straight leg raise with extensor lag.

The three previous chapters introduced the inflammatory response, acute pain, and lasting pain. Those chapters, and this introduction to neuromuscular control, form the foundation for the application of therapeutic modalities. This chapter identifies the causes of impaired neuromuscular control and introduces basic concepts of neuromuscular reeducation. Chapter 10 presents techniques of neuromuscular electrical stimulation, and chapter 15 presents the role of biofeedback in restoring neuromuscular control. Additional treatment strategies are discussed in detail in another text in this series: *Therapeutic Exercise for Musculoskeletal Injuries, Second Edition* (Houglum 2005).

Six components of a progressive rehabilitation program were identified in the first chapter (see figure 1.3 on page 7). Therapeutic modalities are commonly applied to control pain and interrupt the pain–spasm cycle. Pain control and appropriate postinjury care to minimize swelling will help restore range of motion. The next priority in rehabilitation is to return neuromuscular control, the last component of the rehabilitation program affected by modality application (figure 6.2).

## INTEGRATION OF COMPONENTS OF NEUROMUSCULAR CONTROL INTO A REHABILITATION PLAN OF CARE

Restoration of control over volitional contractions, reflex reactions, and complex functional movements were identified in chapter 1 (see figure 1.3) as components of a progressive

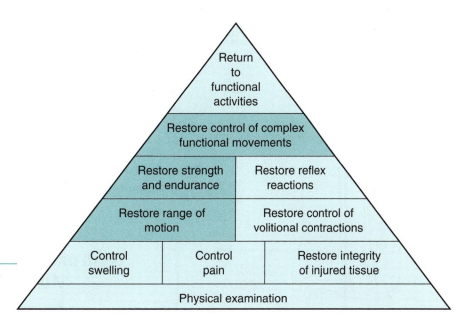

**Figure 6.2** Hierarchy of rehabilitation goals.

Reprinted by permission from Hertel and Denegar 1998.

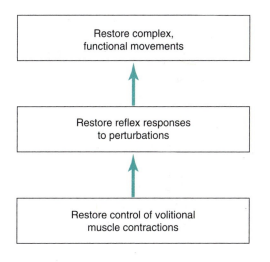

**Figure 6.3** Rehabilitation paradigm for restoring muscular control.

Reprinted by permission from Hertel and Denegar 1998.

rehabilitation plan of care. These components encompass the continuum of neuromuscular control. By recognizing that neuromuscular control consists of three components the certified athletic trainer can integrate activities to restore neuromuscular control throughout the plan of care (figure 6.3).

**Neuromuscular control** is an elusive concept in the rehabilitation paradigm. Unlike pain, range of motion, strength, endurance, and power, neuromuscular control is difficult to measure and quantify. From a practical and clinical perspective, there are three components of neuromuscular control (figure 6.2). The first is consciously controlled, voluntary muscle contraction (or volitional contraction). Individuals who suffer significant knee injuries, experience patellofemoral pain, or undergo knee surgery lose neuromuscular control of the quadriceps as a result of pain and swelling. A loss of volitional control of muscle is illustrated in the opening case study, in which the rugby player was unable to contract the quadriceps muscle (quadriceps set) or perform a straight leg raise. This athlete demonstrated a disruption of the body's ability to recruit strong, volitional muscle contraction because normal neuromuscular control had been compromised.

The second component of neuromuscular control involves restoring reflex responses. For example, when the lateral ligaments of the ankle are stressed, mechanoreceptors in the joint capsules and ligaments respond with a volley of sensory input (see chapter 4). The increase in sensory input recruits the ankle everters to resist ankle inversion. Because the reflex loop synapses are found in the dorsal horn, the reaction is a spinal reflex-generated muscle contraction (figure 6.4). When ligaments are damaged, the sensory input from the mechanoreceptors is altered and the reflex control over the muscles inhibited. This loss of reflex response is most associated with the concept of proprioception. However, proprioception is really the afferent component of neuromuscular control. Furthermore, in tasks such as balancing, the individual's ability to recruit skeletal muscle to maintain stance is based on sensory input from mechanoreceptors, Golgi tendon organs, and muscle spindles. Thus, these assessments really measure neuromuscular control rather than partialing out true proprioception.

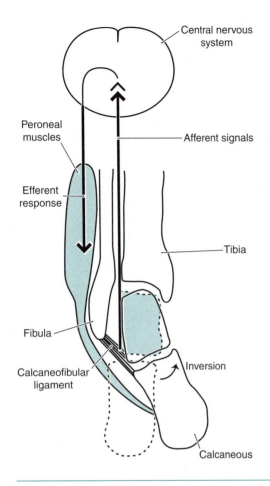

**Figure 6.4** Reflex circuits.

Reprinted by permission from Human Kinetics 2000.

The final component of neuromuscular control relates to complex, functional movements. When one becomes proficient in athletics, complex integration of afferent input is required to precisely control movement through efferent pathways. Conscious effort is absent once the movement begins. For example, when attempting to learn to play golf, the player is consciously aware of each movement. As the player becomes proficient, he or she executes the swing without conscious control. However, injury can disrupt the ability to perform well-practiced, functional movement patterns. The individual who is unable to perform a straight leg raise will also demonstrate abnormal stair climbing patterns and running gait, indicating disrupted neuromuscular control of functional and sport-specific movements.

## Neuromuscular Control and Muscle Atrophy

Muscles generate force when motor nerves send impulses to the muscle fibers they innervate. The more muscle fibers stimulated to contract, the more force is generated. The cross section of muscles also influences the amount of force a muscle can generate. When muscle is not used for a period of time, the cross section diminishes, or atrophies, which is a relatively slow process. When the ability to recruit muscle fiber contraction in a coordinated manner is impaired, neuromuscular control has been lost, a process that can occur quite quickly.

Thus, a loss of neuromuscular control should not be confused with muscle **atrophy.** Several weeks of muscle disuse, such as cast immobilization, will result in atrophy as well as loss of neuromuscular control. Fortunately, the importance of early motion following musculoskeletal injury is widely recognized, and prolonged immobilization is used only when absolutely necessary.

# WHY IS NEUROMUSCULAR CONTROL LOST?

The case study at the beginning of this chapter provides a clinical example of lost neuromuscular control. Inhibition of quadriceps function following knee injury is commonly encountered in clinical practice. The relationship between knee injury and neuromuscular control of the quadriceps has received considerable attention in the medical literature. However, much more study is needed for us to fully understand the impact of musculoskeletal injury on neuromuscular control and refine therapeutic approaches to restoring neuromuscular control.

Clinical observations and scientific investigations suggest that more than one factor contributes to decreased neuromuscular control following musculoskeletal injury. This chapter further explores the impact of swelling, pain, and altered mechanoreceptor input on the ability to consciously perform volitional muscle contractions. Mechanoreceptor input is often altered when the ligaments and the capsule protecting a joint are sprained and the joint becomes unstable. As discussed in chapter 3, pain and swelling are associated with acute inflammation. Furthermore, as discussed in chapter 5, pain may occur in the absence of inflammation. In any case, these factors contribute individually and collectively to impaired neuromuscular control.

Activities to restore pattern-generated movements and reflexive muscle contractions usually do not involve therapeutic modalities. These therapeutic strategies are addressed by Houglum (2005) in *Therapeutic Exercise for Musculoskeletal Injuries, Second Edition.* However, volitional control over isolated muscles, such as occurs when a straight leg raise is used to recruit the quadriceps, or when controlled functional motions such as bending and stair climbing are initiated, can be restored by therapeutic modality application. Furthermore, conscious control of muscle must be restored before reflex patterns and more complex movement patterns can be retrained. Thus, successful rehabilitation often requires that you identify and correct deficits in volitional control over skeletal muscles.

## Swelling

Swelling within the joint capsule of the knee decreases quadriceps function. Certified athletic trainers observe this phenomenon following knee injury, and researchers have studied it. By infusing saline solution into the knee, researchers have been able to inhibit quadriceps function as measured through electromyography (EMG) (Kennedy, Alexander, and Hayes 1982; Spencer, Hayes, and Alexander 1984). Vastus medialis activity can be inhibited by as little as 30 ml of fluid (Spencer, Hayes, and Alexander 1984). This small increase in fluid volume would appear as very mild effusion upon clinical exam. Larger increases in volume affect the function of the other quadriceps muscles. A 200-ml increase can severely limit the ability to perform a straight leg raise even in the absence of knee injury (Kennedy, Alexander, and Hayes 1982). Neuromuscular inhibition appears to persist as long as joint capsule volume remains elevated (Kennedy, Alexander, and Hayes 1982).

The reason joint effusion inhibits quadriceps femoris function is not fully understood. However, much of the knee joint capsule is innervated by articular branches of the femoral nerve (figure 6.5). In particular, the articular branch of the femoral nerve to the vastus medialis supplies a large portion of the anteromedial joint capsule. Swelling within the capsule may stimulate stretch receptors, which in turn trigger reflex inhibition of the motor neuron pool. The suprapatellar pouch accommodates increases in joint fluid volume more than do other parts of the joint capsule. The tendency of fluid to accumulate in this area of the knee may partially explain why the vastus medialis is most affected by swelling within the knee joint.

Tsang (2001) found that the infusion of saline into the joint capsule of the ankle impaired postural control and inhibited recruitment of the peroneal musculature. His results suggest that the phenomenon of swelling-induced loss of neuromuscular control is not isolated to the knee joint. The impact of extracapsular swelling on measures of neuromuscular control has not been examined in a laboratory model and warrants investigation.

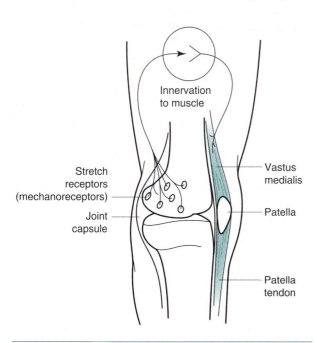

Stretch receptors (mechanoreceptors)

Joint capsule

Innervation to muscle

Vastus medialis

Patella

Patella tendon

**Figure 6.5** Swelling within the capsule may stimulate stretch receptors, which in turn trigger reflex inhibition of the motor neuron pool.

## Pain

Pain also appears to affect neuromuscular control. Individuals who have sustained injury to the lower extremity often limp to protect damaged tissue and minimize pain. The altered movement patterns represent alterations in neuromuscular control. Could the observed gait deviation be due to swelling and altered mechanoreceptor input? Perhaps, but careful observation suggests that pain contributes to neuromuscular control deficits. Individuals with little or no swelling and no history of trauma may exhibit decreased neuromuscular control.

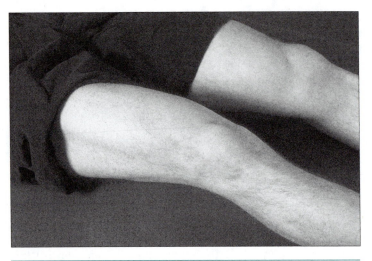

**Figure 6.6**    Decreased tone in quadriceps.

For example, individuals with patellofemoral pain (PFP) experience little or no swelling. The connective tissues housing mechanoreceptors have not been damaged, nor are these receptors stimulated due to swelling. However, if you ask the person with PFP to tighten the quadriceps muscle and you palpate the vastus medialis, it will feel softer than the fully tightened quadriceps of the uninjured leg (figure 6.6) because the individual is unable to effectively recruit the vastus medialis.

Observations such as these support the notion that pain contributes to the loss of neuromuscular control. Unfortunately, it is difficult to study the impact of joint pain on neuromuscular control in a research laboratory. Ethical and methodological considerations restrict the induction of joint pain, so clinical observation remains the best evidence that pain alters neuromuscular control.

Despite the lack of research evidence, clinical observation offers insights into successful clinical practice. The first such insight relates to the discussion of PFP. When knee pain inhibits vastus medialis function, patellar mobility increases. With greater patellar mobility, there is more irritation of the joint tissues and more pain. Thus, a cycle is created that gradually turns into patellofemoral pain syndrome. With sufficient irritation, swelling will also develop, further compromising neuromuscular control and exacerbating the cycle.

This phenomenon explains why some athletes who present with the signs and symptoms of patellofemoral pain syndrome have no history of knee injury. Other factors, such as changes in training routine, and biomechanical problems such as subtalar hyperpronation and genu varus, clearly are contributors. However, these factors do not explain the loss of neuromuscular control of the quadriceps. Thus, it appears that pain decreases neuromuscular control.

The role of pain in the loss of neuromuscular control is an important consideration during therapeutic exercise. When active exercise is painful, normal neuromuscular patterning is disrupted. Painful exercise inhibits muscle groups, perpetuates abnormal motor control, and slows recovery from injury. With the exception of passive stretching of muscle and connective tissue, therapeutic exercise must remain pain free if neuromuscular control is to be reestablished and maintained.

## Altered Input

The proprioceptors in the skin, muscles, tendons, and joints provide the central nervous system (CNS) with a constant flow of **somatosensory information.** The CNS responds by generating appropriate motor commands to allow the body to move safely through a changing environment.

For example, when the ankle is inverted toward the limits of the range of motion, afferent input is generated in three ways: (1) The mechanoreceptors within the ligaments and joint capsule alert the CNS to the precarious position of the ankle; (2) muscle spindles within the muscles that evert the ankle (peroneus longus and brevis) signal that the muscle is rapidly stretching; and (3) skin receptors signal the distortion and stretch of the skin over the lateral ankle. The CNS processes these afferent signals and responds by activating the motor pathways that cause the everters to contract and by inhibiting motor activity in the antagonistic muscles to counteract the sudden inversion of the ankle. Thus, the proprioceptors sense the potential for ankle joint injury, and the CNS responds through a dorsal horn synaptic reflex loop to prevent joint injury.

The sensory input from mechanoreceptors can trigger muscle contractions through the spinal reflex loops. Moreover, the continuous flow of sensory input from mechanoreceptors is essential to the performance of coordinated movements. Mechanoreceptors are most active at the anatomical limits of the physiological range of motion. Damage to ligaments and joint capsules alters mechanoreceptor input in the damaged tissue and subsequently affects neuromuscular control. Swelling that limits full range of motion also alters mechanoreceptor activity. These changes in the pattern of sensory input from mechanoreceptors decrease neuromuscular control. For example, researchers studying quadriceps musculature in patients with anterior cruciate ligament (ACL)-deficient knees found 10% to 30% decreases in pain-free, isokinetic force production despite minor atrophy and little morphological change (Lorentzon et al. 1993).

It has been suggested that following ACL injury, input from capsular mechanoreceptors facilitates hamstring function and inhibits recruitment of the quadriceps (Solomonow et al. 1987). Certainly the observant athletic trainer can detect altered movement patterns in physically active people following knee injuries, as well as in those with more chronic knee instability. The evidence suggests that these changes in neuromuscular control persist after pain and swelling have resolved.

Much of our understanding of the impact of swelling and pain on neuromuscular control has come from the study of knee injury. However, alterations in kinesthetic awareness and slowed reflex contractions have been observed following injury to other joints.

## Ankle Injuries

Neuromuscular control is lost following sprains of the lateral ligaments of the ankle. Researchers have reported deficits in position sense (Freeman 1965) and balance in single-leg stance (Gross 1987). In addition, the response of the peroneal muscles is slowed following ankle sprain (Lofvenberg et al. 1995). One of the goals of treatment following an ankle sprain is to restore neuromuscular control of the muscles surrounding the ankle. This is accomplished through a return to pain-free weight bearing as early as possible, depending on the severity of the injury, and a progressive program of balance and coordination exercises (figure 6.7).

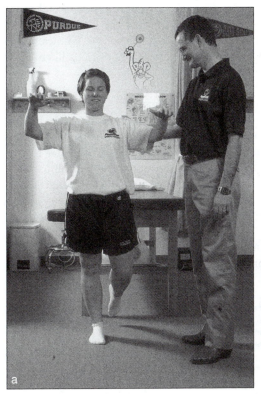

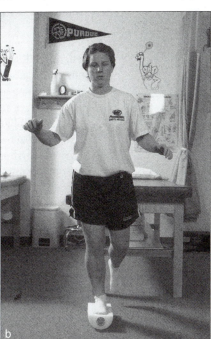

**Figure 6.7**  An example of balance and coordination exercises: Single-leg balance *(a)* and sport cord balance on foam *(b)*.

### Shoulder Injuries

Pain, disruption in ligamentous stability, and swelling appear to inhibit the rotator cuff, especially supraspinatus, and perhaps the scapular stabilizers. The stabilizing function of these two muscle groups is essential for normal, pain-free shoulder function. For many years, individuals with rotator cuff tendinitis and glenohumeral impingement were treated with rotator cuff strengthening exercises. Some improved rapidly, whereas others improved very slowly. Closer examination of those who failed to respond to rotator cuff strengthening revealed that many demonstrated impaired neuromuscular control of the rotator cuff, the scapular stabilizers, or both (figure 6.8).

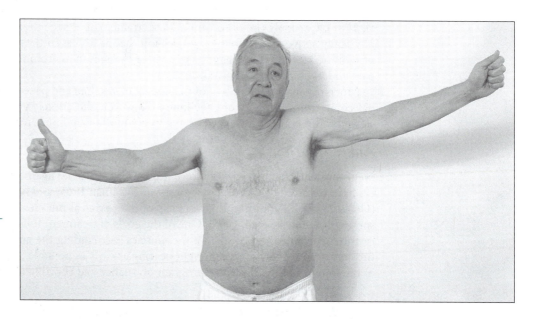

**Figure 6.8** Shoulder hiking in an effort to abduct the arm is a common manifestation of impaired neuromuscular control.

Injury to the ligaments and capsule of the glenohumeral joint compromises the sense of shoulder positioning and movement detection. Clinically these injuries compromise the athlete's ability to keep the shoulder out of positions likely to cause dislocation and further injury.

Training with visual and EMG biofeedback effectively addresses neuromuscular control deficits and speeds recovery. Pain, instability, and swelling appear to affect the shoulder muscles in much the same manner as occurs with the quadriceps following knee injury. Strengthening alone does not relieve shoulder pain or promote recovery following shoulder dislocation. The injured individual must relearn proper control of the glenohumeral and scapular stabilizers—in other words, reestablish neuromuscular control.

The impact of swelling, pain, and instability in other joints on neuromuscular control warrants further study. Certainly, there is a component of neuromuscular retraining following any injury; however, it may be more easily accomplished in some parts of the body than others. One area receiving greater attention is the lower back, where pain may alter neuromuscular function of paraspinal muscles. This loss of neuromuscular control represents a significant challenge in treating a physically active person with a history of back injury and pain.

## THE ROLE OF THERAPEUTIC MODALITIES IN RESTORING NEUROMUSCULAR CONTROL

Subsequent chapters discuss neuromuscular electrical stimulation and EMG biofeedback, the modalities most commonly used to help individuals regain volitional control of muscle contraction. There are no direct modality applications used to retrain protective reflex responses or control of complex movements. However, several therapeutic modalities may be used to permit pain-free exercises aimed at restoring these components of neuromuscular control. When rehabilitation is viewed as a hierarchy of goals and modalities are viewed as a means of achieving specific goals, the relationship between modality application and efforts to restore neuromuscular control becomes evident.

## SUMMARY

1. Identify the three components of neuromuscular control.

   Neuromuscular control can be divided into three components: (1) conscious, volitional control over isolated muscle contraction; (2) protective reflex patterns; and (3) control over complex, functional movements.

2. Differentiate between neuromuscular control deficits and muscle atrophy as causes of muscular weakness.

   Muscles generate force when motor nerves send impulses to the muscle fibers they innervate. The more muscle fibers stimulated to contract, the more force is generated. The cross section of muscles also influences the amount of force a muscle can generate. When muscle is not used for a period of time, the cross section diminishes, or atrophies, which is a relatively slow process. When the ability to recruit muscle fiber contraction in a coordinated manner is impaired, neuromuscular control has been lost; this can occur quite quickly.

3. Discuss the effects of swelling, pain, and altered mechanoreceptor input on neuromuscular control.

   Impaired neuromuscular control is common following musculoskeletal injury. Research has demonstrated that swelling alone can impair neuromuscular control. Most of the work has involved the knee, where relatively small amounts of fluid infused into the joint diminish the ability to contract the quadriceps muscle. Pain results in protective muscle spasm and loss of function. The precise mechanisms by which pain affects neuromuscular control have not been fully explained. However, observations of individuals without demonstrable swelling or instability often reveal inhibition of neuromuscular control. Joint instability resulting from ligament and capsular injury has also been shown to alter neuromuscular control. Injuries to ligaments and joint capsules damage the mechanoreceptors and alter the proprioceptive feedback to the CNS. Control of muscle activity depends on sensory feedback, and disruption of this loop manifests as loss of neuromuscular control.

## CITED SOURCES

Freeman MAR: Instability of the foot after injuries to the lateral ligaments of the ankle. *J Bone Joint Surg* 47B:669-677, 1965.

Gross MT: Effects of recurrent lateral ankle sprains on active and passive judgment of joint position. *Phys Ther* 67:1505-1509, 1987.

Hentel J, Denegar CR: A rehabilitation paradigm for restoring neuromuscular control following athletic injury. *Athletic Therapy Today* 3(5): 12-16, 1998.

Houglum PA: *Therapeutic Exercise for Musculoskeletal Injuries*, 2nd ed. Champaign, IL, Human Kinetics, 2005.

Kennedy JC, Alexander IJ, Hayes KC: Nerve supply to the human knee and its functional importance. *Am J Sports Med* 10:329-335, 1982.

Lofvenberg R, Karrholm J, Sundelin G, Ahlgren O: Prolonged reaction time in patients with chronic lateral instability of the ankle. *Am J Sports Med* 23:414-417, 1995.

Lorentzon R, Elmqvist L, Sjostrom M, Fagerlund M, Fuglmeyer AR: Thigh musculature in relation to chronic anterior cruciate ligament tear: Muscle size, morphology and mechanical output before reconstruction. *Am J Sports Med* 17:423-429, 1993.

Solomonow M, Baratta R, Zhou BH, Shoji H, Bose W, Beck C, D'Ambrosia R: The synergistic action of the anterior cruciate ligament and thigh muscles in maintaining joint stability. *Am J Sports Med* 15:207-213, 1987.

Spencer JD, Hayes KC, Alexander IJ: Knee joint effusion and quadriceps reflex inhibition in man. *Arch Phys Med Rehabil* 65:171-177, 1984.

Tsang KKW: The Effects of Induced Effusion of the Ankle on Neuromuscular Control. Doctoral dissertation, Penn State University, 2001.

## ADDITIONAL READINGS

Basmajian J, Deluca C: *Muscles Alive: Their Function Revealed by Electromyography.* Baltimore, Williams & Wilkins, 1985.

Smith LK, Weiss EL, Lehmkuhl LD: *Brunnstrom's Clinical Kinesiology,* 5th ed. Philadelphia, Davis, 1996.

# CHAPTER 7

# Evidence-Based Application of Therapeutic Modalities

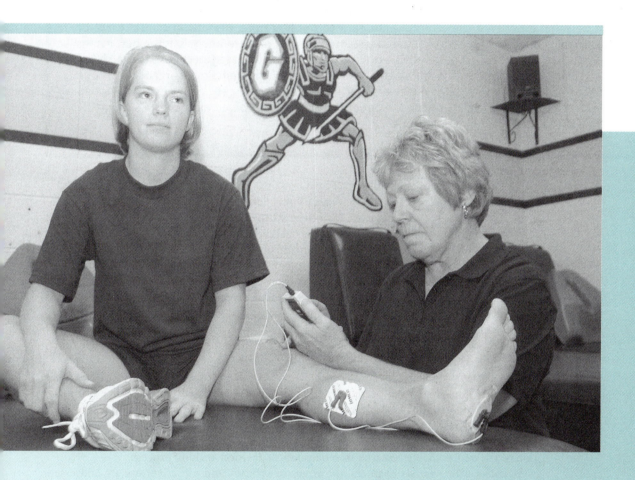

## *Objectives*

After reading this chapter, the student will be able to

1. define the term *evidence-based health care*;
2. discuss the role of outcomes assessment in advancing evidence-based health care;
3. describe how clinical trials are conducted;
4. identify the components of well-designed randomized controlled clinical trials; and
5. identify resources for locating clinical trials of treatments in which therapeutic modalities were used.

An active middle-aged woman is referred for treatment of knee pain due to moderate osteo-arthritis in the medial compartment and patellofemoral joint of her left knee. She was an avid runner but is now cycling and swimming for cardiovascular fitness. Her primary complaint is aching in the joint, most bothersome in the evening. She also reports that her knee pain awakens her several times each week. The attending orthopedic surgeon has requested a trial of transcutaneous electrical nerve stimulation (TENS) with a home unit.

As you instruct the patient in the use of the device, she asks "Is TENS effective in managing knee pain?" How can you best answer this question? You might be able to rely on previous experiences, although most clinicians will have only a few such experiences on which to base a response. Lacking sufficient personal experience the clinician must turn to the literature. Reviewing clinical trials, or being fortunate enough to find a well-prepared systematic review or meta-analysis, is the best means of providing a response based on the available clinical literature. In this case you choose to search the Cochrane Library. The search yields a systematic review of clinical trials employing TENS to manage knee pain caused by osteoarthritis. The reviewers concluded that there is sufficient evidence to recommend the treatment. Now you can provide the patient with an answer based on the results of quality clinical trials rather than your limited experience.

The practice of **evidence-based health care** was defined by Sacket et al. (2000) as the integration of the best research evidence with clinical expertise and patient values. In the previous four chapters, the sequelae to injury and the challenges of lasting pain were presented. This background was provided so that the therapeutic modalities that are to be discussed can be applied with an understanding of the physiology of injury and repair as well as an appreciation for the impairments, functional limitations, and disabilities experienced by injured athletes. In the succeeding six chapters, the physical principles and application techniques of contemporary modalities will be presented. Issues of safety and contraindications will be highlighted. Following the introduction of the modalities, discussion will turn to the "when" and "why" of modality application. These issues are further summarized in the concluding chapters, in which principles of clinical decision making are applied.

The answers regarding the "why" and "when" of therapeutic modalities, as well as other medical interventions, have been and often continue to be based upon practice traditions and theory. Increasingly, health care providers are being called upon to seek out and provide evidence that the interventions they recommend *enhance recovery and improve the outcome of treatment*. This search for evidence may challenge our assumptions but permits the integration of the best available research into our clinical decision-making process.

In each of the next six chapters, the issues of **efficacy** and **effectiveness** are addressed. We provide references to clinical trials and make practice recommendations based on our reviews. Reading these sections should not substitute for individual effort. Each clinician is responsible for the decisions he or she makes based on the information available. Reviewing, analyzing, and applying the evidence found in the existing literature has several potential benefits for the patient, clinician, and health care system. First, critical review may lead to the discontinuation of treatments that may do more harm than good and of ineffective treatments that only delay appropriate care. Furthermore, such efforts identify how effective treatments may be rendered in the most cost- and time-efficient manner. Lastly, this process helps focus attention on what is really important—did the patient get better, and if so, was this really the result of the treatment rendered?

## THE NEED FOR EVIDENCE-BASED PRACTICE

Health care is complex, costly, and essential. The cost of health care can be assessed not only in terms of dollars spent but also in terms of time required of patients and providers. The challenge across health care is to provide the care necessary to optimize treatment outcome in the most efficient manner. The challenges facing the health care system of patients, providers, and payers are no less a concern in athletic training than in other health care disciplines. To meet these challenges, treatment regimens need to be analyzed and compared based on the outcomes and costs of care. Those treatments not demonstrated to improve outcomes should be abandoned from general practice. For example, Deyo et al. (1990a) reported that TENS is ineffective in the management of chronic low back pain. This is does not mean that a particular modality like TENS is of no value. Further study of some treatments may be warranted to identify conditions or populations (patients without contraindications treated for pain associated with acute rib fracture) for which the treatment is effective (Oncel et al. 2002). New evidence should be evaluated and, when appropriate, should change how individuals practice. Moreover, new research and systematic reviews of existing research may also result in new practice recommendations for all clinicians.

Numerous assessment tools have been developed to assess the outcomes of treatment with medications and surgery as well as modality application and therapeutic exercises. Outcome assessments often include clinician-derived measures such as changes in range of motion and strength. However, information provided by patients regarding levels of pain, functional limitations, and perceived disability is also vital. Reports of treatment outcomes based on clinician assessments and patient self-assessments are increasingly available to guide the clinician's selection of effective treatments with therapeutic modalities and exercises. The certified athletic trainer must develop the ability to identify pertinent literature, assess the validity of the conclusions drawn by investigators, and judge the extent to which the results of **clinical trials** generalize to the people they treat.

At this point you may question why published clinical trials are important to modality use specifically and health care in general. When an injured athlete under your care reports improvement, you can be certain that treatment you provided was beneficial. *Unfortunately, that is not the case!* Many factors can lead to improvements associated with care rendered by certified athletic trainers and all other health care providers. In many situations, improvement occurs with the passage of time (natural history of the condition). Simple reassurance that a condition is not serious and that the athlete will recover, and similar efforts to reassure and empathize, can result in perceived improvement. True placebo and the effects of other interventions such as exercise may also explain the perceived benefits of modality application.

Given that many factors may contribute to reports of improvement and demonstrable functional recovery, how does the clinician decide how to best treat the patient? Searching the literature for clinical trials on treatments of various conditions can yield valuable information, and this process is introduced in the next section. The literature, unfortunately, is lacking in many areas of athletic health care; and while success in managing nonathletic patients provides some evidence of efficacy, the generalization to athletic populations may not be possible. Clearly a great deal of research is needed to better define those treatments that are truly beneficial in the management of specific athletic injuries. This is not laboratory research but rather research that must be conducted in the practice setting and must involve the clinicians providing care.

## TOOLS NECESSARY FOR ASSESSING OUTCOMES

It is now apparent that the improvement of an individual patient may or may not be due to the care rendered and that answers regarding what treatments are effective may lie in the clinical literature. The next question is, what should you as a certified athletic trainer be searching for? What data are needed to assess outcomes? The best way to answer these questions may be to consider the desired outcome of intervention from the perspective of the injured athlete. Decreased pain, improved range of motion, and restored strength are often important short-term goals of treatment. It is important that the long-term goals of the athlete-patient also be considered. The ultimate treatment goals are participation in sport and avoidance of reinjury.

Objective measures obtained by the certified athletic trainer may not correlate well with functional limitations and athletic disability and do not reflect the athlete's treatment goals. For example, following knee surgery the strength of the quadriceps and hamstring muscles is often assessed on an isokinetic dynamometer. While strength recovery is important, just having strength does not mean that the athlete will be able to run, cut, jump, and perform in his or her sport. In general, the clinician will find a mix of outcomes measures that include objective measures obtained by clinicians and patient-generated self-reports. The first question to ask in reviewing a clinical trial is whether the measures assessed are of interest and whether the measurement instruments are valid.

## Patient Self-Report Instruments

Patient self-report instruments have been developed and validated for a number of situations. Condition-specific instruments have also been developed. The Lysholm Knee Scale (Lysholm and Gillquist 1982) and Oswestry Back Pain Index (figures 7.1 and 7.2) provide illustrations of these instruments.

The development and validation of self-report instruments is complex and time-consuming. Efforts continue to develop instruments specific to the certified athletic trainer and the athletes we treat. What is apparent is that the use of self-report instruments is needed to adequately assess whether the treatments provided by health care providers really make a difference in the outcome following injury or illness.

## Clinical Trials: Studies of Effectiveness and Efficacy

After you consider the measurement instruments used in a clinical investigation, the next considerations involve study validity and generalization of results into your practice. Clinical trials can address the efficacy or the effectiveness of health care procedures. Effectiveness is defined as the result of interventions applied during routine daily practice. Efficacy is established through randomized controlled clinical trials in which efforts are made to control for all threats to the validity of the results. Well-designed, randomized controlled clinical trials account for the effects of factors such as the passage of time (natural history), placebo, and multiple treatment interactions. Studies of effectiveness and efficacy are both valuable. Studies of effectiveness may be more readily generalized to everyday clinical practice. Studies of efficacy, however, are considered essential for evaluating the effects of therapeutic modalities because of the necessity of controlling for factors including placebo, natural history, and examiner bias.

What are randomized controlled clinical trials? This type of study randomly assigns a group of patients with a condition of interest to treatment groups. Efforts are taken to blind subjects, clinicians, and evaluators, to the greatest degree possible, to the treatment received. Control of natural history and subject and investigator bias is necessary to truly assess the effect of therapeutic modality application on the outcome of treatment. High-quality randomized controlled clinical trials are few in athletic health care, but we can turn to the management of lateral epicondylitis (tennis elbow) for an example of the process. Iontophoresis, discussed in detail in chapter 10, is often administered by certified athletic trainers and physical therapists in the treatment of lateral epicondylitis. Each of the authors of this text has done this procedure. Our collective observation has been that some athletes treated for lateral epicondylitis with iontophoresis get better, suggesting that the treatment is, to some extent, effective. However, when the hypothesis that iontophoresis with a steroidal medication is effective in the treatment of lateral epicondylitis was tested in a high-quality randomized controlled clinical trial, the result was that the treatment did not improve outcome (Runeson and Hacker 2002). Such studies provide far stronger evidence of benefit, or lack thereof, than individual observations that improvement was noted after one or more treatments. It is quite possible that benefits we have observed in response to iontophoresis were attributable to factors other than that specific intervention, factors we could not control for at the time of treatment.

# Lysholm Knee Scale

## Limp (5 points)

| | | |
|---|---|---|
| None | 5 | _____ |
| Slight or periodic | 3 | _____ |
| Severe and constant | 0 | _____ |

## Support (5 points)

| | | |
|---|---|---|
| Full support | 5 | _____ |
| Cane or crutch | 3 | _____ |
| Weight bearing impossible | 0 | _____ |

## Stair climbing (5 points)

| | | |
|---|---|---|
| No problems | 5 | _____ |
| Slightly impaired | 3 | _____ |
| One step at a time | 2 | _____ |
| Unable | 0 | _____ |

## Squatting (5 points)

| | | |
|---|---|---|
| No problems | 5 | _____ |
| Slightly impaired | 3 | _____ |
| Not past 90 degrees | 2 | _____ |
| Unable | 0 | _____ |

**Total** _____

# Walking, Running, and Jumping

## Instability (30 points)

| | | |
|---|---|---|
| Never gives way | 30 | _____ |
| Rarely gives way except for athletic or other severe exertion | 25 | _____ |
| Gives way frequently during athletic events or severe exertion | 0 | _____ |
| Occasionally in daily activities | 10 | _____ |
| Often in daily activities | 0 | _____ |
| Every step | 0 | _____ |

## Swelling (10 points)

| | | |
|---|---|---|
| None | 10 | _____ |
| With giving way | 7 | _____ |
| On severe exertion | 5 | _____ |
| On ordinary exertion | 2 | _____ |
| On severe exertion | 5 | _____ |
| Constant | 0 | _____ |

## Pain (30 points)

| | | |
|---|---|---|
| None | 30 | _____ |
| Inconstant and slight during severe exertion | 25 | _____ |
| Marked on giving away | 20 | _____ |
| Marked during severe exertion | 15 | _____ |
| Marked on or after walking more than 1-1/4 miles | 10 | _____ |
| Marked on or after walking less than 1-1/4 miles | 5 | _____ |
| Constant and severe | 0 | _____ |

## Atrophy of thigh (5 points)

| | | |
|---|---|---|
| None | 5 | _____ |
| 1-2 cm | 3 | _____ |
| > 2 cm | 0 | _____ |

**Total** _____

**Figure 7.1** Lysholm Knee Scale.

Reprinted by permission from Lysholm and Gillquist 1982.

# Oswestry Low Back Pain Scale

Please rate the severity of your pain by circling a number below:

No pain | 0 | 1 | 2 | 3 | 4 | 5 | 6 | 7 | 8 | 9 | 10 | Unbearable pain

Name_____     Date _____

Instructions: Please circle the ONE NUMBER in each section which most closely describes your problem.

### Section 1—Pain Intensity
0. The pain comes and goes and is very mild.
1. The pain is mild and does not vary much.
2. The pain comes and goes and is very moderate.
3. The pain is moderate and does not vary much.
4. The pain comes and goes and is severe.
5. The pain is severe and does not vary much.

### Section 2—Personal Care (Washing, Dressing, etc.)
0. I would not have to change my way of washing or dressing in order to avoid pain.
1. I do not normally change my way of washing or dressing even though it causes some pain.
2. Washing and dressing increase the pain but I manage not to change my way of doing it.
3. Washing and dressing increase the pain and I find it necessary to change my way of doing it.
4. Because of the pain I am unable to do some washing and dressing without help.
5. Because of the pain I am unable to do any washing and dressing without help.

### Section 3—Lifting
0. I can lift heavy weights without extra pain.
1. I can lift heavy weights but it gives extra pain.
2. Pain prevents me from lifting heavy weights off the floor.
3. Pain prevents me from lifting heavy weights off the floor, but I can manage if they are conveniently positioned, e.g., on a table.
4. Pain prevents me from lifting heavy weights but I can manage light to medium weights if they are conveniently positioned.
5. I can only lift very light weights at most.

### Section 4—Walking
0. I have no pain on walking.
1. I have some pain on walking but it does not increase with distance.
2. I cannot walk more than 1 mile without increasing pain.
3. I cannot walk more than 1/2 mile without increasing pain.
4. I cannot walk more than 1/4 mile without increasing pain.
5. I cannot walk at all without increasing pain.

### Section 5—Sitting
0. I can sit in any chair as long as I like.
1. I can sit only in my favorite chair as long as I like.
2. Pain prevents me from sitting more than 1 hour.
3. Pain prevents me from sitting more than 1/2 hour.
4. Pain prevents me from sitting more than 10 minutes.
5. I avoid sitting because it increases pain immediately.

### Section 6—Standing
0. I can stand as long as I want without pain.
1. I have some pain on standing but it does not increase with time.
2. I cannot stand for longer than 1 hour without increasing pain.
3. I cannot stand for longer than 1/2 hour without increasing pain.
4. I cannot stand for longer than 10 minutes without increasing pain.
5. I avoid standing because it increases the pain immediately.

### Section 7—Sleeping
0. I get no pain in bed.
1. I get pain in bed but it does not prevent me from sleeping well.
2. Because of my pain my normal nights sleep is reduced by less than one quarter.
3. Because of my pain my normal nights sleep is reduced by less than one half.
4. Because of my pain normal nights sleep is reduced by less than three quarters.
5. Pain prevents me from sleeping at all.

### Section 8—Social Life
0. My social life is normal and gives me no pain.
1. My social life is normal but it increases the degree of pain.
2. Pain has no significant effect on my social life apart from limiting my more energetic interests, e.g., dancing.
3. Pain has restricted my social life and I do not go out very often.
4. Pain has restricted my social life to my home.
5. I have hardly any social life because of the pain.

### Section 9—Traveling
0. I get no pain when traveling.
1. I get some pain when traveling but none of my usual forms of travel make it any worse.
2. I get extra pain while traveling but it does not compel me to seek alternate forms of travel.
3. I get extra pain while traveling, which compels me to seek alternative forms of travel.
4. Pain restricts me to short necessary journeys under 1/2 hour.
5. Pain restricts all forms of travel.

### Section 10—Changing Degrees of Pain
0. My pain is rapidly getting better.
1. My pain fluctuates but is definitely getting better.
2. My pain seems to be getting better but improvement is slow.
3. My pain is neither getting better nor worse.
4. My pain is gradually worsening.
5. My pain is rapidly worsening.

**Figure 7.2**  Oswestry Back Pain Index.
Reprinted from Spine Research Institute of San Diego.

Interestingly, some of the third-party health insurance providers we work with, with including Medicare, no longer reimburse for iontophoresis treatment because of the lack of evidence of efficacy. Evidence-based medicine is not only a strategy used by individuals to improve the responses of the patients they treat but also one through which public health policies are being revised. This is also a dynamic process. As new randomized controlled clinical trials and other studies are published, clinical practice guidelines (discussed later) and health care policies can be revised. Ultimately, the most beneficial treatments will become the standard for care, and ineffective treatment will be abandoned. Studies of the therapeutic modalities discussed in this text are particularly needed.

## FINDING AND ASSESSING THE EVIDENCE

How was the Runeson and Hacker paper cited in the preceding section identified? Following discussions on how to best manage lateral epicondylitis in a monthly staff meeting, a computer search was conducted. Prior to the development of computerized databases, such a search would have required a trip to the library to find potential sources in volumes such as *Index Medicus*, a search for the desired article, and frequently a delay while the paper was retrieved through interlibrary loan. Today abstracts and, increasingly, full-text papers are available immediately. In this case the entire search and review process was completed from a desktop computer.

There are several databases available to the certified athletic trainer (see "Sample of Databases of Interest to the Certified Athletic Trainer" below), and more will emerge. With experience, the databases most appropriate for a particular search can be easily identified. Each database permits searches based on subjects and key words. Once a list of relevant papers is identified, copies are obtained online or through libraries.

Locating relevant literature is easier than ever, but the volume of material available must be read and analyzed. The adage "Don't believe everything you read" still holds true. Students and clinicians are faced with two challenges. The first is the evolution of science. New research brings new understanding, and old "truths" are replaced. The solution to this challenge is to be a clinician/scholar throughout your professional career. Strive to stay current.

## Sample of Databases of Interest to the Certified Athletic Trainer

- Medline and Pubmed: comprehensive online medical database compiled by the National Library of Medicine; free public access from any internet connection is available via Pubmed (Domholdt 2005)
- CINAHL: nursing and allied health cumulative index
- EMBASE: a comprehensive bibliographic database covering the worldwide literature on biomedical and pharmaceutical fields
- Physiotherapy Evidence Database: an Australian-based initiative to catalog systematic reviews and clinical trials and grade the methodological quality of clinical trials
- Cochrane database: a collaboration that is a multicenter international project providing high-quality systematic reviews and analyses of clinical trials across a broad spectrum of medicine
- SPORTDiscus: database of published papers related to sports medicine; includes journals not currently contained in *Index Medicus,* including *The Journal of Athletic Training*

# Understanding Study Design

The second challenge is more complex and comes down to understanding study design. Investigations that best control for factors that could influence the results are far more likely to draw conclusions portraying reality than are poorly controlled investigations. For example, an athlete might elect to apply a flexible magnet over a lateral ankle sprain. The athlete may recover and return to play basketball. A report detailing the case (case study) is prepared and concludes that the flexible magnet was effective in promoting recovery from the lateral ankle sprain. The natural history, placebo, and the effect of other interventions were not controlled for. It is really not possible to draw a conclusion regarding the efficacy of treatment of lateral ankle sprains with flexible magnets. Such a case study might lead to the development of a randomized controlled clinical trial that involves the random assignment of a series of athletes with lateral ankle sprains to treatment with real or placebo magnets. Objective and self-report data could then be collected to assess outcomes by evaluators blinded to treatment group to eliminate investigator bias. Other aspects of the treatment regimen could be kept as consistent as possible. From such a study, a far clearer picture regarding the efficacy of treatment of lateral ankle sprains with flexible magnets would emerge.

Table 7.1 details a hierarchy of study designs in order of control of confounding variables (see MacCauley and Best 2002 and Domholdt 2005 for greater detail). In "Assessing the Methodological Quality of RCTs" (p. 103), the criteria for grading clinical trials developed by the Physiotherapy Evidence Database are provided and discussed. These guidelines identify those factors that minimize the risk of falsely attributing favorable treatment outcomes to specific interventions. Ultimately, certified athletic trainers must be able to evaluate the quality of clinical trials, as such studies are necessary to define the efficacy of the therapeutic modalities and other interventions applied in the treatment of the injured athlete.

The 11 points identified permit a critical appraisal of the quality of controlled clinical trials. When there is conflicting information regarding an intervention, higher-quality studies are much more likely to reflect the truth. Readers should be careful, however, not to dismiss a study due to the absence of one or more of the criteria listed. In some cases it is not possible, even under ideal circumstances, to meet all criteria. This guide will assist you in sorting out those studies most likely to help you make sound clinical decisions.

## Table 7.1    Hierarchy of Study Designs in Order of Control of Confounding Variables

| Type of study | Important characteristics |
| --- | --- |
| Randomized controlled clinical trial (RCT) | Prospective assignment of subjects/patients to two or more treatment groups |
| Case-control study* | Begins with focus on effect of interest and then seeks to identify causes |
| May be prospective or retrospective | |
| Cross-sectional study* | Documents health status at a single point in time |
| Seeks to compare associations across groups | |
| Case study/case report/case series* # | Reports on one or more cases including condition, treatments, and outcomes |

* Studies lack prospective random assignment and generally have less control over factors that threaten validity of study results.

# In cases of relatively rare and more chronic conditions, case series reports may be useful in identifying effective treatments, especially when variables of interest are objective and highly reproducible.

# Assessing the Methodological Quality of RCTs

Here are the guidelines for assessing the methodological quality of randomized controlled clinical trials (RCTs):

1. **Eligibility criteria were specified.** Investigators should include specific information regarding criteria for entry into and exclusion from a study. This is critical when the certified athletic trainer ponders whether the results of a study can be generalized to an individual case.

2. **Subjects were randomly allocated to groups.** Studies in which subjects are assigned to groups by investigators and studies involving self-select group membership introduce the potential for bias on the part of the researcher or subject.

3. **Allocation was concealed.** Treatment group assignment should not be shared among participants, providers, and evaluators.

4. **The groups were similar at baseline regarding the most important prognostic indicators.** Investigators should adequately describe the composition for each of the treatment groups. For most characteristics there is a normal distribution across the population, and this distribution is reflected in all treatment groups. Random chance can, however, result in unequal distributions and should be identified and when possible controlled for.

5. **There was blinding of all subjects.** When subjects are unaware whether they received a "real" or placebo treatment, subject bias is eliminated. Blinding subjects to treatment may sound simple and in some cases may be. One could provide real and placebo magnets that look identical. In other cases, however, such as with TENS (discussed in chapter 10), it may not be possible to adequately blind subjects to the treatment they receive. This issue is discussed in detail by Deyo (1990b).

6. **There was blinding of all clinicians who administered therapy.** When possible, the clinician providing the treatment (e.g., instructing the subject in the application of a flexible magnet) should not be aware whether the magnet is active or placebo. This process prevents the clinician from introducing bias into the study. As with blinding of subjects, blinding of clinicians is easily accomplished in some studies and impossible in others.

7. **There was blinding of all assessors who measured at least one key outcome.** When assessors—whether they are taking measurements such as range of motion or collecting self-report information—are unaware of the treatment received, the potential of the assessor to bias the results is removed.

8. **Measures of at least one key outcome were obtained from more than 85% of the subjects initially allocated to groups.** Loss of subjects to follow-up or dropout can occur for a number of reasons. When dropout exceeds 15%, however, the validity of the results is threatened. For example, suppose that 100 subjects are randomly assigned to receive ultrasound or sham ultrasound treatments for Achilles tendinopathy. The authors indicate that at follow-up, 20 of 24 in the treatment group reported significant improvement while 20 of 40 in the sham group improved. The investigators conclude that the 80% recovery in those treated is significantly better than the 50% in the sham treatment group and that ultrasound enhances recovery in athletes suffering from Achilles tendinopathy. A closer look, however, reveals that 20 of 50 in each of the original treatment groups are improved. Did dropout bias the results?

9. **All subjects for whom measures were available received the treatment or control condition as allocated.** Or, where this was not the case, data for at least one key outcome were analyzed by intention to treat.

10. **The results of between-groups statistical comparisons are reported for at least one key outcome.** Statistical analysis controls for random fluctuations in the populations and provides estimates of the extent to which outcomes attributed to treatment effects were due to chance. A low probability that results were chance events strengthens the validity of study conclusions.

11. **The study provides both point measures and measures of variability for at least one key outcome.** Reports of clinical trials should provide information regarding change over time and estimates of variability in outcomes measures and thus responses to treatments.

## Using Evidence-Based Practice Guidelines

The ability to search and critically appraise the research literature is an essential skill for the practicing clinician. Individual clinicians cannot, however, devote the time to collecting and critically reviewing the literature on each diagnostic test performed or each therapeutic intervention rendered. This is reality also for other health care professionals. In an effort to apply and disseminate new information, several professional groups have authored evidence-based practice guidelines. Evidence-based practice guidelines are developed by groups of authors that systematically review the existing literature using preestablished criteria. The Cochrane Collaboration is an example of this process. The group then makes recommendations for the use or discontinuation of specific interventions and identifies areas where further research is needed.

The development of evidence-based practice guidelines in sports medicine and athletic training has lagged behind that of some other disciplines. The development of new evidence-based practice guidelines will permit practicing certified athletic trainers to remain abreast of a greater range of research related to athletic health care than can individual investigation of topics of interest. Clearly, evidence-based practice guidelines will affect practice patterns. However, the reader should not interpret these guidelines as complete truths, recipes, or protocols. A consensus of experts independently reviewing the available literature does offer a strong measure of credibility; but, as noted previously, evidence-based practice and therefore practice guidelines are dynamic. New research may emerge that will cause individuals to change how they practice before practice guidelines can be revised. This takes us back to the primary issue addressed in this chapter: Be prepared to integrate, and base your decisions on, the best currently available evidence.

Clinical practice will never be based exclusively on practice guidelines and the critical review of clinical trials. To conclude this chapter, we need to return to the beginning and the definition of evidence-based practice: *the integration of the best research evidence with clinical expertise and patient values.* Each patient and each clinician is unique. Patients vary in terms of health histories, coexisting conditions, and personal preferences. Clinicians vary in experiences and skills. Ultimately each clinician has a responsibility to provide care that effectively addresses the patient's condition at a reasonable cost. The integration of the best available evidence into daily practice facilitates achievement of these objectives.

In the succeeding chapters we will make reference to some of the published clinical trials, systematic reviews, and practice guidelines available. It is not possible to complete a thorough analysis of all of the available literature within a single volume. Furthermore, new studies have been published since the revisions to this text. Most important, it is not desirable for readers to rely solely on our interpretations. What is vital is that the student and practicing clinician use the literature, engage in evidence-based health care, and provide the most effective treatments available.

## SUMMARY

1. Define the term *evidence-based health care*.

   Evidence-based health care, as defined by Sacket et al. (2000), is the integration of the best research evidence with clinical expertise and patient values.

2. Discuss the role of outcomes assessment in advancing evidence-based health care.

   Outcomes assessment is necessary to determine if the treatments rendered to patients result in greater or more rapid recovery or reduce the incidence of reinjury. Some outcomes measures can be obtained by clinicians, but patients' self-reports provide important insights into the effects of the treatments they receive.

3. Describe how clinical trials are conducted.

> Clinical trials involve the study of patients with specific conditions and their change in health status over time. Randomized controlled clinical trials randomly select patients into one or more treatment groups. One or more groups usually are treated with a placebo or serves as a no-treatment control.

4. Identify the components of well-designed randomized controlled clinical trials.

> The methods of a randomized controlled clinical trial can introduce bias that may ultimately affect the conclusions of the investigators. Potential bias can be minimized through true random assignment to treatment groups; blinding of subjects, clinicians, and assessors to the treatment delivered; analysis of data as though all subjects completed the study; assessment of differences between groups at the start of the study; provision of valid measures of treatment outcomes; and comparison of the results from the various treatment groups.

5. Identify resources for locating clinical trials of treatments in which therapeutic modalities were used.

> While there is a need for more quality randomized controlled clinical trials in sports medicine, there are several databases that can assist the certified athletic trainer in the practice of evidence-based health care. These include, but are not limited to, CINAHL (nursing and allied health cumulative index), EMBASE (a comprehensive bibliographic database covering the worldwide literature in biomedical and pharmaceutical fields), Physiotherapy Evidence Database (an Australian-based initiative to catalog systematic reviews and clinical trials and grade the methodological quality of clinical trials), Cochrane database (the Cochrane Collaboration is a multicenter international project providing high-quality systematic reviews and analyses of clinical trials across a broad spectrum of medicine), and SPORTDiscus (database of published papers related to sports medicine).

## CITED SOURCES

Deyo RA, Walsh NE, Martin DC, Schoenfeld LS, Ramamurthy S: A controlled trial of transcutaneous electrical nerve stimulation and exercise for chronic back pain. *N Engl J Med* 322:1627-1634, 1990a.

Deyo RA, Walsh NE, Martin DC, Schoenfeld LS, Ramamurthy S: Can trials of physical treatments be blinded? The example of transcutaneous electrical nerve stimulation for pain. *Am J Phys Med Rehabil* 69: 6-10, 1990b.

Domholdt E: *Physical Therapy Research: Principles and Applications*, 3rd ed. Philadelphia, Saunders, 2000.

Evans T: The Reliability, Validity, Sensitivity and Standard Values of the Athletic Training Outcome Assessment Self-report Instrument. Doctoral dissertation, Penn State University, 2002.

Lysholm J, Gillquist J: Evaluation of knee ligament surgery results with special emphasis on use of a scoring scale. *Am J Sports Med* 10:150-154, 1982.

MacCauley D, Best T: *Evidence-based Sports Medicine*. London, UK, BMJ Books, 2002.

Oncel M, Sencan S, Yildiz H, Kurt N: Trancutaneous electrical nerve stimulation for pain in patients with uncomplicated minor rib fractures. *Eur J Cardiothorac Surg* 22:13-17, 2002.

Runeson L, Hacker E: Iontophoresis with cortisone in the treatment of lateral epicondylalgia (tennis elbow)—a double blind study. *Scand J Med Sci Sports* 12:136-142, 2002.

Sacket DL, Straus SE, Richardson WS, Rosenberg W, Haynes RB: *Evidence-Based Medicine: How to Practice and Teach EBM*, 2nd ed. Philadelphia, Churchill Livingstone, 2000.

## ADDITIONAL READINGS

Sacket DL, Haynes RB, Guyatt GH, Tugwell P. Clinical Epideniology: *A Basic Science for Clinical Medicine*, 2nd ed. Philadelphia, Lippincott, Williams & Wilkins, 1991.

Katz DL: Clinical Epideniology and Evidence-based Medicine. Thousand Oaks, CA, Sage Publications, 2001.

# CHAPTER 8

# Cold and Superficial Heat

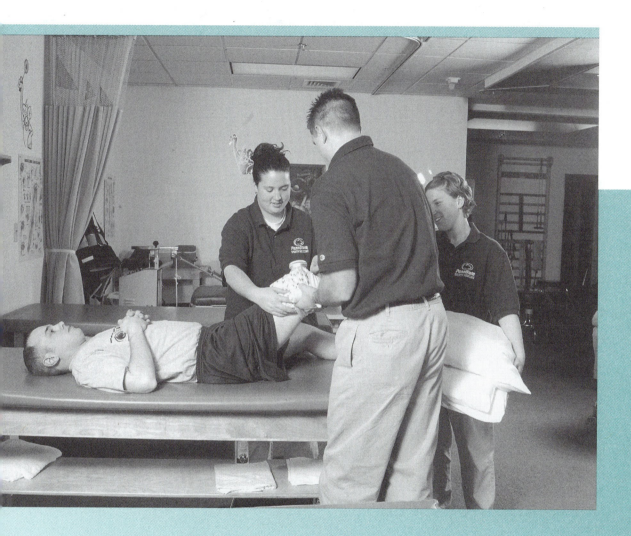

## Objectives

After reading this chapter, the student will be able to

1. describe the four energy transfer mechanisms related to therapeutic modalities;

2. describe the common methods of applying superficial heat and therapeutic cold;

3. describe the thermal changes that occur with superficial heat and local cold application;

4. discuss the effect of superficial heat and local cooling on blood flow, muscle, and the nervous system;

5. discuss the indications for cold application and the impact of cooling on acute inflammation;

6. describe the common indications for the application of superficial heat;

7. describe the application of cold in a program of cryokinetics;

8. identify contraindications and precautions in applying superficial heat and therapeutic cold;

9. differentiate between superficial heating and deep heating modalities; and

10. describe contrast therapy.

A 43-year-old club hockey player is referred to your care for treatment of an acute recurrence of low back pain. The player states that he twisted his back when he collided with two opponents in a game early this morning. He experienced immediate pain and chose not to continue playing because there were only a few minutes left in the game. He was evaluated by his personal physician because he began experiencing increased pain and muscle spasm while at work. He was provided with analgesic medications and referred for treatment of "mechanical low back pain."

On presentation he is in obvious discomfort but states that the pain is well localized to the mid-lumbar spine. He denies radicular symptoms or significant medical problems except for one previous episode of back pain that he experienced while cutting wood last year. He received treatment on three occasions consisting of superficial heat, manual therapies, and therapeutic exercise, and his back pain resolved within 2 weeks.

You determine that relieving pain and muscle spasm is the first priority. Which modality is the best choice? Are any treatments contraindicated? Which treatments will facilitate completion of therapeutic exercises at home? This chapter addresses the application of cryotherapy and superficial heat as therapeutic modalities.

Cold and superficial heat are probably the most commonly applied therapeutic modalities. These modalities conduct heat to or away from the body. The application of cold decreases temperature of the skin and deeper tissues; however, the application of heat increases temperature only in the superficial tissue. Deeper heating can be accomplished with ultrasound and diathermy, which are discussed in chapter 11. This chapter is limited to modalities that cool tissue or warm superficial tissue.

Despite the simplicity and widespread use of cold and superficial heat, the evidence of clinical benefit is somewhat limited, and the results of clinical trials are often contradictory. Furthermore, the mechanisms that bring about the desired effects are not fully understood. Although these modalities are applied to help individuals recover from injury, they can also cause injury. Thus, this chapter presents fundamental concepts of energy transfer, the indications and contraindications of cryotherapy and superficial heat, and physiological responses to these modalities. A review of clinical trials investigating the use of cold and superficial heat is also provided.

## ENERGY TRANSFER

Thermal energy can be transferred to or from the body by four mechanisms: conduction, convection, radiation, and conversion. **Conduction** is the transfer of heat through the direct contact between a hotter and a cooler area (Michlovitz 1990). When heat or cold is applied directly to the skin, the amount of temperature change depends primarily on the temperature difference between the two surfaces and the length of time the two surfaces are in contact. Surface cooling begins immediately; however, the deeper the tissue, the longer cooling takes. When a larger surface area is heated or cooled, temperature at the center of the area being treated changes somewhat more rapidly than when smaller areas are treated.

**Convection** is the transfer of heat by the movement of air or liquid between regions of unequal temperature. For example, a convection oven circulates heated air around the food that is being cooked. In athletic training, a whirlpool or a fluidotherapy unit can be used to heat or cool via convection. As with conduction, the rate and extent of temperature change are determined primarily by the differences in temperature between the medium and the tissue, the length of exposure, and the size of the area treated.

Radiant energy is emitted from surfaces with temperatures above absolute 0° (Michlovitz 1990). Thus, the body emits radiant energy. However, the body can also absorb radiant energy, and radiant energy can heat the superficial tissues. The obvious example of **radiation** is sunbathing. At one time infrared or baker's lamps were commonly used for superficial heating in athletic training and physical therapy. Although less common today, these modalities are quite useful for warming large areas. The amount of heating caused by radiant energy relates primarily to the output of the infrared bulb, the distance between the bulb and the skin, and the length of exposure.

The relationship between the heating effect and the distance between the bulb and the skin is stated as the inverse square law (figure 8.1). The inverse square law implies that the change in heating effect varies with the inverse square of the distance between the bulb and skin. For example, if a lamp were lowered from 60 cm above the skin to 30 cm, the distance would be reduced by 1/2. The inverse of 1/2 is 2, and the square of 2 is 4. Thus, the heating effect is increased fourfold when the height of the lamp is reduced by 1/2.

This relationship assumes that the radiant energy strikes the skin perpendicularly. If the light strikes the skin at an angle, some is reflected, reducing the heating effect. This relationship is defined by the cosine law, which states that the heating effect varies with the cosine of the angle formed between the beam of radiant energy and the perpendicular (figure 8.2). For example, if the light forms a 30° angle with the perpendicular, the reduction in heating effect is calculated by multiplying the cosine of 30°, which is 0.86. Thus, only 86% as much heating occurs when light strikes a surface at an angle 30° from

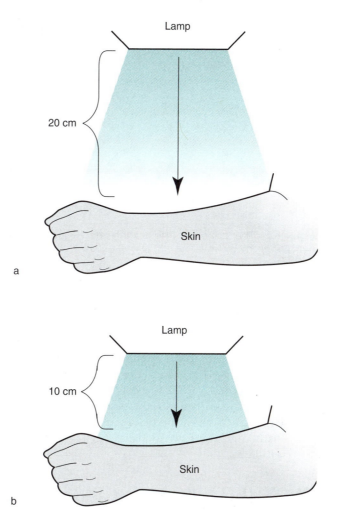

**Figure 8.1**   The inverse square law: Heating effect equals *x (a)*. When the distance between the lamp and the skin is reduced by half *(b)*, the heating effect is increased to *4x* (the inverse of 1/2 equals 2, and $2^2$ equals 4).

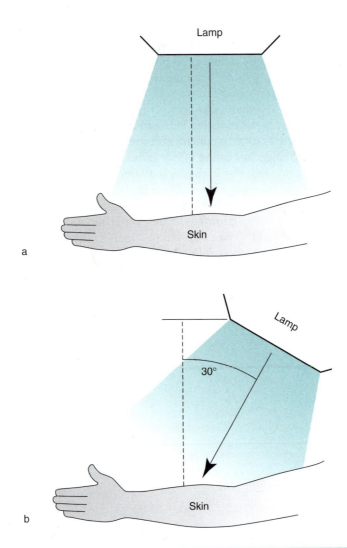

**Figure 8.2** The cosine law: The heating effect equals *x (a)*. The angle of the light does not deviate (= 0°) from the vertical. The cosine of 0 equals 1; thus, the heating effect equals 1*x*. The light strikes the skin at a 30° angle *(b)*. The cosine of 30° is 0.86. Thus, the heating effect is only 86% of the effect when the light was beaming straight down.

perpendicular as when it strikes perpendicular to the surface. In other words, the heating effect is reduced 14%.

**Conversion** implies that energy is changed from one form to another, so this concept does not relate to the application of cold and superficial heat. However, it does relate to two modalities discussed later and is included here for completeness. Ultrasound machines deliver acoustic (sound) energy to tissues where it is reflected and absorbed. When sound energy is absorbed into the tissues, it is converted to thermal energy. A similar phenomenon occurs when the tissues are exposed to continuous electromagnetic energy as with diathermy. These two modalities increase tissue temperature through conversion of energy within the body.

# CRYOTHERAPY AND CRYOKINETICS

The application of cold for therapeutic purposes, termed **cryotherapy,** and the therapeutic combination of cold and exercise, **cryokinetics,** are common in athletic training. These treatments are inexpensive and commonly applied. Cryotherapy has also been extensively studied by athletic trainers, and much of what we know can be attributed to Dr. Ken Knight

(1995). His text reviews and summarizes many studies that have investigated the extent of cooling that occurs, compared cooling devices, investigated responses in healthy individuals, or studied injury models. However, further investigation into the extent of benefit of these and other modalities on treatment outcomes through randomized, controlled clinical trials is clearly needed (Bleakley, McDonough, and MacAuley 2004).

## Methods of Application

Therapeutic cooling can be accomplished by several means. The most simple is an ice pack (figure 8.3), whereby crushed ice in a waterproof bag is placed or wrapped on the skin to cool tissues. This is an inexpensive treatment that also allows for compression and elevation of the injured part. Commercial cold packs can also be applied; however, crushed ice applied directly to the skin is preferable for several reasons. Some commercial cold packs do not conform well to the skin. In addition, cold packs stored in a freezer may be considerably colder than crushed ice, which is maintained at 32° F (0° C). Because of the greater temperature difference between the cold pack and the skin, cooling is greater and more rapid and may result in cold injury to the skin (frostbite). Because of the differences between ice and the materials used in commercial cold packs, an insulating layer of plastic or cloth must be used between commercial cold packs and the skin in order to protect it. Ultimately, greater cooling is achieved with crushed ice, especially if an elastic bandage is applied over the ice pack (Knight 1995).

Cold water circulating units (figure 8.4), also called cryocuffs (a term derived from the trade name Cryo/Cuff), are similar to ice packs in that a cold surface is placed on or near the skin. Cold water is pumped into a cuff, which is then placed on or near the skin to withdraw heat from the tissue. However, a cuff filled with cold water results in less tissue cooling than the direct application of an ice pack. Perhaps the best use of cryocuffs is under wraps and braces used postoperatively. Although the wound dressing insulates the skin against the cold, the cold water circulating unit may lessen postoperative pain and the need for analgesic medications. These devices have also been reported to lessen blood loss following total knee

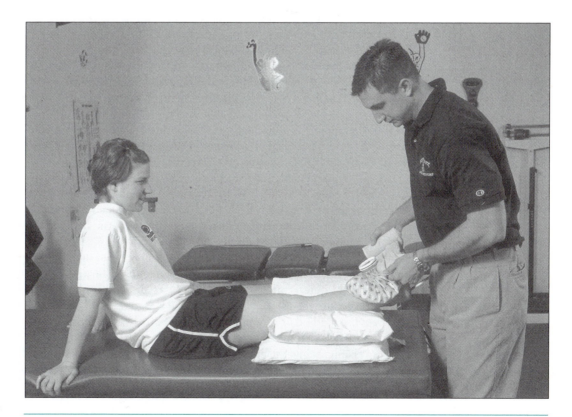

**Figure 8.3**  Application of an ice pack.

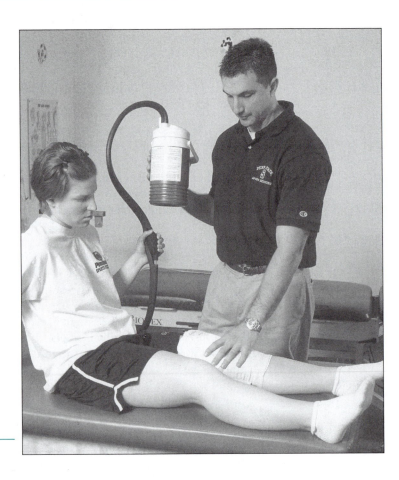

**Figure 8.4**  Cold water circulating unit.

arthroplasty (knee replacement surgery) (Levy and Marmar 1993; Leutz and Harris 1995). The cold water circulating unit provides hours of mild cooling without the need to remove braces and wraps and without the mess of ice packs.

Ice massage offers another inexpensive form of cryotherapy (figure 8.5), whereby water frozen in a paper or Styrofoam cup can be used to cool and massage the skin. Ice massage should not be applied as a first aid treatment or during the acute inflammatory response, because ice massage is incompatible with compression. However, ice massage reduces pain prior to therapeutic exercise and relieves postexercise discomfort. This technique can also be used to desensitize trigger points in individuals who have myofascial pain syndrome and is readily available for home-based treatment.

Cold water immersion and cold whirlpools are also used to administer cryotherapy (figure 8.6). Immersion in 40° to 50° F (4-10° C) water or a 50° to 60° F (10-15° C) whirlpool will cool tissue as well as an ice pack will. Warmer water is used in a whirlpool because the movement of the water continually breaks down the thermopane, the boundary layer of water around the foot that is warmer than the cold bath (figure 8.7). Loss of the thermopane allows tissues to cool more rapidly. These application methods offer a couple of advantages: The entire limb or joint can be cooled, and active exercise can be performed during the cooling process. However, cold water immersion is not ideal for first aid or during the acute inflammatory response, because the injured limb cannot be elevated.

One more method of cold application warrants brief mention. Vapocoolant sprays result in very superficial, rapid cooling through evaporation (figure 8.8). There is virtually no temperature change below the epidermis; however, vapocoolant sprays numb an area briefly and may be effective in the management of tender trigger points associated with myofascial pain syndrome (Travel and Simons 1983).

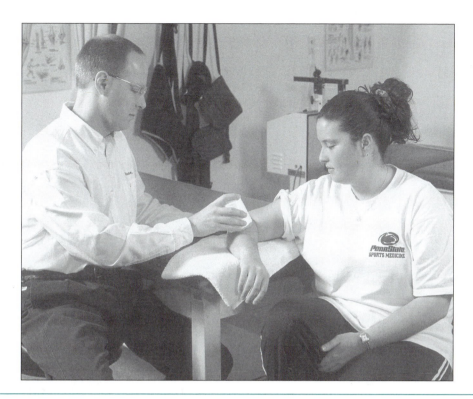

**Figure 8.5**  Ice massage.

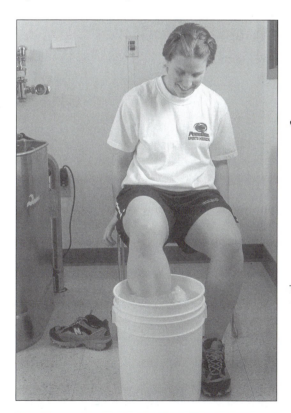

**Figure 8.6**  Cold water immersion/cold whirlpool.

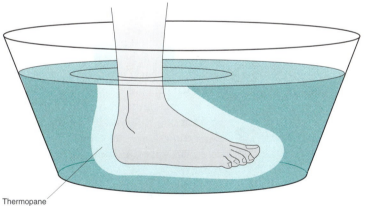

Thermopane

**Figure 8.7**  The foot immersed in cold water. The skin warms the surrounding water, forming a thermopane on the boundary layer, which is warmer than the cold bath.

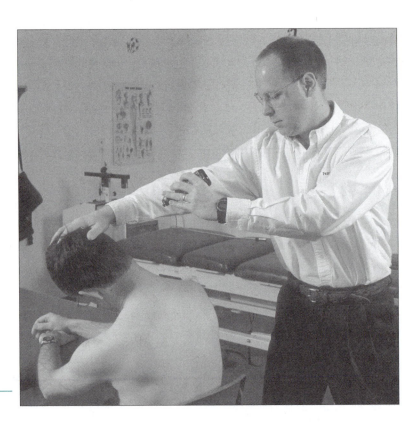

**Figure 8.8**    Vapocoolant spray.

## Temperature Decreases and Physiological Reponses

Localized cooling results in a number of physiological responses.

### Cooling and Rewarming Skin

When an ice pack is applied or a limb is immersed in an ice bath, the skin cools rapidly. After a few minutes, the rate of cooling slows and finally levels off at a few degrees above the temperature of the ice pack or ice bath (Knight 1995). When a compression wrap is applied over the ice pack, greater decreases in skin temperature are observed (Knight 1995).

When the cold is removed, a similar pattern of rewarming occurs. There is an initial rapid rise in temperature (which is of lesser magnitude than the sudden drop that occurs with cold application), followed by a more gradual return to preapplication temperature. At rest, the skin temperature can remain below preapplication levels for over 1 h following 30 min of cold pack application. More rapid rewarming occurs when cooling is followed by physical activity.

### Cooling and Rewarming Deeper Tissues

In general, deeper tissues cool more slowly and to a lesser extent than skin. Measures of gastrocnemius muscle tissue temperature at a depth of 2.3 cm revealed slow cooling during a 22-min ice pack application (Hartviksen 1962). However, temperatures continued to drop for several minutes following the removal of ice pack in subjects at rest, and cooling plateaued at approximately 28° C.

Research suggests that changes in intra-articular temperature follow a pattern similar to that observed in muscle (Haimovici 1982; Oosterveld et al. 1992). However, there is a greater temperature decrease in the joint than in the surrounding muscle (Wakin, Porter, and Krusen 1951). When the joint is held at rest, temperatures continue to drop after cold is removed (Bocobo et al. 1991; McMaster, Little, and Waugh 1978). Cold water immersion results in greater cooling of the intra-articular space than an ice pack (Bocobo et al. 1991), because a greater surface area of the joint is exposed to cold.

Deep tissues maintained at rest rewarm very slowly, and the rewarming of muscle and intra-articular spaces has been reported to exceed 2 1/2 h (Knight 1995; Knight et al. 1980). The research into rewarming has implications for athletic training. For example, in treating an individual who will remain at rest following knee surgery, you can use ice to control pain and swelling. Research suggests that a 20- to 30-min ice pack application will cool tissues for 2 h or more. Reapplication during the rewarming period will result in cooler tissue temperatures. Although there are not enough data to recommend a specific cooling–rewarming ratio, Knight (1995) recommended a rewarming period of at least twice the cooling period with application of ice directly to the skin. This is excellent advice.

Clinicians have frequently used commercial (e.g., Cryo/Cuff; Aircast Inc., Summit, NJ) cold water circulating units following surgery. Although the cuff is applied over the surgical dressing, these devices have been reported by some investigators to relieve pain (Ohkoshi et al. 1999) and to decrease the use of pain medication (Ohkoshi et al. 1999; Barber, McGuire, and Click 1998). Because there is less tissue cooling, the unit can be applied for an extended period of time. However, further study is needed to substantiate these reports and assess the costs to benefit of these cooling units.

When the individual is active following cryotherapy, rewarming occurs much more quickly. Physical activity rapidly increases body temperature. Thus, deep tissue temperatures return to normal much more rapidly when cryotherapy is followed by exercise.

## Impact on Blood Flow

Localized cooling results in a number of physiological responses. Cooling lowers the metabolic activity and oxygen demand of cells. Vasoconstriction and decreased local blood flow occur in superficial and deep tissues, although different mechanisms are involved. Superficial vasoconstriction occurs primarily through reflex mechanisms, whereas decreased metabolic activity is responsible for decreased blood flow in deep tissues.

## Impact on the Nervous System and Muscle Function

Cold application also affects the nervous system, and individuals have described a progression of sensations during cold application. Initially, intense cold is perceived. This is followed by an aching pain, which gives way to sensations of pins and needles or warmth and finally numbness. Although not every individual will experience these sensations, this general description suggests that cold initially stimulates cold and pain receptors. Cooling of nerve fibers slows the conduction of neural impulses. Thus, after several minutes of cold, sensation is diminished because impulses cannot be transmitted from the periphery to the sensory cortex. The numbness or analgesia experienced during cryotherapy results in the first goal of rehabilitation: pain relief.

## Impact on Muscle Spasm and Function

Muscle function is controlled by the nervous system. However, we will examine muscle spasm and function separately because of their importance in athletic training. In addition to relieving pain and thus breaking the pain–spasm cycle, cold also reduces muscle spasm by directly affecting the muscle spindle.

Muscle spindles sense the stretch of a muscle. The spindles are innervated by gamma efferent fibers, which allow the spindle to adjust to changes in muscle length. When injury occurs, the body responds through reflex contraction of surrounding muscles. These involuntary contractions or spasms splint the injured area and prevent further injury. However, spasm occludes blood flow and exacerbates the pain–spasm cycle.

Cold application appears to decrease spasm through direct and reflex mechanisms. When cooled, the muscle spindles are less sensitive; thus, the muscle relaxes and spasm is relieved. However, decreases in muscle spasm begin to occur before the muscle cools significantly, suggesting that a reflex response to cold also occurs. Certainly, the antispasmotic effects of cryotherapy are an important consideration when one is selecting a therapeutic modality to treat musculoskeletal injuries.

Force production of muscle is decreased by cooling. Knight (1995) summarized the find-ings of several investigators and concluded that maximum isometric and isotonic strength and rate of force development are reduced when the muscle tissue is cooled below 15° to 18° C. Cooling to this level requires at least 20 min of application. Following cryotherapy, an individual should rewarm muscle tissue through rhythmic exercises before returning to activities that require maximal muscular efforts.

### Impact on Proprioception and Sensation

Although cooling slows nerve conduction velocity and relieves pain and muscle spasm, the effects on proprioception, postural stability, and sensation are less evident. Studies on the effect of cryotherapy on balance and postural stability have presented conflicting conclusions. Ice bath immersion of the ankle and lower leg appears to temporarily reduce postural stability and balance (Gerig 1990; Rivers et al. 1995; Steinagel et al. 1996). However, ice pack application to the ankle and knee does not result in similar changes (McDonough et al. 1996; Thieme et al. 1996). Open kinetic chain repositioning is not altered following cold water immersion (LaRiviere and Osternig 1994). Cold application (15-min, 10° C ice bath) was not found to affect control of force production or two-point discrimination in the hand, although pressure sensitivity was reduced (Rubley et al. 2003). A similar treatment was found not to affect the haptic system responsible for nonvisual perception, for example when an implement is held in the hand (West 1998).

Performance of maximal-effort jumping and agility tasks may also be affected by tissue cooling, although the results of studies are conflicting. Some investigators (Cross, Wilson, and Perrin 1995; Greicar et al. 1996) reported that cold adversely affects jumping and agility performance, whereas others (Evans et al. 1996; Shuler et al. 1996) found no performance differences after cryotherapy.

The previously mentioned research may appear confusing, and you may question when to apply cold in light of the potential to affect sport performance. However, when cold is used to treat athletic injury, these issues are of minimal concern. Individuals treated with cryotherapy are rarely capable of maximal-effort, functional exercise. For the few who are capable of such exercise but need to apply cold for pain management, a period of rewarming with safe, rhythmic exercises is advised. One must question, however, if jumping and agility exercises are appropriate for injured individuals requiring cryotherapy for pain management.

There is also conflicting information on the effect of cold on cutaneous sensation. Cool-ing of the forearm and hand appears to alter cutaneous sensation in the fingers and thumb (Provins and Morton 1960; Rubley 2003). However, cooling of the foot does not affect cutaneous sensation on the plantar surface. The differences in these findings are probably due to the greater sensitivity of the hand. Rewarming of the hand appears warranted before performance of fine motor tasks.

## Indications for Therapeutic Cold

The primary reason cold is applied in clinical practice is pain relief. Cold likely affects sec-ondary tissue injury (introduced in chapter 3 and discussed in more detail in the next section here), although much more study is needed to fully understand this phenomenon. Cryotherapy is a simple, portable, and inexpensive means of relieving pain and muscle spasm following musculoskeletal injury. Cryotherapy can be used to manage pain during the acute inflam-matory response, to allow for pain-free therapeutic exercise, and to manage some persistent pain patterns, particularly myofascial pain syndrome.

### Cryotherapy and Acute Inflammation

During the acute inflammatory response, use of an ice pack or cold pack should be com-bined with compression, elevation, and protection of the injured tissues. This combination of treatments controls pain, limits swelling, and prevents further injury. Each component plays a role in increasing the injured individual's comfort and in speeding recovery. However, these treatments should be combined for maximum effect. Cold should be applied early in the treatment process, and application must be repeated. A 20- to 30-min cold application repeated every 2 h is a reasonable and well-tolerated use of cold in the management of acute musculoskeletal injuries.

During the acute inflammatory response following tissue injury, cold is applied to reduce pain and minimize secondary tissue injury. Pain relief is most likely due to a slowed nerve conduction velocity. Clinical observation and investigation suggest that cold decreases secondary injury. Knight (1995) suggested that secondary injury is due to *hypoxic cell death*. He theorized that during an acute inflammatory response, disruption of capillaries and congestion due to edema decrease oxygenation of healthy cells close to the tissue damage. **Hypoxia** leads to further cell death. Thus, following musculoskeletal injury there is a period of additional tissue damage, or secondary injury, due to hypoxia.

Certainly cooling of tissue lowers the metabolic activity and reduces oxygen demand. When oxygen demand is reduced through cooling, cells can survive a period of hypoxia. Because more cells survive, there is less total tissue damage, a more rapid resolution of the signs and symptoms of acute inflammation, and a more rapid recovery.

In light of the hypoxic cell death model, the benefits of cold following acute injury are obvious. However, the phenomenon of secondary cell death is likely more complicated than hypoxic cell death. Merrick (2002), in an extensive review of the subject, stated that from a research perspective, it is not possible to distinguish between primary and secondary cell death. While some cells die almost immediately, others may be damaged. Some of the damaged cells die over a period of time due to the traumatic event. It is believed, however, that other cells die as the result of the physiological events associated with inflammation (secondary cell death).

Secondary cell death, furthermore, is likely not due solely, if at all, to hypoxia. Merrick (2002) identified multiple potential contributors to secondary cell death. He identified ischemia, oxidative injury (action of free radicals), and calcium influx into cells as factors in the secondary cell injury process.

In figure 3.5, cyclooxygenase was identified as the enzyme that converts arachidonic acid to endoperoxide. This conversion and neutrophil activity generate large quantities of oxygen free radicals. These free radicals and lysosomal enzymes are present to break down the damaged cells so that the area can be cleared for tissue repair. However, the free radicals also damage healthy cells. It is possible that secondary tissue injury is due more to the actions of free radicals and cell-damaging enzymes than to hypoxia. According to Merrick (2002, pg. 214), "Most authors agree that more damage actually occurs after the return of perfusion and oxygen to the previously hypoxic area."

Merrick (2002, 2003) further suggested that failure of the mitochondria is the central mechanism behind secondary cell death. He stated that calcium influx disrupts mitochondrial function and represents a unique contributor to secondary cell death. The phenomenon of secondary cell death is very complex, and thus the full effect of cold application on the process is not fully understood.

The application of cold is a widely accepted and practiced treatment. Some may view the issue of secondary tissue injury and cell death as academic, having little clinical relevance. However, given that the clinician cannot influence primary tissue injury (cell death occurring immediately after trauma) and that no intervention has been proven to speed tissue repair, further investigation into the phenomenon of secondary tissue injury is clearly needed. A better understanding of secondary tissue injury *may* identify the most effective use of cold applications. Further investigation *may* also lead to additional therapeutic adjuncts, such as antioxidant therapy, that the sports medicine team can use to help injured athletes.

The use of compression and elevation in conjunction with cold applications is commonly recommended in acute injury management. Elevation lowers capillary hydrostatic pressure. Chapter 3 introduced a capillary filtration pressure system. When tissue injury occurs, osmotic pressure exerted by free proteins in the interstitium disrupts normal pressure. Swelling will increase until a new pressure balance is reached. When the injured body part is elevated and capillary hydrostatic pressure is lowered, less fluid escapes from the capillary and a new filtration pressure balance is reached sooner.

Compression also can influence swelling by exerting an external force that tends to hold fluid within the capillary system. However, the pressure exerted by elastic wraps probably has little impact on swelling. Felt pads and tape exert greater pressures but may increase pain as tissue is squeezed between the force of the interstitial fluid volume and the external compression.

Although elastic wraps do not exert a great deal of pressure, the wraps do remind the individual to protect injured tissues and may reduce pain and protective muscle spasms. Protecting the injured tissues is very important through the first two phases of the inflammatory process. Others have used terms such as *rest* and *stabilization* rather than *protection*. Whichever term is used, the injured individual should avoid activity that increases pain during the acute inflammatory response.

## Cryotherapy and Therapeutic Exercise: Cryokinetics

Knight (1995) described the application of cold before or during exercise and coined the term *cryokinetics* ("cold and motion"). Cryokinetics involves cold application, usually consisting of cold water immersion, cold whirlpool, or ice massage, and active exercise. Cold is applied until analgesia is achieved (10-15 min). Once the painful area is numbed, a careful progression of exercises is initiated. When the numbing effects of the cold wear off, cold is reapplied. Several repetitions of cold application and exercise can be performed.

Cryokinetics can speed functional recovery. A pain–spasm cycle can persist beyond acute inflammation, and you may have to break the cycle before therapeutic exercises can progress. In addition, injury sensitizes the tissues. Following an injury, normal stresses may be perceived as painful despite ample time for tissue repair. Peppard (personal communication 1977) described using cryokinetics to reset central bias. By using cold to control pain, you can progress the individual through increasingly demanding activities. When you carefully control the injured individual's activity progression, previously painful movements become pain free, central bias is reset, and normal, painless functional movement patterns are restored.

Sound clinical judgment must be used in initiating cryokinetics. With relatively minor injuries such as a Grade I lateral ankle sprain with injury isolated to the anterior talofibular ligament, cryokinetics can be initiated 1 to 2 days following injury. Activities such as walking and jogging do not stress the ligament. Thus, the injured person can return to play when his or her function allows, provided that the ankle is protected from forced inversion. However, if the ankle injury is more severe and involves, for example, injury to the syndesmosis (articulation between the distal tibia and fibula), walking and jogging must be delayed until the damaged ligaments heal. These activities greatly stress the syndesmotic ligaments, and would delay healing and result in an unstable ankle.

In general, cold decreases sensation and relieves pain but does not provide **anesthesia.** If exercise during cryotherapy is painful, it should be discontinued. You can reapply the cold and resume exercises after numbness has returned or can end the exercise session. Likewise, if the injured individual becomes too aggressive with a therapeutic regimen, pain, spasm, and swelling will increase the following day, and rehabilitation will be slowed for 1 to 3 days while the newly inflamed tissue recovers. Two good rules in any rehabilitation exercise program are as follows: (1) Pain that alters normal movement patterns indicates that the individual is not ready to perform the exercise and (2) the individual should be able to do tomorrow what was done today. Clinical experience will refine your ability to judge the appropriateness of an exercise for each individual, but these rules are commonsense guidelines for the progression of therapeutic exercise, especially cryokinetics.

## Cryotherapy in the Treatment of Persistent Pain

Cryotherapy may also be effective in managing some persistent pain problems. For individuals with myofascial pain syndrome, characterized by very sensitive trigger points, cryotherapy offers a safe, cost-effective home treatment. Travel and Simons (1983) described the used of ethyl chloride spray and stretch in treating myofascial pain. Ice massage using brief stroking can produce similar responses.

Brief, intense cold to sensitive points may decrease pain by stimulating descending spinal pathways described in chapter 4. A more prolonged ice massage decreases the sensitivity of free nerve endings and slows conduction velocity of afferent fibers. The numbing effect of the ice breaks local pain–spasm cycles, relieving the symptoms of myofascial pain.

Cryokinetics may also be useful in the management of myofascial pain. Therapeutic exercises to restore motion, improve posture, and reestablish pain-free, functional movement patterns are often better tolerated following cryotherapy.

Cold is not indicated in the treatment of all persistent pain problems. Complex regional pain syndrome may be exacerbated by cryotherapy; the intense stimulus of the cold can result in excruciating pain and worsen the problem.

## Cautions and Contraindications

Although therapeutic modalities are applied to make injured individuals more comfortable and speed rehabilitation, these treatments can also cause harm. Before applying any therapeutic agent, be certain that relevant equipment is in proper working order, ensure that any electrical equipment (e.g., whirlpool) is powered by a circuit served by a ground fault interrupter, and identify known contraindications or conditions that warrant special caution.

Some medical conditions result in significant adverse reactions and contraindicate the application of cold (table 8.1). The most common condition in this category is vasospastic disorders, of which Raynaud's phenomenon is in turn the most common. Raynaud's phenomenon is characterized by constriction of arteries and arterioles in an extremity. The restriction in blood flow results in a blue, gray, or purplish discoloration of the skin accompanied by burning or tingling sensations or numbness. Raynaud's phenomenon is most common in women. The symptoms and signs are transient; however, many individuals with Raynaud's phenomenon experience such discomfort that cold cannot be applied long enough to have a beneficial effect. Thus, cryotherapy is contraindicated.

Cold urticaria, an allergic reaction to cold exposure, also contraindicates cryotherapy. When cold is applied to someone susceptible to cold urticaria, an anaphylactic reaction occurs. Hives break out in the cooler area and are accompanied by intense itching. Failure to recognize the problem and discontinue the cryotherapy could result in a more systemic reaction and could affect respiration and consciousness.

Cold-induced hemoglobinuria (paroxymal cold hemoglobinuria) and cryoglobinemia are two rare conditions that also contraindicate cryotherapy. Hemoglobinuria occurs when the rate of red blood cell breakdown exceeds the rate at which hemoglobin combines with other proteins. The excess hemoglobin is excreted in the urine. The condition is characterized by darkened urine and back pain. Cryoglobinemia is a condition in which an abnormal clumping of plasma proteins (cryoglobins) is stimulated by cold application. The symptoms include skin discoloration and dyspnea. These conditions may occur in conjunction with Raynaud's phenomenon or cold urticaria. Although these conditions are rare, you must keep them in mind. Initially cryotherapy is uncomfortable, but most individuals accommodate and tolerate it well. Be certain that discomfort during cryotherapy is not associated with any of these conditions.

## Table 8.1    Indications, Contraindications, and Precautions for Cold

| Indications | Contraindications | Precautions |
|---|---|---|
| Relieve pain | Raynaud's phenomenon | Application over superficial nerves |
| Control swelling and protect injured tissues (when combined with rest, elevation, and compression) | Cold urticaria | Diminished sensation |
| Decrease muscle spasm | Cryoglobinemia | Poor local circulation |
| | Paroxymal cold hemoglobinuria | Slow-healing wounds |
| | | Medically unstable |

Some other situations warrant caution. Some large nerves emerge from deep tissue and pass just below the skin and fatty layer. Because there is less tissue to insulate the nerve, it can be injured by cold or pressure during ice pack application. These injuries, referred to as cold-induced nerve palsy, are preventable. The ulnar nerve as it passes through the ulnar groove, and the peroneal nerve as it passes through the posterior lateral aspect of the knee, are most susceptible. The lateral femoral cutaneous nerve can also be injured by cold applied in the area of the femoral triangle. Protect these nerves by applying a dry cloth over the nerve, and limit cold application in the area to 20 to 30 min.

Special caution is warranted when using cryotherapy to treat individuals who are frail, are suffering from significant medical problems, have slow-healing wounds, or have diminished circulation or sensation. The first law of therapeutics is "Do no harm." Thus, if you are uncertain about the safety of any modality application, do not administer the treatment.

## Does Cold Application Improve Treatment Outcomes?

In chapter 7, issues of treatment outcome and evidence-based practice were introduced. This chapter has introduced the application techniques, theoretical basis, indications, and contraindications for therapeutic cold application. However, the question "Does cold application speed or enhance recovery from injury or surgery?" has not been addressed from an evidence perspective. Interestingly, the quantity of published reports that provide evidence of benefit or lack of benefit from cold application is not large. Belanger (2002) lists fewer than 15 references to clinical trials involving cold application for musculoskeletal conditions (ankle sprain and knee surgery) of interest here.

Bleakley, McDonough, and MacAuley (2004) completed a systematic review of randomized controlled trials related to cold therapy. Their summary suggests that cryotherapy is better than superficial heating or contrast in the treatment of acute ankle injuries. However, a single application of ice and compression was reported to be of little or no benefit. Cold following arthroscopic knee procedures, combined with exercise, was reported to reduce pain and facilitate weight bearing when compared to performing exercise alone. There is little evidence, however, to support cold therapy following anterior cruciate ligament reconstruction. Moreover, Daniel, Stone, and Arendt (1994) reported no benefit of cold wrap adjusted to as low as 45° on pain, medication use, or other outcome measures following arthroscopically assisted anterior cruciate ligament reconstruction. Dervin, Taylor, and Keene (1998), Edwards, Rimmer, and Keene (1996), and Konrath et al. (1996) reported similar results using a continuous flow of cool water through Cryocuff cooling pads and ice packs. Ohkoshi et al. (1999), Cohn, Draeger, and Jackson (1989), and Barber, McGuire, and Click (1998) reported, however, that cooling reduced reports of pain and analgesic use after surgery. Lessard et al. (1997) reported similar findings after arthroscopic knee surgery. These conflicting findings highlight concerns over the insulating effects of postoperative dressings and the need for investigators to be very specific when describing treatment protocols.

There is agreement (Levy et al. 1993; Leutz et al. 1995) that cold therapy lessens blood loss following total knee arthroplasty, but these groups of investigators differed as to whether any additional benefits are realized with cold application. Levy et al. found small differences in pain report and medication use in patients receiving cold therapy, while Leutz et al. reported no additional benefit.

Hubbard, Aronson, and Denegar (2004, p. 93) completed a systematic review of the effects of cold treatments on return to work or sport. The focus on functional return resulted in location of only four clinical trials. The authors found that "most of the research related to cryotherapy has focused on the physiologic response to cold application" and that "there is a current void in the literature related to clinically relevant treatment outcomes." They concluded that "based on the evidence of the four studies we critically examined for this study, . . . cryotherapy had a positive effect on return to participation." Sloan, Hain, and Pownall (1989) reported that immediate cold therapy patients treated in an emergency department with compression and nonsteroidal anti-inflammatory medication plus early cold application were not significantly better at 7-day follow-up than those treated with medication and compression only. Thus, repeated applications are necessary to achieve the more rapid return to work and sport identified by Hubbard, Aronson, and Denegar.

These reviews of treatment outcomes demonstrate the need for additional study. Many clinicians routinely apply cold therapy or other modalities based on what they were taught and the practice habits they have developed. At this time we conclude that when patients are free of contraindications, cold can be safely applied. It is likely to reduce pain and decrease secondary tissue injury and may speed recovery following ankle sprains and knee surgery. The evidence for expedited recovery, however, is not compelling.

## SUPERFICIAL HEAT

Because the fatty layer of tissue beneath the dermis insulates the deeper tissues, modalities that heat the skin are classified as superficial heating modalities. These modalities have little to no effect on the temperature of deeper tissues (Draper et al. 1998, Holcomb 2003), and therefore metabolism, or blood flow, except in areas with little fat, such as over the joints of the hand. Despite the limited effects on deep tissue temperature, these modalities are commonly used to decrease pain and muscle spasm. The remainder of this chapter addresses methods of application, physiological effects, safety issues, and evidence of effectiveness related to the application of superficial heat.

### Methods of Application

The most common form of superficial heat is the moist heat pack, usually a hydrocollator pack (figure 8.9). Hot water tanks called hydrocollator units are found in most athletic training rooms and sports medicine clinics. These heat packs are filled with a gel that retains heat. By placing the packs into a hydrocollator tank (170° F, or 76.6° C), you have ready access to superficial heat. At that temperature, direct contact would burn the skin, so you should wrap the packs in terry cloth covers and towels for protection. When using heat packs with individuals who are at risk for skin injury (i.e., those with circulatory compromise) and in circumstances when a person lies on a hot pack, be certain to provide sufficient insulation.

Warm water whirlpools are another common form of superficial heat (figure 8.10). Whirlpools permit heating around an entire limb or joint. The motion of the water also massages the tissue, which may add to the analgesic and antispasmotic effects of superficial heating. Whirlpools also allow for active or passive motion during heating.

The temperature of the water must be maintained within a safe range. Water that is too hot can scald the skin, and whirlpool temperatures should never exceed 115° F (46° C). Because treatment in a whirlpool also stresses the body's ability to dissipate heat, whirlpool treatment can result in hyperthermia and heat illness. The larger the portion of the body immersed in the whirlpool, the greater the heat stress. Table 8.2 provides reasonable guidelines for maximum whirlpool temperatures for various areas of the body. If the whirlpool is located in a poorly ventilated area, greater caution is advised. The whirlpool should be visible from all areas of the athletic training room or clinic, and no one should use a whirlpool unsupervised. Use extra caution when treating individuals prone to heat illness or with medical conditions that compromise the body's ability to withstand hot, humid environments.

Thermal injury is not the only concern associated with whirlpool use. Bacteria thrive in warm, moist environments. Whirlpools should be thoroughly cleaned and disinfected after each use. Because in some facilities many individuals are treated, the whirlpool may not be properly cleaned between uses. Under these circumstances, identify

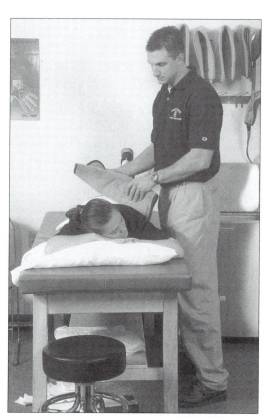

**Figure 8.9** A hydrocollator pack application.

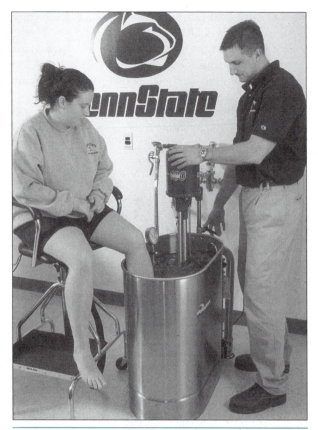

**Figure 8.10**    A warm water whirlpool.

individuals with open wounds and take extra precautions to prevent the spread of infections.

Moist heat packs and warm whirlpools are the most commonly applied superficial heating modalities. However, paraffin baths, heat lamps, and fluidotherapy are also classified as superficial heating devices.

Paraffin baths are filled with seven parts paraffin wax and one part mineral oil heated to 125° to 127° F (51.6-52.7° C). Because of the lower specific heat of the wax compared to water, higher temperatures are used than with whirlpool baths. Paraffin is most commonly used in treating the hand and wrist. The treated hand should be washed and then dipped into the paraffin (figure 8.11). The hand is then removed until the wax hardens. This procedure is repeated four to five times until there is a thick layer of warm wax around the treated area. The hand is placed in a plastic bag or an oven mitt; the plastic bag allows you to remove the wax at the end of treatment without making a mess, but the oven mitt holds heat longer. Generally the paraffin is left on for 20 to 30 min. Paraffin has limited application in athletic training but is valuable in treating hand pain and loss of hand function. Paraffin cannot be used if there is an open wound and should be used with caution if the individual has sensory or vascular compromise in the area to be treated.

Heat lamps were once commonly used to provide superficial heat. Because of cost and convenience, heat lamps have been replaced by moist heat packs. A heat lamp positioned over a moist towel will increase the temperature of the skin. The amount of heating depends on the strength of the bulb and the distance between the lamp and the towel (see inverse square law, p. 107). The heat lamp provides the same benefits as a moist heat pack. However, each lamp can be used on only one person at a time, whereas many individuals can be treated simultaneously with inexpensive moist heat packs.

Fluidotherapy has been referred to as a dry whirlpool (figure 8.12). A fluidotherapy unit contains ground cellulose material that can be heated to 120° to 125° F (48.8-51.6° C) and then blown around the chamber with forced air. The result is heating through convection and a massage. Fluidotherapy allows passive or active movement during treatment. Individuals with properly dressed open wounds can be treated with fluidotherapy without the risk of contamination. In contrast to what happens in treatment of an extremity in a whirlpool, with fluidotherapy the treated limb does not sit in a gravity-dependent position.

## Table 8.2   Maximum Whirlpool Temperature by Body Part*

| Body part | Degrees F | Degrees C |
| --- | --- | --- |
| Wrist and hand | 112 | 44.4 |
| Foot and ankle | 110 | 43.3 |
| Elbow | 108 | 42.2 |
| Knee | 106 | 41.1 |
| Thigh | 104 | 40.0 |

*Assuming well-ventilated whirlpool area and absence of medical conditions that require precaution in warm, humid environments.

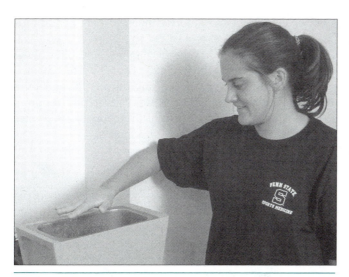

**Figure 8.11** A paraffin bath.

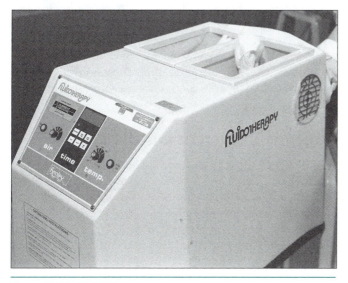

**Figure 8.12**   Fluidotherapy.

## Temperature Increases and Physiological Responses

Superficial heating increases the skin temperature several degrees. The intra-articular temperature of small joints such as the interphalangeals can be increased to therapeutically beneficial levels. The temperature of deeper tissues such as large muscles and deep joints rises insignificantly. Draper et al. (1998) reported a 3.8° C temperature rise at 1-cm depth but only a 0.74° rise at 3 cm following a 15-min hot pack application. Holcomb (2003) reported no change in temperature at 3.75cm at the same hot pack temperature and application time used by Draper. Thus superficial heat placed over the hamstrings or the glenohumeral joint of a muscular individual will not raise the temperature of those tissues sufficiently to have a therapeutic benefit.

If superficial heat has little effect on the temperature of injured tissue, why is it so commonly applied in athletic training and physical therapy? Much as with cold, the primary clinical benefits of superficial heat are pain control and relief of muscle spasm. However, the mechanisms responsible for these physiological responses are not well understood.

The sensation of heat is carried by small-diameter fibers (A-delta and C fibers). Thus, it is unlikely that pain modulation occurs through a gating mechanism. Is it possible that a descending pain modulation mechanism is involved? Input into the central nervous system via small-diameter afferent input may stimulate descending pain control mechanisms. Clinical observation suggests that this theory may have merit. Superficial heat applied for 20 to 30 min often has a calming, sedating effect. The mechanisms behind the calming, analgesic effects of superficial heat are not well understood; however, the answers lie in the advances in neuroscience described in chapter 4.

The mechanism behind the antispasmodic effect of superficial heating is equally speculative. One explanation is that by relieving pain, superficial heating breaks the pain–spasm cycle. However, other factors may be involved. When heat is applied, the sensitivity of muscle spindles decreases, even though the temperature of the spindle is not affected. Thus, superficial heating may alter muscle spindle activity through a spinal reflex mechanism. Although speculative, this is the best explanation for the decrease in spindle sensitivity and relief of spasm associated with superficial heating.

Other physiological responses are associated with tissue heating, including increased metabolic activity, increased circulation, increased inflammation, increased tissue elasticity and decreased viscosity, and sweating. Although these responses occur in the dermis, deeper tissues are much less affected because of the insulating effects of adipose tissue. Except in superficial joint structures, superficial heating does not alter deeper tissues. Thus, superficial heating does little to the metabolism or blood flow of deeper damaged tissues.

## Indications for Superficial Heating

Certified athletic trainers primarily apply superficial heat to relieve pain and muscle spasm prior to therapeutic exercise. Superficial heating in a whirlpool or fluidotherapy unit also permits passive or active range of motion exercises. Active motion increases lymphatic drainage, which will reduce swelling.

Superficial heat can also be used to treat restrictions in superficial joints. The joints of the hand, wrist, foot, and ankle respond best because there is little adipose tissue over these joints. However, ultrasound and diathermy result in a more vigorous heating and are the modalities of choice for heating tissue prior to mobilization and stretching. Knight et al. (2001) reported that the application of superficial heat did not enhance the effect of stretching of the plantar flexor muscles while a 7-min ultrasound treatment was an effective adjunct.

## Cautions and Contraindications

Unlike the situation with cold, there are no rare complications associated with superficial heat (table 8.3). This does not imply, however, that superficial heat is completely safe. In fact, burns from superficial heating are far more common than cold-induced injuries. Burns, the primary risk of superficial heating, can be prevented by providing adequate insulation around moist heat packs, controlling whirlpool and fluidotherapy temperatures, and screening out individuals at risk for burns due to loss of sensation or circulatory problems. In addition, caution is needed when anyone lies on a moist heat pack, because heat cannot escape and builds up more rapidly than it would otherwise. Extra insulation with toweling is necessary if the injured person is to lie on the heat pack.

Heat also stresses the cardiovascular system. The heat stress from a superficial heat application combined with a warm, humid environment can be lethal for someone with coronary artery disease or multiple medical problems. These problems are rarely encountered in athletic training. But you need to be ever mindful that modalities routinely used with young, healthy individuals are not safe for everyone.

## Does Superficial Heat Improve Treatment Outcomes?

The literature related to outcomes of treatment with superficial heat, like that related to cold therapy, is limited. What is available, however, suggests that superficial heat does have a clinically useful analgesic effect. Nadler et al. (2002) reported that continuous heat wrap application was more effective in reducing pain than oral administration of acetaminophen or ibuprofen. Akin et al. (2001) found similar treatment as effective as ibuprofen in treatment of dysmenorrhea. Nadler et al. (2003a, 2003b) reported on two trials of continuous heat wrap in the treatment of acute low back pain. In both trials the heat wrap was more effective

## Table 8.3    Indications, Contraindications, and Precautions for Superficial Heat

|  | Indications | Contraindications | Precautions |
|---|---|---|---|
| Superficial heating in general | Decrease pain | Diminished sensation | Medically unstable |
|  | Decrease muscle spasm | Poor local circulation | Coronary heart disease |
| **Modality specific** | | | |
| Whirlpool | Heat very superficial joint capsules | Open wounds |  |
| Fluidotherapy | Heat very superficial joint capsules |  |  |
| Paraffin | Heat very superficial joint capsules | Open wounds |  |

than placebo medication or oral ibuprofen. Superficial heat applied for 20 min has also been reported to reduce the sensitivity of active myofascial trigger points. Robinson et al. (2002) concluded that superficial moist heat can be used as palliative therapy in the treatment of rheumatoid arthritis.

On the basis of the available literature we can conclude that long-duration (8 h), low-level heat can be recommended in the management of acute low back pain, and that shorter-duration moist heat can be used clinically to reduce myofascial pain as part of a more comprehensive treatment session. More investigation is needed to examine the effect of the use of superficial heat on recovery from other musculoskeletal conditions. When it is used safely, however, the clinician can expect that 20 or more minutes of superficial heat will reduce pain and thus likely stiffness in patients with musculoskeletal injuries and arthritic conditions.

## HEAT AND COLD: CONTRAST THERAPY

Contrast therapy, which consists of alternating applications of heat and cold, is also used to treat athletic injuries. The most common approach to contrast treatment consists of alternately immersing the foot, ankle, and leg in a cold water whirlpool or bath and a warm whirlpool (figure 8.13). The temperature of the cold bath and warm whirlpool should be within the ranges previously described in this chapter. The literature provides several recommendations (Walsh 1996; Bell and Prentice 1998) as to the length of time cold and heat should be applied, as well as the number of cycles of heat and cold that should be completed during a treatment. A cold-to-warm ratio of 1 to 3 min or 1 to 4 min appears reasonable based upon clinical observations and experience.

Several physiological effects have been proposed to explain the benefits of contrast therapy. Many have suggested that contrast therapy results in cycles of vasodilation and vasoconstriction, thus creating a pumping action to reduce swelling. However, tissue temperatures are not affected by contrast treatments (Myrer et al. 1994, 1997; Higgins and Kaminski 1998). The brief exposure to cold and the fact that superficial heating has minimal effect on deep blood flow suggest that there is little vascular response to contrast therapy.

Even though there is no good explanation for the effects of contrast therapy, this approach has been used to treat some physically active individuals. For example, contrast therapy may be effective in reducing edema in subacute foot and ankle injuries. When swelling limits range of motion several days after injury, contrast therapy along with active range of motion appears to reduce swelling. The sharp sensory contrast between heat and cold appears reduce pain and therefore muscle spasm. Models of descending influence over dorsal horn processing of nociceptive input certainly offer a plausible explanation for the analgesic response to contrast. A decrease in pain and spasm, combined with active, pain-free range of motion, would in turn increase lymphatic drainage from the area and decrease swelling.

As with many therapies, there has been little investigation of the effectiveness of contrast treatments. Cote et al. (1988) reported that swelling increased in sprained ankles after contrast therapy administered over 3 days after acute lateral ankle sprain. Certainly, these results suggest that contrast therapy should not be administered early in the plan of care. Kuligowski et al. (1998), however, found that contrast or cold therapy had more effect on pain and loss of motion associated with delayed onset muscle soreness than superficial heat. Further investigation is needed on this treatment approach to identify if and when it should be applied.

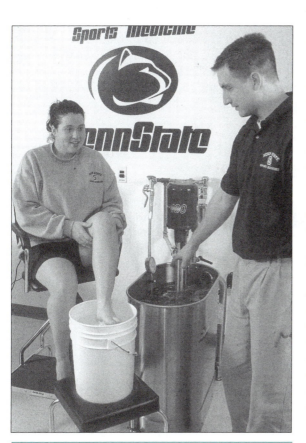

**Figure 8.13** Contrast therapy.

# HEAT, COLD, AND CONTRAST THERAPY: DECIDING WHAT TO APPLY

Pain and muscle spasm indicate the use of cryotherapy, superficial heat, and contrast treatment. This raises the question, which is best? There is no simple answer, and you must consider several factors when selecting a modality, weighing the potential benefits against potential risks.

Contraindications are the first consideration in selecting a therapeutic modality. If the injured person suffers from Raynaud's phenomenon (cryoglobinemia, hemoglobinuria) or cold urticaria, then cold and contrast cannot be used.

Traditionally heat has been thought to be contraindicated following acute injury because of the associated increase in blood flow. However, superficial heat has little effect on deep tissue temperature and blood flow, and there is little evidence to suggest that heat combined with rest, compression, and elevation slows recovery. Nonetheless, cold is the treatment of choice in the management of acute injuries because it is an effective analgesic and antispasmotic and may minimize secondary tissue injury. In the management of acute injuries, cold should be combined with protection of the healing tissues, compression, and elevation. Thus, cold pack application is preferred over cold water immersion or cold whirlpool, because these treatments place the limb in a gravity-dependent position.

If neither heat nor cold is contraindicated and the condition is not acute, you must consider other factors in choosing between cryotherapy, superficial heat, and contrast therapy. The most important considerations are the severity of pain and muscle spasm and patient preference. Cold is a better choice when pain and muscle spasm are severe. However, the preference of the individual is also important. If a certain treatment has helped a person in the past, he or she is likely to believe that the treatment will work again and is likely to actively participate in a plan of care that includes the specific treatment.

Compliance by the injured individual is especially important in a sports medicine clinic. The certified athletic trainer often must develop home treatment programs for athletes who are treated in the clinic only once or twice per week. Certainly someone who prefers not to be treated with cryotherapy is unlikely to use cold at home unless provided with a very convincing argument as to why such treatments are essential to his or her recovery. Thus, the ease of application and the probability of compliance with home use are also considerations when you are choosing between cryotherapy and superficial heat.

## A Word on Counterirritants

The subject of counterirritants (analgesic balm) designed for superficial application does not fit with any specific chapter on therapeutic modalities. Although the topical application of some of these agents results in a sensation of heating, topical counterirritants do not result in clinically meaningful changes in tissue temperature.

The lack of a thermal response does not mean, however, that these agents are useless. The chemical stimulation of cutaneous sensory receptors will alter sensory input into the dorsal horn of the spinal column. The pain theories presented in chapter 4 offer some explanation for the soothing, analgesic benefits of counterirritants. The rubbing required for application and the stimulating effects of the counterirritant will increase large-diameter afferent input. Thus, the stimulation of large-diameter first-order afferent nerves offers a plausible explanation for a favorable response to topical counterirritants.

# SUMMARY

1. Describe the four energy transfer mechanisms related to therapeutic modalities.

   Thermal energy can be transferred to or from the body by four mechanisms: conduction, convection, radiation, and conversion. Conduction involves direct contact between a warm and a cool surface. Convection involves heating or cooling through movement of air or a liquid. Radiation involves exposure of a surface to radiant energy such as occurs with lying in the sun or under a heat lamp. Conversion involves converting one form of energy, such as ultrasound, to thermal energy.

2. Describe the common methods of applying superficial heat and therapeutic cold.

   Superficial heat can be applied with a hot pack, a heating lamp, a warm whirlpool, paraffin, or fluidotherapy. Therapeutic cold can be applied with an ice pack, ice massage, a cold whirlpool, cold water immersion, or a vapocoolant spray.

3. Describe the thermal changes that occur with superficial heat and local cold application.

   Superficial heat increases the temperature of the skin. Due to the insulating effects of adipose tissues, the superficial joint structures are the only deep tissues that are heated to a clinically significant degree. Cold application cools the skin and deeper tissues. Cooling of the skin occurs more rapidly than cooling of deeper tissues, and the skin is cooled to lower temperatures than the deeper tissues. However, a 20-min cold pack application will decrease muscle temperature approximately 7° F at a depth of over 2 cm.

4. Discuss the effect of superficial heat and local cooling on blood flow, muscle tone, and the nervous system.

   Superficial heat increases cutaneous blood flow. However, because blood flow to deeper tissues such as muscle is regulated by metabolic demand rather than temperature, superficial heating has little effect on blood flow in deeper tissues. Therapeutic cold causes vasoconstriction in cutaneous and deep tissues. Both therapeutic cold and superficial heat can decrease muscle spasm. Therapeutic cold decreases the temperature of muscle spindles, relieving muscle spasm. Superficial heat has a similar effect; however, because superficial heating does not raise deep tissue temperature, the decrease in muscle spindle activity is thought to occur through reflex mechanisms. A 15- to 20-min application of cold will decrease nerve conduction velocity. Because the rate at which impulses are carried by small-diameter primary afferent nerves is slowed, fewer pain messages reach the central nervous system and less pain is perceived. Superficial heat stimulates thermal receptors, from which increased input may trigger descending analgesic mechanisms mediated by the release of beta endorphin.

5. Discuss the indications for cold application and the impact of cooling on acute inflammation.

   Cold is primarily used to relieve pain and muscle spasm. Cold may also limit swelling following musculoskeletal injury. Cold application will be maximally effective when combined with compression, elevation, and protection of injured tissues.

6. Describe the common indications for the application of superficial heat.

   Superficial heat is used to relieve pain and muscle spasm. The choice between using heat and cold depends on a number of factors including contraindications, degree of pain and muscle spasm, and preference.

7. Describe the application of cold in a program of cryokinetics.

   Cryokinetics is a treatment technique that combines cold application and active exercise. Cold is used to decrease pain and muscle spasm and allow for pain-free therapeutic exercise.

8. Identify contraindications and precautions in applying superficial heat and therapeutic cold.

Some medical conditions result in significant adverse reactions and contraindicate the application of cold (table 8.1). The most common condition in this category is vasospastic disorders, among which Raynaud's phenomenon occurs the most frequently. Cold urticaria, an allergic reaction to cold exposure, also contraindicates cold application. Cold-induced hemoglobinuria (paroxymal cold hemoglobinuria) and cryoglobinemia are two rare conditions that also contraindicate cryotherapy. Hemoglobinuria occurs when the rate of red blood cell breakdown exceeds the rate at which hemoglobin combines with other proteins. Cryoglobinemia is a condition in which an abnormal clumping of plasma proteins (cryoglobins) is stimulated by cold application. In addition, cold can injure superficial nerves such as the ulnar and common peroneal. Thus, extreme caution is required when cold is applied near or over these structures.

Burns are the primary risk of superficial heating. These can be prevented by providing adequate insulation around moist heat packs and by properly adjusting fluidotherapy and whirlpool temperatures. Heat and cold stress the cardiovascular system, so special caution is warranted when superficial heat or cryotherapy is used to treat individuals who are frail, have significant medical problems (such as coronary artery disease), or have diminished circulation or sensation.

9. Differentiate between superficial heating and deep heating modalities.

The superficial heating modalities described in this chapter have little effect on the temperature of deeper tissues such as muscle. Ultrasound and diathermy, however, can increase the temperature of deeper tissues by converting acoustic or electromagnetic energy to thermal energy in the tissues.

10. Describe contrast therapy.

Contrast therapy involves alternating therapeutic cold and superficial heating modalities. Most often this technique is used to treat the foot, leg, and ankle by alternating immersion in a warm and a cold whirlpool or water bath.

## CITED SOURCES

Akin MD, Weingand KW, Hengehold DA, Goodale MB, Kinkle Rt, Smith RP: Continuous low-level topical heat in the treatment of dysmenorrhea. *Obstet Gynecol* 97:343-349, 2001.

Barber FA, McGuire DA, Click S: Continuous-flow cold therapy for outpatient anterior cruciate ligament reconstruction. *Arthroscopy* 14:130-135, 1998.

Belanger AY: *Evidence-based Guide to Therapeutic Physical Agents.* Philadelphia, Lippincott Williams & Wilkins, 2002.

Bell GW, Prentice WE: Infrared modalities. In Prentice WE (Ed), *Therapeutic Modalities for Allied Health Professionals.* New York, McGraw-Hill, 1998, 201-239.

Bleakley C, McDonough S, MacAuley D: The use of ice in the treatment of acute soft-tissue injury: A systematic review of randomized controlled trials. *Am J Sports Med* 32:251-261, 2004.

Bocobo C, Fast A, Kingery W, Kaplan M: The effect of ice on intraarticular temperature in the knee of the dog. *Am J Phys Med Rehabil* 70:181-185, 1991.

Cohn BT, Draeger RI, Jackson DW: The effects of cold therapy in the postoperative management of pain in patients undergoing anterior cruciate ligament reconstruction. *Am J Sports Med* 17:344-349, 1989.

Cote DJ, Prentice WE Jr., Hooker DN, Shields EW: Comparison of three treatment procedures for minimizing ankle sprain swelling. *Phys Ther* 68:1072-1076, 1988.

Cross KM, Wilson RW, Perrin DH: Functional performance following ice immersion to the lower extremity. *J Athl Train* 30:231-234, 1995.

Daniel DM, Stone ML, Arendt DL: The effect of cold therapy on pain, swelling, and range of motion after anterior cruciate ligament reconstructive surgery. *Arthroscopy* 10:530-533, 1994.

Dervin GF, Taylor DE, Keene GC: Effects of cold and compression dressings on early postoperative outcomes for the arthroscopic anterior cruciate ligament reconstruction patient. *J Orthop Sports Phys Ther* 27:403-406, 1998.

Draper DO, Harris ST, Schulthies S, Durrant E, Knight KL, Richard M: Hot-pack and 1 MHz ultrasound treatments have an additive effect on muscle temperature increase. *J Athl Train* 33: 21-24,1998.

Edwards DJ, Rimmer M, Keene GC: The use of cold therapy in the postoperative management of patients undergoing arthroscopic anterior cruciate ligament reconstruction. *Am J Sports Med* 24: 193-195, 1996.

Evans TA, Ingersoll C, Knight KL, Worrell TW: Agility following the application of cold therapy (Abstract). *J Athl Train* 31:S-53, 1996.

Gerig BK: The effects of cryotherapy on ankle proprioception (Abstract). *J Athl Train* 24:S-119, 1990.

Greicar M, Kendrick Z, Kimura I, Sitler M: Immediate and delayed effects of cryotherapy on functional power and agility (Abstract). *J Athl Train* 31:S-33, 1996.

Haimovici N: Three years experience in direct intra-articular temperature measurement. *Prog Clin Biol Res* 107:453-461, 1982.

Hartviksen K: Ice therapy in spasticity. *Acta Neurol Scand* 38(Suppl 3):79-84, 1962.

Higgins D, Kaminski TW: Contrast therapy does not cause fluctuations in human gastrocnemius intramuscular temperature. *J Athl Train* 33:336-340, 1998.

Holcomb WR: The effects of superficial heating before 1 MHz ultrasound on tissue temperature. *J Sport Rehabil* 12:95-103, 2003.

Hubbard TJ, Aronson SL, Denegar CR: Does cryotherapy improve treatment outcome? A systematic review. *J Athl Train* 29:88-94, 2004

Knight CA, Rutledge CR, Cox ME, Acosta M, Hall SJ: Effect of superficial heat, deep heat, and active exercise warm-up on extensibility of the plantar flexors. *Phys Ther* 81:1206-1214, 2001.

Knight KL: *Cryotherapy in Sport Injury Management.* Champaign, IL, Human Kinetics, 1995.

Knight KL, Aquino J, Johannes SM, Urban CD: A re-examination of Lewis' cold-induced vasodilation in the finger and ankle. *J Athl Train* 15:238-250, 1980.

Konrath G, Lock T, Goitz H, Scheider J: The use of cold therapy after anterior cruciate ligament reconstruction; a prospective randomized study and literature study. *Am J Sports Med* 24:629-633, 1996.

Kuligowski LA, Lephart SM, Giannantonio FP, Blanc RO: Effect of whirlpool therapy on the signs and symptoms of delayed-onset muscle soreness. *J Athl Train* 33:222-228, 1998.

LaRiviere J, Osternig LR: The effect of ice immersion on joint position sense. *J Sport Rehab* 3:58-67, 1994.

Lessard LA, Scudds RA, Amendola A, Vaz MD: The efficacy of cryotherapy following arthroscopic knee surgery. *J Orthop Sports Phys Ther.* 26:14-22, 1997.

Leutz DW, Harris H: Continuous cold therapy in total knee arthroplasty. *Am J Knee Surg* 8:121-123, 1995.

Levy AS, Marmar E: The role of cold compression dressings in the postoperative treatment of total knee arthroplasty. *Clin Orthop* 297:174-178, 1993.

McDonough E, Strauss K, Apel T, Ingersoll C, Knight KL: Cooling the ankle, lower leg and both affects dynamic postural sway (Abstract). *J Athl Train* 31:S-10, 1996.

McMaster WC, Little S, Waugh TR: Laboratory evaluations of various cold therapy modalities. *Am J Sports Med* 6:291-294, 1978.

Merrick MA: Secondary injury after musculoskeletal trauma: A review and update. *J Athl Train* 37: 209-217, 2002.

Merrick MA: *Inflammation and Secondary Injury.* Paper presented at the Penn State Athletic Training Conference, March 28, 2003.

Michlovitz SL: *Thermal Agents in Rehabilitation,* 2nd ed. Philadelphia, Davis, 1990.

Myrer JW, Draper DO, Durrant E: Contrast therapy and intramuscular temperature in the human leg. *J Athl Train* 29:318-322, 1994.

Myrer JW, Measom G, Durrant E, Fellingham GW: Cold- and hot-pack contrast therapy: Subcutaneous and intramuscular temperature change. *J Athl Train* 32:238-241, 1997.

Nadler SF, Steiner DJ, Erasala GN, Hengehold DA, Abeln SB, Weingand KW: Continuous low-level heatwrap therapy for treating acute nonspecific low back pain. *Arch Phys Med Rehabil* 84:329-334, 2003a.

Nadler SF, Steiner DJ, Erasala GN, Hengehold DA, Hinkle RT, Beth Goodale M, Abeln SB, Weingand KW: Continuous low-level heat wrap therapy provides more efficacy than Ibuprofen and acetaminophen for acute low back pain. *Spine* 27:1012-1017, 2002.

Nadler SF, Steiner DJ, Petty SR, Erasala GN, Hengehold DA, Weingand KW: Overnight use of continuous low-level heatwrap therapy for relief of low back pain. *Arch Phys Med Rehabil* 84:335-342, 2003b.

Ohkoshi Y, Ohkoshi M, Nagasaki S, Ono A, Hashimoto T, Yamane S: The effect of cryotherapy on intraarticular temperature and postoperative care after anterior cruciate ligament reconstruction. *Am J Sports Med* 27:357-362, 1999.

Oosterveld FGJ, Rasker JJ, Jacobs JWG, Overmars HJA: The effect of local heat and cold therapy on the intraarticular and skin surface temperature. *Arthritis Rheum* 35:146-151, 1992.

Peppard A: Personal Communication. Brockport, NY (1997).

Provins KA, Morton R: Tactile discrimination and skin temperature. *J Appl Phys* 15:155-160, 1960.

Rivers D, Kimura I, Sitler M, Kendrick Z: The influence of cryotherapy and Aircast bracing on total body balance and proprioception (Abstract). *J Athl Train* 30:S-15, 1995.

Robinson V, Brosseau L, Casimiro L, Judd M, Shea B, Wells G. Tugwell P. Thermotherapy for treating rheumatoid arthritis (Cochrane Review) Cochrane Library, Issue 1, 2002.

Rubley MD, Denegar CR, Buckley WE, Newell KM: Cryotherapy, sensation and isometric force variability. *J Athl Train* 38:113-119, 2003.

Shuler DE, Ingersoll C, Knight KL, Kuhlman JS: Local cold application to the foot and ankle, lower leg, or both effects on a cutting drill (Abstract). *J Athl Train* 31:S-35, 1996.

Sloan JP, Hain R, Pownall R: Clinical benefits of early cold therapy in accident and emergency following ankle sprain. *Arch Emerg Med* 6:1-6, 1989.

Steinagel MC, Szczerba JE, Guskiewicz KM, Perrin DH: Ankle ice immersion effect on postural sway (Abstract). *J Athl Train* 31:S-53, 1996.

Thieme HA, Ingersoll CD, Knight KL, Ozmun JC: Cooling does not affect knee proprioception. *J Athl Train* 31:8-10, 1996.

Travel JG, Simons DG: *Myofascial Pain and Dysfunction: The Trigger Point Manual.* Baltimore, Williams & Wilkins, 1983.

Wakin LG, Porter AN, Krusen FH: Influence of physical agents and certain drugs on intraarticular temperature. *Arch Phys Med Rehabil* 32:714-721, 1951.

Walsh MT: Hydrotherapy: The use of water as a therapeutic agent. In Michlovitz SL (Ed), *Thermal Agents in Rehabilitation*, 3rd ed. Philadelphia, Davis, 1996, 139-167.

West TF: The Role of Diminished Cutaneous Sensory Information and Cryotherapy on Haptic Determination of Rod Length. Doctoral dissertation, Penn State University, 1998.

## ADDITIONAL READINGS

Knight KL: *Cryotherapy.* Champaign, IL, Human Kinetics, 1995.

Lehman JF: *Therapeutic Heat and Cold,* 4th ed. Baltimore, Williams & Wilkins, 1990.

Michlovitz SL: *Thermal Agents in Rehabilitation*, 3rd ed. Philadelphia, Davis, 1996.

# CHAPTER 9

# Principles of Electrotherapy

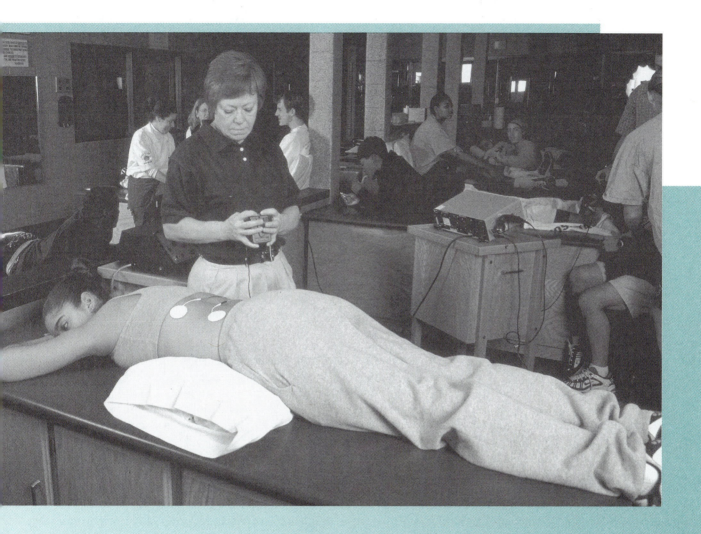

## Objectives

After reading this chapter, the student will be able to

1. define volt, ampere, impedance, and resistance;
2. describe the differences between alternating, direct, and pulsatile currents;
3. define parameters of pulsatile current including phase duration, amplitude, phase charge, and frequency;
4. describe the capacitance of nerve and muscle tissue and how it affects the strength–duration curve;
5. understand the law of Dubois Reymond with respect to the application of electrical current; and
6. describe the types of electrode configurations used with electrical stimulation application.

The therapeutic use of electricity dates back to ancient times, when the Greeks used electric eels to treat physical ailments (Kahn 1987). Electrotherapy has continued to evolve and is very commonly applied by certified athletic trainers. Electrical stimulation has many uses ranging from pain modulation to assisting muscle contraction. The waveforms and parameters available can be confusing. The goal of this chapter is to introduce the principles of electrotherapy and provide a sound foundation for using electrical stimulation in clinical decision making.

# BASICS OF ELECTRICITY

Electrical current is the flow of electrons. To have current, there must be (1) a source of electrons, (2) a material that allows passage of electrons or a conductor, and (3) a driving force of electrons (voltage). Current (identified by the symbol $I$) is measured in **amperes.** One ampere (abbreviated A) is equal to the flow of $6.25 \times 10^{18}$ electrons per second. Amperage is the rate of electron flow past a given point. Because electrons possess a negative charge, a difference in concentrations creates positive and negative polarity. Electrons flow from negative to positive, creating the electrical current.

Electrical charge is measured in **coulombs** (C). One coulomb equals $6.25 \times 10^{18}$ electrons. Thus, 1 A equals the delivery of 1 C of electrical charge per second. Electrical current and electrical charge are both important for an understanding of the principles of electrotherapy. In electrotherapy, the amount of electricity delivered is very small, usually in microamperes ($\mu$A or 1/1,000,000 of an ampere) or milliamps (mA or 1/1,000 A).

**Voltage** (V) is a measure of **electromotive force** and is also referred to as the electrical potential difference. In order for electrons to flow, there must be a difference in the quantity of electrons between two points. The magnitude of the difference between the positive and negative poles is the electromotive force that will drive the current.

Resistance *(R)* is the opposition to the flow of electrons by the material through which the current travels. Resistance is measured in **ohms** ($\Omega$). When the driving force is present (voltage), the amount of resistance determines the amount of current flow (amperage). Thus, current, voltage, and resistance are closely related. An electromotive force of 1 V is required to drive 1 A of current across a resistance of 1 $\Omega$. This relationship, known as Ohm's law, states that current = voltage/resistance, or $I = V/R$. Thus, if resistance increases, a greater voltage is required to drive the same current.

Before voltage can be quantified, impedance must be defined. Impedance is often equated with the term *resistance* in that it is the force that resists the flow of electrons. Impedance is the sum of resistance, inductance, and capacitance. Resistance is the opposition that a substance offers to the flow of current. Inductance is opposition created by eddy currents that form around materials conducting current. Inductance is of little importance in the discussion of electrotherapy in this chapter but is important for an understanding how another modality, diathermy (discussed in chapter 11), works. Capacitance is the ability of a material to store an electrical charge. Capacitors are important in the function of many electrical devices. The human body can store electrical charge, and the concept of capacitance will be very important in understanding transcutaneous electrical nerve stimulation (TENS). (You will read about the application of this modality in chapter 10.) Of the three components of impedance, resistance has the greatest influence in the application of electrotherapy.

# Definitions

- coulomb (C)—Measure of electrical charge or a quantity of electrons. One coulomb = $6.25 \times 10^{18}$ electrons.
- ampere (A)—Measure of electrical current. One ampere equals the movement of 1 C per second.
- volt (V)—Measure of potential difference or electromotive force. One volt equals the electromotive force required to drive 1 A of current across 1 $\Omega$ of resistance.
- ohm ($\Omega$)—Measure of resistance to the flow of electrons.
- impedance—Resistance + inductance + capacitance.
- resistance—Opposition to the flow of electrical current by a material (measured in ohms).
- inductance—Opposition to electrical current created by electromagnetic eddy currents that are generated when current passes through a wire.
- capacitance—Ability of a material to store an electrical charge.

# Ohm's Law

Ohm's law states that voltage = current × resistance. As resistance increases, more voltage is required to pass the same current through an electrical circuit. If resistance is held constant, a greater voltage will result in greater current.

# Relationship of Current, Resistance, and Voltage

The components of electrical current can be analogized to water flowing in a river. The electrons are drops of water (there are *a lot* of water drops in a river, just like electrons in current). The current—the flow of electrons—is like the flow of the river. The voltage is like a waterfall. As the height of the water-fall is increased, the potential energy is greater. Likewise, as the difference in concentration of electrons increases between two points in a circuit, the voltage is higher. Finally, the flow of the river depends on the resistance. If the water is forced through a thin pipe, the pressure is increased, but the total flow of water is lessened. Electrical resistance is affected by the nature of the conductor and increased with the length of the conductor, the cross-sectional area of the conductor, and the temperature. Resistance is lessened when a short, smooth, and large-diameter pipe is used for water flow.

When a certified athletic trainer applies electrotherapy, the body becomes part of an electrical circuit as the current travels from one electrode to the other (figure 9.1). The electrical stimulator generates a voltage to overcome the resistance of the wires and tissues, and a current passes through the body along the path of least resistance. Among the various tissues in the body, the skin has the greatest resistance to current flow. Once the current has penetrated the skin, the electricity has numerous paths—through the vascular system, through the nerves, through the adipose, muscle, tendon, and bone. Current travels best through tissues with the least amount of resistance, such as the nerves. By understanding electrical charge, current, voltage, resistance, and capacitance, you are prepared to explore the differences between the types of electrical stimulators.

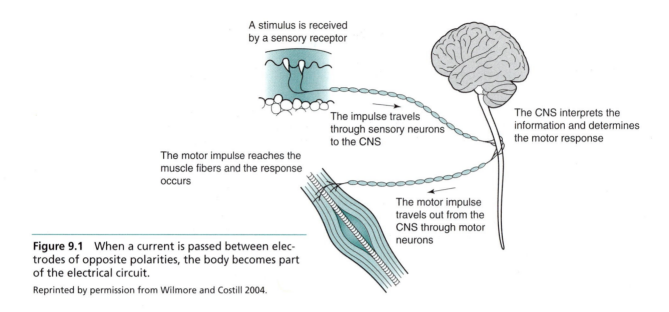

A stimulus is received by a sensory receptor

The impulse travels through sensory neurons to the CNS

The CNS interprets the information and determines the motor response

The motor impulse reaches the muscle fibers and the response occurs

The motor impulse travels out from the CNS through motor neurons

**Figure 9.1** When a current is passed between electrodes of opposite polarities, the body becomes part of the electrical circuit.

Reprinted by permission from Wilmore and Costill 2004.

# TYPES OF ELECTRICAL CURRENT: ALTERNATING, DIRECT, AND PULSATILE

To understand the different types of electrical stimulators available, it is important to be aware of the characteristics of the current applied to the body. The waveform describes the configuration of the pulses of the electrical current. Very specific definitions have been assigned to waveforms, such as **alternating current (AC)** and **direct current (DC),** to provide consistent terminology within physical medicine and to minimize confusion in communication with other professions. There are two major classifications of waveforms: monophasic and biphasic. DC and AC currents can be categorized as monophasic and biphasic, respectively; but DC and AC currents have no interruption between each pulse and continue indefinitely. **Monophasic currents** have uniquely positive and negative electrodes while **biphasic currents** shift polarity continually and each electrode has identical effects if the waveform is symmetrical. Polarity effects to the tissues are minimized or eliminated with a biphasic current (figure 9.2).

Modulation of the waveform within the unit produces **pulsatile currents,** which have temporary interruptions between each pulse. Pulsatile currents have various shapes, phase durations (usually short), and interpulse intervals (figure 9.3). The space between each pulse eliminates the normal inverse relationship between frequency and wavelength as with AC and all natural electromagnetic energy. This allows the clinician to independently control the number of pulses per second **(frequency)** and the phase duration of pulsatile currents (figure 9.4).

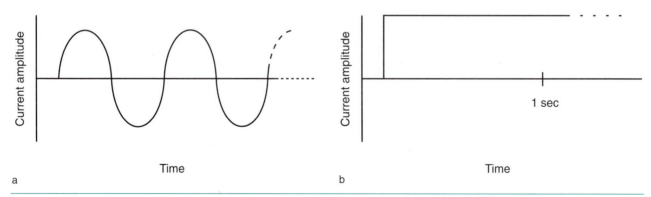

a — Current amplitude / Time

b — Current amplitude / 1 sec / Time

**Figure 9.2** Continuous currents. Alternating current (AC): continuous sinusoidal, biphasic current with no interruption between each pulse. There is an inverse relationship between the phase duration and the pulse frequency *(a)*. Direct current (DC): monophasic current that flows in one direction for longer than 1 sec *(b)*.

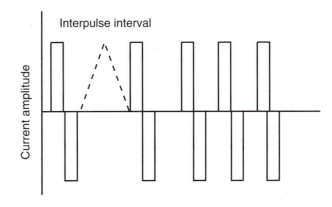

Figure 9.3    Relationship of frequency to pulse duration. A pulsatile current has interruptions called interpulse intervals between each pulse that eliminate the relationship between pulse duration and frequency.

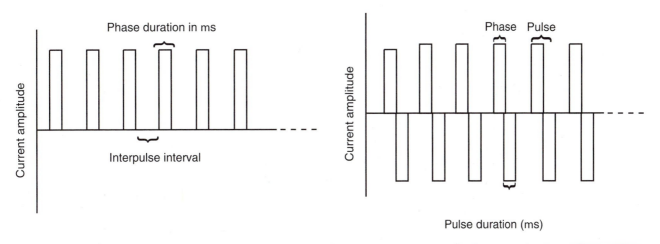

Figure 9.4    Pulsatile monophasic and biphasic currents. Monophasic current flows in one direction only. One electrode is always positive (+) and the other is always negative (–). The interpulse interval allows independent control of phase duration and pulse frequency. Pulsatile biphasic current flows in one direction, then the other. Neither electrode is exclusively positive (+) or negative (–) since they constantly switch. Each pulse (two phases) is separated by an interpulse interval, and there is independent control of pulse duration and frequency.

It is important to understand these waveforms and use proper terminology when discussing electrical stimulators. Consider the following true story. A member of the electrical engineering faculty at a college was referred for treatment by the team physician. This man had experienced an acute onset of mechanical low back pain while playing tennis. The certified athletic trainer elected to use TENS to treat the pain and muscle spasm. When the professor inquired what the athletic trainer was using, he was told that the unit was a high-volt, pulsed galvanic stimulator. This patient informed the athletic trainer that **galvanic** and DC are synonymous and that there was no such thing as pulsed, continuous current. He was, of course, correct. To be considered DC, the current must flow in one direction for at least 1 sec, making it impossible to be pulsed (i.e., it cannot have more than one cycle in 1 sec). The high-volt, pulsed galvanic stimulator was incorrectly named.

In addition to helping you use proper terminology, understanding the various electrical waveforms will help you use TENS in the athletic training room and clinic. Finally, and most importantly, understanding the basics of electricity and the physiological response to TENS will help you understand the differences between stimulators producing different forms of pulsatile currents. The clinical effect and application of electrical stimulation are the focus of chapter 10.

# PARAMETERS OF ELECTRICAL STIMULATION

When electricity is therapeutically applied to the body, certain effects are expected. A thermal effect is created when the frequency of the current is very high (over 100,000 Hz) and is associated with diathermies. A **physiochemical effect** occurs when there is a pH change in the tissues. Galvanic stimulation is required to alter the chemical composition under the electrodes and occurs because of the ionizing effects. And finally, a **physiological effect** occurs when the electrical stimulation causes a **depolarization** of a nerve and an action potential results. The physiological effect is desired with TENS and with neuromuscular electrical stimulation and will be the focus of this chapter. The specific effect is determined by the manipulations of the electrical current, the waveform, and the clinical parameters available on most machines. The parameters of electrical stimulation determine the effect of current on the body.

The characteristics of electrical current that will be considered are the following:

1. Amplitude
2. Phase duration
3. Frequency
4. Rise time (rate of rise of the leading edge of the pulse)
5. Duty cycle

## Amplitude (Intensity)

The amplitude refers to the intensity or magnitude of the current. The **peak current** is the maximum amplitude of the current at any point during the pulse without regard to its duration. The peak current must be high enough to exceed threshold for the nerve or muscle fiber. Generally, large-diameter sensory and motor nerves (A-beta and A-alpha) have low thresholds, and smaller intensities of electrical current are needed to cause an action potential. The A-beta nerves are closer to the skin, so when the intensity on an electrical stimulator is turned up, a sensory response occurs before a motor response. A high peak current causes a greater depth of penetration of the electrical stimulation, which allows more fibers to be recruited. More nerves are stimulated with a higher amplitude, resulting in a stronger sensory or motor response.

Peak current is the measure from the isoelectric line (zero) to the maximum positive or negative point without regard to the time duration that the pulse is maintained (figure 9.5).

**Average current,** however, refers to the amount of current supplied over a period of time, which takes into consideration both the peak amplitude and the phase duration. The average current may be described as the phase charge and is associated with the ability of the stimulator to produce physiochemical effects such as pH changes under each electrode, or the ability to perform denervated nerve stimulation or iontophoresis. These clinical uses require galvanic current that maximizes the phase charge. Depending on the waveform, it is possible to have a high peak but low average current. These features are characteristic of a high-voltage stimulator. The average current can damage tissue, and manufacturers limit the maximum amplitude on galvanic stimulators and minimize the phase duration on high-voltage stimulators for safety reasons. This is further discussed in chapter 10.

Peak current and root-mean-square values are used to describe the intensity of various waveforms. Peak intensity is measured from the isoelectric line to the highest point of the waveform.

**Root mean square (RMS)** is a means of determining phase charge or the effective area contained in the waveform that results in the physiochemical effects. It corresponds to an equivalent amount of direct current in the waveform and requires a complex calculus computation. The term

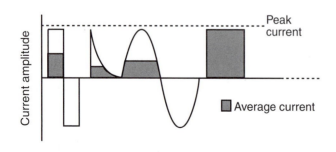

**Figure 9.5**   Peak current and average current.

"average current" is often used to describe the same effect. The RMS measure is preferred over the average current, especially as more complicated waveforms are being used. The RMS is a more accurate measure of the effective current available with a specific waveform.

The RMS of a sinusoidal wave (alternating current) is 0.707 times the peak value. The average current of the same alternating current is 0.639 times the peak value.

## Phase Duration

The duration of the individual phase of a current is the time it takes to leave the isoelectric (zero) line to when it returns to the isoelectric line. If the current is biphasic, then there are two phase durations for each pulse. In monophasic currents, the phase duration and the pulse duration are the same. Tissues respond only to the phase duration, not the pulse duration. Biphasic currents do minimize the net charge by reversing the charge within each waveform (figure 9.6).

The phase duration must be long enough to overcome the capacitance of the targeted nerve to cause an action potential. Each fiber type, depending on its characteristics of size and degree of myelination, has capacitance, that is, the ability to store charge before discharging. Large-diameter nerve fibers have low capacitance. They cannot store the charge, and an action potential results very quickly (within microseconds). Smaller nerve fibers and the muscle membrane itself have more capacitance and store the charge. In these tissues, there is minimal disruption in the membrane with a short phase duration. When the current is applied, if the current does not flow in one direction long enough, there will not be an action potential (figure 9.7).

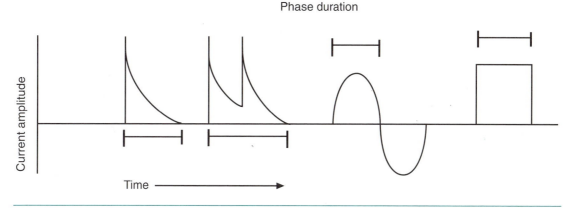

**Figure 9.6**   Phase duration: length of time current flows in one direction before turning to the isoelectric line.

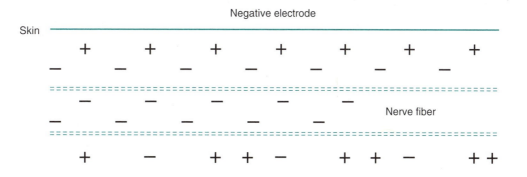

**Figure 9.7**   When the area surrounding a nerve becomes negatively charged by electrical current, the nerve fiber is no longer polarized in relation to the surroundings. When the nerve is depolarized, an impulse travels along the nerve to a synaptic junction.

The strength–duration curve is important for describing the relationship of amplitude (strength) of the electrical current and the duration (phase duration). These two parameters are linked in the phase charge.

Why is phase charge so important? As mentioned previously, nerve fibers act as capacitors and store an electrical charge. If the electrical charge delivered is sufficient to overcome the capacitance of a nerve fiber, it will depolarize (figure 9.7). If the electrical charge does not exceed the capacitance of a nerve fiber, the electrical charge will leak out of the fiber during the interpulse interval and the nerve will not depolarize. Likewise, if the amplitude is not high enough despite the duration, threshold will not be reached. Again, there will not be an action potential.

Figure 9.8 depicts the capacitance of the nerve fiber types introduced in chapter 4. Using a monophasic square wave, figure 9.9 illustrates the concept of phase charge being increased to overcome the capacitance of each nerve fiber. Thus, in TENS application you can select the nerve fiber type or types to be depolarized.

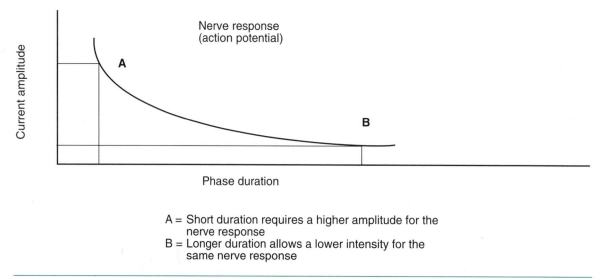

A = Short duration requires a higher amplitude for the nerve response
B = Longer duration allows a lower intensity for the same nerve response

**Figure 9.8**    Strength–duration curve.

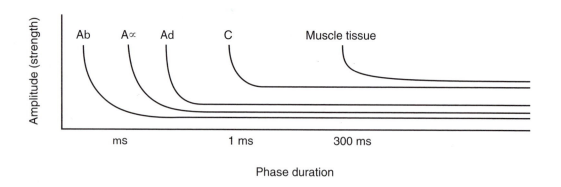

**Figure 9.9**    Strength–duration curves for various tissues. Because of the capacitance of the tissues, sensory nerves are the most easily excitable and can reach an action potential with a short phase duration. C fibers and the muscle membrane are difficult to excite and require much longer phase durations.

If phase charge is so important, why is it not important to know the precise phase charge? If you adjust the phase duration and amplitude of TENS to cause a tingling sensation without muscle twitch, you have adjusted the phase charge to exceed the capacitance of A-alpha and A-beta afferent nerve fibers, but not A-alpha motor nerves. A muscle contraction indicates that the capacitance of the A-alpha motor nerves has also been exceeded. If TENS application results in a burning, needling sensation, you have exceeded the capacitance of A-delta afferents. Thus, by soliciting feedback from the individual and observing for muscle twitch, you can alter phase charge by adjusting amplitude and phase duration (figure 9.10).

Two concepts related to the adjustment of amplitude and phase duration are rheobase and chronaxie (figure 9.11). These terms are used primarily in electrodiagnostic evaluation of nerve regeneration. **Rheobase** is the minimum amplitude needed to depolarize a nerve fiber when the phase duration is infinite (DC current). If the peak amplitude of an electrical current fails to exceed rheobase, the nerve will not depolarize regardless of phase duration.

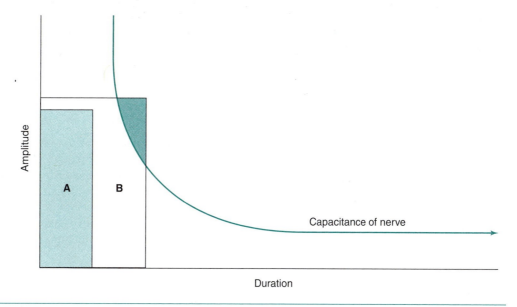

**Figure 9.10**    Capacitance is the ability of a nerve to store an electrical charge. The pulse charge must exceed capacitance to depolarize the nerve. Pulse A lacks sufficient charge to overcome capacitance of the nerve. However, by increasing amplitude and phase duration, you increase phase charge to overcome capacitance and cause depolarization.

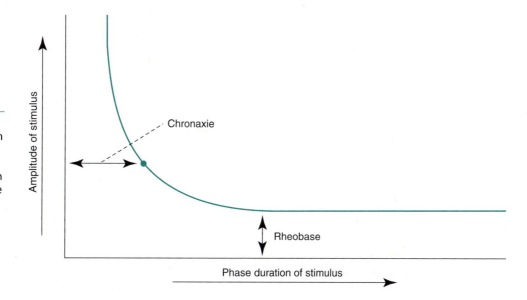

**Figure 9.11**    Rheobase is the minimum amplitude required to depolarize a nerve fiber, given an infinitely long phase duration. Chronaxie is the phase duration required to depolarize a nerve fiber when the amplitude is 2 × rheobase.

**Chronaxie** is the time or phase duration required to depolarize a nerve fiber when the peak current is twice rheobase. Chronaxie is thought to occur at the break in the capacitance curve. Stimulation parameters with an amplitude twice rheobase and a phase duration slightly greater than chronaxie result in greatest comfort for the recipient of TENS. Later this chapter provides guidelines for parameter adjustment to elicit the desired response with the greatest comfort.

---

## Experimental Relationship of Intensity and Phase Duration of Electrical Stimulation

As an exercise, you may experiment with manipulation of the amplitude and duration of the electrical current. Note the minimal intensity needed to elicit a sensory response when the phase duration is preset to 50 microseconds. Increase the phase duration and again note the intensity at a minimal motor response. To achieve the same clinical effect, each of these parameters can be manipulated. However, if the machine does not allow a phase duration of greater than 1 millisecond (ms), it will not be able to depolarize C fibers or the muscle membrane directly. Another type of stimulator is necessary for these uses.

---

## Frequency

The frequency of the stimulation is the number of pulses generated per second (pps or Hz). The frequency affects the number of action potentials elicited during the stimulation. Although the same number of fibers is recruited, a higher frequency causes them to fire at a more rapid pace, which ultimately increases the tension generated. Nerve membranes must repolarize, however, after discharging. There is an absolute refractory period in which the resting membrane potential is reinstated, and another action potential cannot be elicited during this time. The absolute refractory period is the rate-limiting factor of the number of impulses that can be generated by a nerve.

The classical delineations of current frequencies in the electromagnetic spectrum are low, medium, and high:

- Low frequency is 1,000 Hz (cycles per second) and below.
- Medium frequency is 1,000 to 100,000 Hz.
- High frequency is greater than 100,000 Hz.

Typically low-frequency stimulators are used to produce the physiologic effect of action potential generation. When the frequency is raised beyond this range, the stimulation encroaches on the refractory period of the sensory nerve and actually causes inhibition by bombarding the membrane with continual stimulation. This is called **Wedenski's inhibition,** or action potential failure and clinically it can result in anesthesia between the electrodes.

Some confusion occurs with the terminology for the categories of stimulators when referring to frequency. The TENS applications refer to treatment frequencies as high (60-100 pps) and low (1-10 pps), but these stimulators may fall into the low and medium frequency stimulator (generator) categories.

Medium-frequency generators are used as TENS devices as well, but their current is modulated to produce a resultant burst rate that the individual nerve fibers are able to respond to. For example, interferential current typically uses carrier frequencies of 4,000 to 5,000 Hz. However, two slightly different medium-frequency currents are crossed, or interfered, to create a net "beat" frequency. More about interferential therapy is discussed in chapter 10. Another example of manipulation of a medium-frequency current is with Russian stimulation. The carrier current of Russian stimulation is 2,500 Hz, and there is an intrinsic duty cycle of 10 ms on and 10 ms off. The result is "bursts" of stimulation at a rate of 50 per second.

High-frequency generators are used for thermal purposes and to elicit an electromagnetic field. High-frequency current is used with diathermies and has minimal sensory effects.

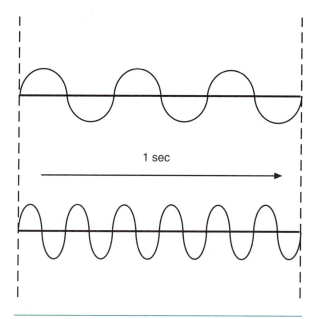

**Figure 9.12** Alternating current has an inverse relationship of pulse duration and frequency. When the frequency is known (4,000 Hz or 5,000 Hz, for example), the pulse duration can be calculated: 1 sec / 4,000 Hz = 0.00025 sec (250 μs) and 1 sec / 5,000 Hz = 0.0002 sec (200 μs). Since the *pulse* duration is for both phases, the *phase* duration is half of the pulse duration. For example, 250-μs pulse duration = 125-μs phase duration.

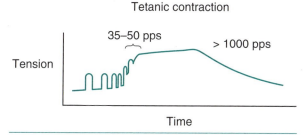

**Figure 9.13** Temporal summation occurs when the frequency of stimulation increases and the sensory nerve and muscle contraction cannot differentiate each individual stimulation. The impulses add together.

The frequency or pulse rate can be varied depending on the purpose of the application of the stimulation. When an AC current is used, there is an inverse relationship between the frequency and the wavelength (phase duration), and either can be calculated when one is known. With pulsatile currents, the interpulse interval allows independent control of phase duration and pulse rate, so the potential variations are broader.

If the frequency does not affect the phase charge, then why is there a stronger sensation of stimulation when the pulse rate increases? Increasing the pulse rate adds more waveforms and ultimately more total charge within a given amount of time (1 sec), but the charge in each pulse is unaffected (figure 9.12).

When the pulse rate is increased with TENS, the higher frequencies cause the nerve fibers recruited to fire more rapidly, allowing summation of the stimulation to occur. The body cannot differentiate when one pulse ends and another begins, and a continuous sensory effect is noted when the pulse rate exceeds 20 pps (figure 9.13). When the frequency is increased, a **tetanic muscle contraction** may result. This usually occurs with a frequency of 35 to 50 Hz. Below this frequency, a twitch response occurs.

## Rate of Rise of the Leading Edge of the Pulse

The rate of rise of the leading edge of the pulse, also known as rise time, is a parameter that is incorporated into a waveform, but it will also affect the type of nerve targeted. The rate of rise refers to the time it takes to get from zero to maximal amplitude within each pulse. Fast rates of rise times are necessary especially with low-capacitance tissues such as large motor nerves. The low-capacitance membrane cannot store much charge and quickly accommodates to a stimulus. These nerves can dissipate the charge from a pulse with slow rates of rise times, and the ion flux needed to alter the voltage to exceed threshold is never reached. Sensory nerves that carry light touch, for example, have low capacitance and easily accommodate. This explains how a person is aware of clothing when it is first put on but then stops paying attention to the sensation

## Clinical Applications of Various Stimulation Frequencies

1. Pain modulation techniques use different frequencies to elicit their desired response.
   - Motor TENS uses frequencies of 2 to 10 Hz to elicit the neurohormonal response.
   - Sensory TENS uses frequencies from 60 to 120 Hz to elicit the enkephalinergic and gating effects.
2. Neuromuscular stimulation for passive exercise uses modulated frequencies of 35 to 50 Hz that create a tetanic contraction.
3. To increase blood flow or lymphatic drainage, a pulsing effect may be desired. A pulse rate of less than 10 pps causes twitching.

(Phase charge determines which nerve fiber will depolarize during stimulation, and frequency determines how often the nerve fibers will depolarize.)

at the skin; **accommodation** to this minimal stimulus has occurred. Generally, tissues with low capacitance accommodate to a stimulus easily whereas high-capacitance tissues, because they store the charge, do not accommodate or dissipate the charge readily.

When you are determining whether there will be a physiological response within the tissues, the law of Dubois Reymond describes three important factors within each pulse of an electrical current that you must consider. First, the stimulus must be of adequate amplitude to reach the threshold level of excitatory tissues. Second, the rate of voltage change (rate of rise of the leading edge of the pulse) must be rapid enough that tissue accommodation cannot take place. Third, the length of stimulus or phase duration must be great enough to overcome the capacitance of the tissue to allow an action potential.

## Law of Dubois Reymond

The effectiveness of a current to target specific excitable tissues is dependent on three major factors:

1. Adequate intensity to reach threshold
2. Current onset fast enough to reduce accommodation
3. Duration long enough to exceed the capacitance of the tissue

The rate of rise of the leading edge of the pulse is the preferred term to describe the onset of the stimulation, since "rise time" is often confused with "ramp." Ramp time has to do with a gradual increase in the amplitude of subsequent pulses so that the intensity does not come on abruptly when a duty cycle is used (figure 9.14).

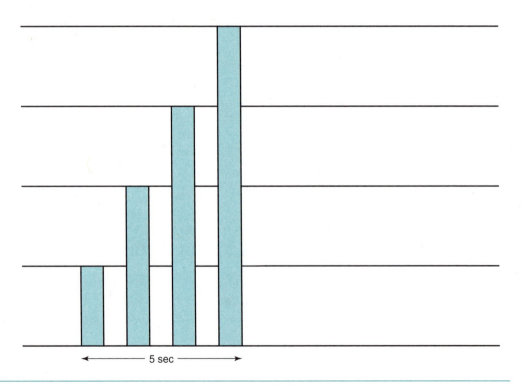

**Figure 9.14**   Ramping is a programmed increase in amplitude over several pulses (1-5 sec).

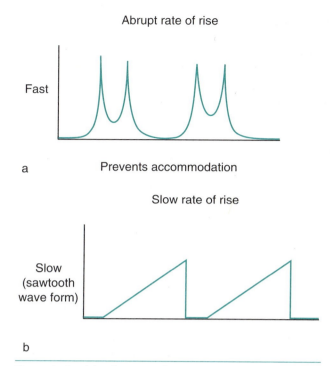

Abrupt rate of rise

Fast

Prevents accommodation

a

Slow rate of rise

Slow
(sawtooth
wave form)

b

**Figure 9.15** *(a)* A fast rate of rise of the leading edge of the pulse minimizes the chance of exciting high-capacitance fibers. *(b)* A long rate of rise causes less stimulation of high-accommodation fibers while stimulating high-capacitance fibers.

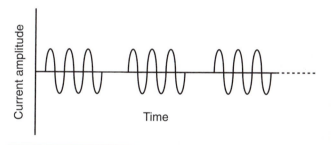

**Figure 9.16** Time-modulated AC. An inherent duty cycle is imposed to create "bursts" of electricity. Each burst has a carrier frequency that is determined by the machine, and there are several bursts in 1 sec. This example shows 3 bursts per sec.

Waveforms with an immediate onset of the pulse or fast rate of rise of the leading edge of the pulse (figure 9.15a) are used when the goal of stimulation is to excite the sensory nerve fibers. A long onset, such as with a sawtooth waveform (figure 9.15b), is used when sensory excitation is undesirable but a long phase duration is required to stimulate the muscle membrane directly. This treatment is used, for example, when a motor nerve has lost innervation but there is good sensation over the area, a common occurrence with Bell's palsy. A long phase duration is required to stimulate the denervated muscle, but the stimulation is noxious. A slow onset helps to minimize sensory excitation.

## Duty Cycle

The final parameter of electrical stimulation to discuss is the duty cycle. **Duty cycles** are imposed by the clinician to interrupt the current periodically for several seconds. This "on–off" timing creates a rest time that is variable on most units. Another form of duty cycles occurs when pulses are packaged into small clusters. These duty cycles interrupt the current at specific intervals so that the manufacturer can produce "time-modulated AC" currents, otherwise known as "burst mode." The carrier frequency is usually AC and is interrupted at regular intervals, often in the millisecond range. Interruptions are generally imperceptible, but they enable the clinician to take advantage of the characteristics of the carrier frequency, such as deeper penetration or greater total current. The classical Russian stimulators utilize this method to modulate medium-frequency sinusoidal waves into bursts of 10 ms on and 10 ms off. Clinical use of Russian stimulation is discussed in chapter 10. The duty cycle reduces the high total current of the medium frequency generators by introducing an "off" time in the current delivery, making this a safer modality (figure 9.16). The duty cycle also modulates the net frequency of medium frequency generates to physiologically active frequencies (e.g., 2500 Hz carrier frequency to 100 burst frequency).

Duty cycle can also be adjusted by the clinician to impose a "rest" period. This is often done when applying TENS to stimulate alpha motor neurons to cause muscle contraction. The duty cycle refers to the pattern of on–off sequencing. For example, you may want to stimulate the quadriceps muscles following knee injury or surgery because the individual has lost volitional control due to pain and swelling. The stimulation must be patterned to allow the muscles to recover between contractions. You might select a 12-sec "on" time during which the quadriceps contract and a 12-sec rest between contractions. The duty cycle would then be 12 sec on and 12 sec off or 1:1. When maximal contractions are attempted with electrical stimulation, a 1:5 duty cycle is recommended to prevent fatigue.

# ELECTRODE CONSIDERATIONS

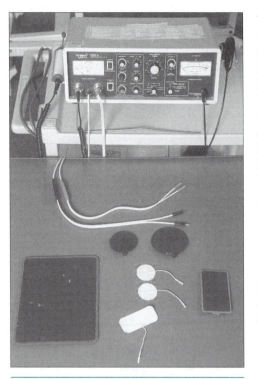

**Figure 9.17**   Small and large electrodes.

To complete a circuit in electrical stimulation, at least one electrode from each output lead must be in contact with the athlete's skin. There will always be resistance to the current from the air–skin interface; and to increase efficiency and consistency of the treatment, the clinician should minimize the resistance.

There are many types of electrodes available for electrical stimulation. Portable TENS units often have "single-use" or disposable electrodes that are self-adhesive. These electrodes are convenient, minimize the irritation of the skin that often occurs with tape adherents, and make the application simple. The electrodes may be remoistened with water when moved to a new location. The expense of these electrodes may prohibit their use when volume is heavy.

Most electrodes for commercial or clinical use are either metal backed or carbon rubber. Various sizes of electrodes are illustrated in figure 9.17. These require an interface such as moistened sponges or gauze. Gel may be used with the carbon rubber electrodes; however, this may reduce the longevity of the electrodes if they are not cleaned properly. Sponges are the most convenient, but gauze is more sanitary. The interface should be thoroughly wet, with no dry spots, but not dripping.

## Minimizing Electrode Resistance

- Use large electrodes.
- Maintain even, firm contact with skin.
- Use clean electrodes and sponges.
- Keep the sponge interface well moistened.
- Remove excess hair and oil from skin.

The electrodes should be firmly attached to the athlete using elastic straps. Weights may be used to secure the electrodes to the low back; however, the current density will change drastically if the electrodes move or become displaced during the treatment. This may cause discomfort to the athlete. The intensity should be adjusted after the electrodes have been secured, since any adjustment in the air–skin interface will affect the resistance and can potentially increase the current or amplitude dramatically. Electrodes should be flexible to conform to body parts such as the ankle or knee.

Any lead can be **bifurcated,** or divided. It is imperative that each lead be used, since a common mistake in applying electrical stimulation is to use one bifurcated lead (two electrodes), which does not complete the circuit and therefore delivers no stimulation. Whenever bifurcated leads are used, current density becomes an issue. Each lead may be bifurcated as many times as needed (figure 9.18).

Current density depends on the size of the electrodes and the distance they are apart. There is an equal amount of current in each of the two essential leads. When unequal-sized electrodes are used, the current is more concentrated in the smaller electrode (figure 9.19). This causes a perception of increased intensity under the smaller electrode. When electrodes are very

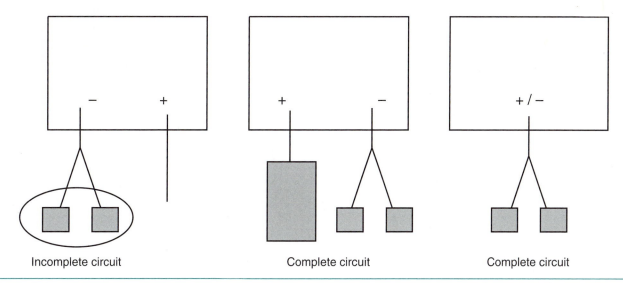

Incomplete circuit                    Complete circuit                    Complete circuit

**Figure 9.18** Monophasic versus biphasic stimulators. Make sure that there are at least two leads to complete the circuit to allow stimulation. The electrode configuration on the left does not complete the circuit.

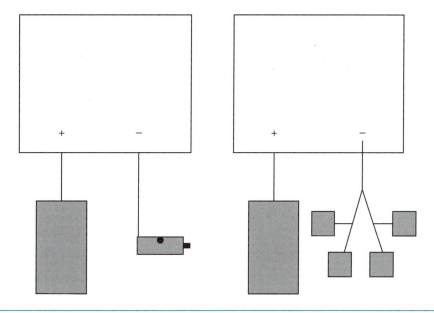

**Figure 9.19** Current density concentrates current in the lead that has the smallest total surface area.

different in size, such as with a point stimulator, the patient may not be able to perceive current in the larger electrode. The larger electrode becomes the dispersive electrode since the current is dispersed over a broad area. When bifurcating leads, it is important to determine the total size of all electrodes that arise from each lead and to compare that total electrode surface area to the opposite lead surface area to determine if current density differences are present.

Current density can also refer to the concentration of current within the tissues. Current always flows in the path of least resistance. If the electrodes are placed very close together, the current is most dense or concentrated in the superficial tissues. If the electrodes are distant to each other, then the current has the potential to take a deeper path through the nerve and blood vessels that have less resistance (figure 9.20).

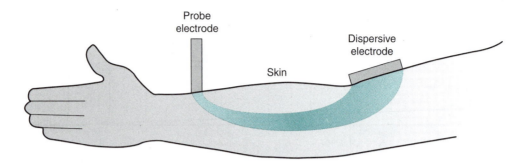

**Figure 9.20**   The small surface area of the probe electrode creates an area of high current density, resulting in perception of an intense electrical stimulus. The relatively large surface area of the dispersive electrode results in low current density and an excellent dispersion of the electrical stimulus.

## Active and Dispersive Leads

All stimulators utilize either a monophasic or a biphasic current. By examining the stimulator, the clinician can determine the polarity. If the stimulator has a polarity switch, then the stimulator is monophasic and the toggle will determine the polarity of the *active* lead. The active lead is demarcated on the unit as well. Additionally, most monophasic machines have leads that arise from different locations on the stimulator, whereas most biphasic units have the two essential leads arising from the same location or socket from the stimulator. In a biphasic machine, there is no physiological difference between the electrodes, and therefore it is not necessary to distinguish the leads (figure 9.21).

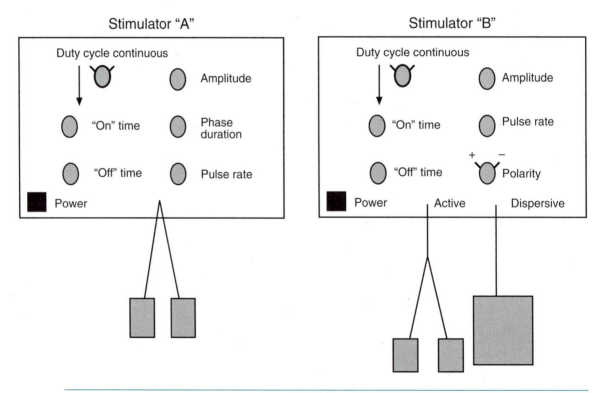

**Figure 9.21**   Determine the polarity of these stimulators. Stimulator A has no polarity switch and both leads arise from the same location. Stimulator B has a polarity switch and each lead is distinct.

The dispersive electrode is necessary to complete the circuit, but is not relevant to the particular treatment. For example, it is not important to have sensory perception under the dispersive electrode, but electrical stimulation cannot be delivered without this pad in place.

## Electrode Configurations

There are two general types of electrode configurations: monopolar and bipolar. Either type may be used with monophasic or biphasic currents. Quadripolar electrode configurations are often used with interferential current.

### *Monopolar Electrode Configuration*

With a monopolar electrode configuration, two or more unequal-sized electrodes are used. One lead is designated as "active" and the other is designated as "dispersive." The leads are placed at different locations, with the active lead at target site and the dispersive placed away from the treatment site (figure 9.22). There are three primary reasons for using a monopolar electrode configuration. One is to place the electrodes farther apart so that penetration is deeper. As an example, with underwater stimulation there is less resistance in the water, so the current would preferentially go through the water instead of through the skin. When a monopolar configuration is used, the current has to travel through the body in order to reach the other electrode that is at a site distant to the treatment location. The second reason for using a monopolar electrode configuration is with a point stimulator. The small electrode with a high current density is desired at the treatment site, but it is more comfortable to use a larger electrode to complete the circuit. Often the patient does not perceive current under the larger electrode. Finally, a monopolar electrode configuration is required when a polarity effect is desired. A monophasic current must be used to differentiate the polarity at the treatment site from the other lead. The polarity is indicated by the "active" lead. Examples of this method are iontophoresis or in situations in which when one is creating an electrical field of a particular polarity, such as with wound healing.

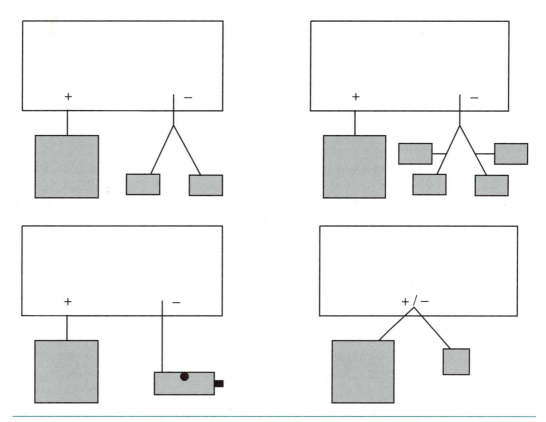

**Figure 9.22**  Monopolar electrode configuration. Note that either a monophasic or biphasic machine can be used. Each example uses different-sized electrodes.

## Bipolar Electrode Configuration

Bipolar electrode configurations can also be used with either monophasic or biphasic currents. In this case, equal-sized electrodes are used, with both placed over the treatment site (figure 9.23). This setup is the most commonly used method in TENS.

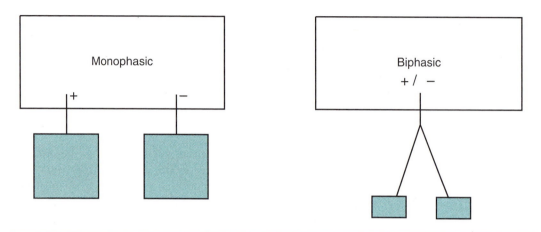

**Figure 9.23**    Bipolar electrode configuration. Similar-sized electrodes are used with either a monophasic or a biphasic machine.

## Quadripolar Electrode Configuration

The quadripolar electrode configuration is often used with interferential current. Two completely separate medium-frequency generators are used, and the electrodes are placed to cross the currents. Ideally, the current is *interfered* in the center of the two currents; however, since the body is not homogeneous, the current may vary. Many interferential stimulators have an adjustment that allows variation in the amplitude of one of the currents so that the location of the perceived current can be adjusted. Interferential current can also be placed on a flat surface such as the low back. The quadripolar arrangement implies a three-dimensional configuration of current; however, because the channels are not placed surrounding the tissues in this example, the current is aligned according to the alignment of the channels. Each channel has a red and a black lead. The concentration of the electrical field generated is in alignment with the same-color lead (figure 9.24).

Quadripolar electrode configuration is not the same as using two channels of TENS with four electrodes. Using two channels with TENS increases the number of stimulation points, which may be advantageous when one is treating a large surface area; however, the currents do not cross and cause interference.

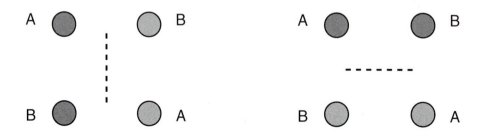

**Figure 9.24**    Quadripolar electrode configuration used with interferential current. The current is aligned so that it is concentrated between the electrodes to localize the stimulation depending on the pathology. A and B are the two channels.

# SUMMARY

1. Define volt, ampere, impedance, and resistance.

   Voltage is a measure of potential difference or electromotive force. One volt is required for 1 A of current to pass through 1 ohm of resistance. Electrical current, measured in amperes, is the flow of electrons. One ampere equals the flow of 1 C ($6.25 \times 10^{18}$ electrons) per second. Resistance, measured in ohms, is the opposition to the flow of electrical current through a material.

2. Describe the differences between alternating, direct, and pulsatile currents.

   There are two classifications of continuous currents: alternating (AC) and direct (DC). TENS units deliver electrical currents that are noncontinuous or pulsed. Pulsatile currents are classified as monophasic or biphasic.

3. Define parameters of pulsatile current including phase duration, amplitude, phase charge, and frequency.

   Pulsatile currents are characterized by pulses of electrical current interrupted by interpulse intervals. Phase duration refers to the length of time required to complete each phase of the waveform. Amplitude is the current or voltage (voltage equals the current if resistance is unchanged) in the electrical circuit. Phase charge, the number of electrons moved during each phase of an electrical pulse, is the primary determinant of which nerve fibers will be depolarized during TENS. Frequency is the number of pulses delivered per second.

4. Describe the capacitance of nerve and muscle tissue and how it affects the strength–duration curve.

   Excitable tissue has a resting membrane potential and can carry an action potential. When electrical stimulation is applied, an action potential can be elicited in these types of tissues. Each tissue type has capacitance, which is the ability to store charge. If the capacitance is high, the electrical stimulation must have a higher phase charge to elicit an action potential. Means of increasing phase charge are to increase either the phase duration or the amplitude of the stimulation or both. Thus the strength or intensity of the stimulation and the phase duration are related to create phase charge. The minimal amount of intensity or phase duration required to elicit a response depends on the capacitance of the targeted tissue.

5. Understand the law of Dubois Reymond with respect to the application of electrical current.

   To create an action potential with electrical stimulation, three factors in the waveform are necessary. The intensity has to be greater than the threshold of the tissue; the phase duration must be long enough to overcome the capacitance of the tissue; and the rate of rise of the leading edge of the pulse has to be fast enough to prevent accommodation.

6. Describe the types of electrode configurations used with electrical stimulation application.

   Electrodes can be placed in a variety of configurations depending on the goal of the treatment. A monopolar electrode configuration uses two unequal-sized electrodes with the smaller, active electrode over the treatment site and the larger, dispersive electrode over a distant site. The electrode configuration is bipolar when two equal-sized electrodes are placed over the treatment site.

# CITED SOURCE

Kahn J: *Principles and Practices of Electrotherapy.* New York, Churchill Livingstone, 1987.

## ADDITIONAL READINGS

Alon G: *High Voltage—a Monograph.* Chattanooga Corp., 1984.

Alon G: Principles of electrical stimulation. In Nelson DP, Currier RM (Eds), *Clinical Electrotherapy.* Norwalk, CT, Appleton & Lange, 1991, 1-10.

Griffin JE, Karselis TC: *Physical Agents for Physical Therapists.* Springfield, IL, Charles C Thomas, 1982.

Guyton AC: *Medical Physiology.* Philadelphia, Saunders, 1981, 41-54.

Kloth L: Electrotherapeutic alternatives for the treatment of pain. In Gersh MR (Ed), *Electrotherapy in Rehabilitation.* Philadelphia, Davis, 1992.

Kukulka CG: Principles of neuromuscular excitation. In Gersh MR (Ed), *Electrotherapy in Rehabilitation.* Philadelphia, Davis, 1992.

Newton RA: *Electrotherapeutic Treatment: Selecting Appropriate Waveform Characteristics.* JA Preston Corp., 1984.

Robinson AJ: Basic concepts and terminology in electricity. In Snyder-Mackler L, Robinson AJ (Eds), *Clinical Electrophysiology.* Baltimore, Williams & Wilkins, 1989, 1-20.

Robinson AJ: Physiology of muscle and nerve. In Snyder-Mackler L, Robinson AJ (Eds), *Clinical Electrophysiology.* Baltimore, Williams & Wilkins, 1989, 59-94.

Urbscheit NL: Review of physiology. In Nelson DP, Currier RM (Eds), *Clinical Electrotherapy.* Norwalk, CT, Appleton & Lange, 1991, 1-10.

# CHAPTER 10

# Clinical Uses of Electrical Stimulation

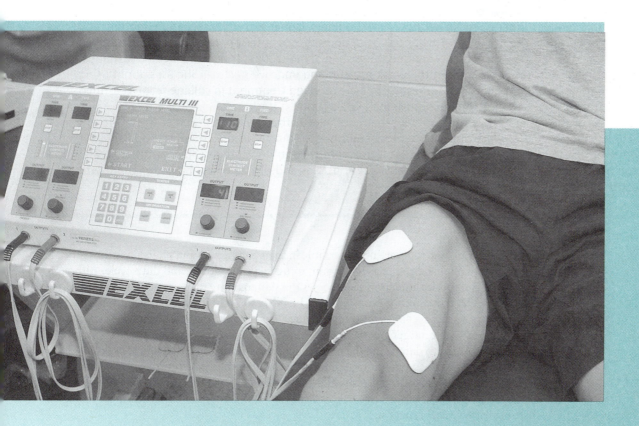

## *Objectives*

After reading this chapter, the student will be able to

1. understand the clinical uses for electrical stimulation in the rehabilitation process;

2. analyze the waveform of the available device and determine whether the treatment goal can be met using that stimulator;

3. incorporate pain modulation theories with the electrical stimulation principles to determine the amplitude, phase duration, and pulse frequency necessary for a variety of clinical purposes;

4. describe the use of neuromuscular electrical stimulation, including Russian stimulation, for muscle reeducation;

5. describe the uses of a galvanic stimulator;

6. understand the use of microcurrent electrical stimulation; and

7. identify contraindications for the application of electrotherapy.

A 30-year-old triathlete is referred to a sports medicine clinic for treatment of myofascial pain syndrome in the neck and shoulders. She has had recurring trouble with her neck and shoulder, mostly associated with prolonged training on her bicycle. Her pain became acutely worse 6 weeks after an accident in which the car she was driving was rear-ended. Her primary complaints are increased pain radiating into the right arm with cycling and with working at her desk for prolonged periods (she is a practicing corporate lawyer). She also reports occasional headaches associated with her neck and shoulder pain, which have become more frequent. X-rays were taken of her neck recently, and the orthopedic surgeon who referred her was unable to identify a structural cause for her pain. Examination reveals a fit, physically active woman with a forward-head, protracted-shoulder posture. There are multiple tender trigger points in her neck and shoulders. Upper extremity sensation, motion, and strength are normal. The middle and lower trapezius and serratus anterior are weaker than expected for her fitness level. A treatment plan is designed consisting of modalities for pain management, manual therapies, and exercises to strengthen the weak muscles and improve posture. She asks about using electrical stimulation for pain control and says that she received treatment in college from a certified athletic trainer for a back and hip injury sustained while running track.

Because of the patient's previous positive experience, electrotherapy is identified as the treatment of choice. Which type of electrotherapy is most appropriate to achieve the treatment goals? What are the optimal parameters of treatment? Is electrotherapy contraindicated? This chapter addresses these types of questions and provides the physical principles and physiological bases for the use of electrotherapy in sport rehabilitation.

Electrical stimulation units are often versatile in their parameters and often allow the clinician freedom to manipulate the phase duration, frequency, amplitude, and duty cycle. Although any type of electrical stimulation that crosses the skin to excite the nerve is considered **transcutaneous electrical nerve stimulation (TENS),** some units are marketed for a specific clinical purpose such as "muscle strengthening." A savvy clinician, knowing the capacitance and ability to excite target fibers, should be able to critically analyze the waveform and parameters offered to determine the cost benefit of a stimulator. The clinical uses of electrical stimulation are for pain, muscle stimulation through the alpha motor nerve, stimulation of denervated muscle, iontophoresis, and some subtle effects such as edema reduction and wound healing. For the purposes of this text, the stimulators are categorized according to their primary clinical function.

The athletic trainer should *not* use electrical stimulation if there are known myocardial problems or arrhythmias. TENS should not be used if there is a pacemaker or if pregnancy is suspected. Electrical stimulation should not be delivered through the chest or over the carotid sinus. Stimulation in the anterior neck elicits activity in the carotid sinus or may cause a contraction of the pharyngeal muscles. This can affect the blood pressure and pulse.

## PAIN RELIEF: TRANSCUTANEOUS ELECTRICAL NERVE STIMULATION

Electrical stimulation for pain modulation is the primary reason for TENS. The student should review the pain modulation theories presented in chapter 4, since the techniques described in this section will follow the guidelines associated with those theories. Specifically, the sensory, noxious, and motor pain modulation theories should be reviewed. Understanding how TENS relieves pain requires integration of the pain control models, as well as the concept of nerve fiber capacitance presented in chapter 9. Examples of TENS units include biphasic low-voltage stimulators, portable TENS units, interferential units, and high-voltage stimulators.

One can achieve variations of TENS by adjusting the current parameters (figure 10.1). The proposed mechanisms of pain modulation appropriate for each type of electrical stimulation are discussed in this chapter. Because therapy with electrical stimulation treats the symptoms of an ailment and generally not the cause, proper evaluation of the etiology of the injury and rectification of the cause are important. Ideally, the pain modulation allows the athlete to perform therapeutic exercise, which will contribute to the alleviation of the problem.

| Goal: TENS pain control | Phase duration | Amplitude | Pulse Frequency | Target nerve fiber |
|---|---|---|---|---|
| Sensory | <150 μs | Submotor | 60-120 pps | A-beta |
| Motor | 200-300 μs | Strong motor | <10 pps | A-delta |
| Noxious | >300 ms | Painful | High or low | C fiber |
| Neuromuscular stimulation | 250 μs | Motor | 50 pps | A-alpha |
| Iontophoresis | n/a (DC) | ≤5 mamp | n/a (DC) | n/a |
| Stimulation of denervated muscle | n/a (DC) | ≤5 mamp | n/a (DC) | Muscle membrane |
| Microcurrent | Variable | Subsensory | Variable | Sympathetic fibers |

**Figure 10.1** Examples of parameters used in the clinical application of electrical stimulation. The clinician can use a variety of machines to deliver the correct parameters.

## The Efficacy of TENS in the Reduction of Pain

Evidence-based research is inconclusive regarding whether TENS reduces pain with a variety of stimulation parameters. Several studies demonstrated that TENS was effective compared to sham treatment in relieving pain (Abelson 1983; Hseuh 1997; Kumar 1997; Moystad 1990; Smith 1983; Thorsteinsson 1977; Vinterberg 1978; Moore and Shurman 1997; Taylor, Hallet, and Flaherty 1981; Jensen 1991). Other investigators found no analgesic effect with TENS (Grimmer 1992; Lewis 1994; Moystad 1990). Databases have been created to identify randomized clinical trials to evaluate the use of TENS for both chronic pain and osteoarthritis. Most studies were eliminated from the evidence-based database because of poorly controlled or confounding variables.

Considerable variation in the site of stimulation and electrode placement was reported across the different studies. Some investigators reported that the electrodes were placed directly over the site of pain (Abelson 1983; Hsueh 1997; Mannheimer 1979; Taylor 1981; Vinterberg 1978). Others stimulated traditional acupuncture points (Ballegaard 1985; Grimmer 1992; Jensen 1991; Kumar 1997; Lewis 1984, 1994). Two reports did not specify the site of electrode placement in the study (Moore 1997; Nash 1990). Other investigators (Moystad 1990a, 1990b; Smith 1983; Thorsteinsson 1978) applied TENS stimulation to acupuncture points and trigger points directly involved in the area of pain.

Considering the money that is spent on the treatment of pain, there is a significant need to further study the analgesic effects of TENS. Large, multisite randomized clinical trials are necessary to evaluate the efficacy of TENS treatments and to validate clinical practice. Transcutaneous electrical nerve stimulation is theorized to improve function through the central nervous system and peripheral mechanisms. These factors, in addition to the acute nature of most athletic injuries that have been shown to respond more favorably to TENS, indicate that electrical stimulation is a viable treatment option. These hypothesized mechanisms and applications are addressed here.

# Mechanisms of Pain Modulation

The mechanisms of pain modulation for electrical stimulation parallel the pain modulation theories discussed in chapter 4.

## *Sensory TENS*

Sensory TENS is also called high-rate TENS and can be used for any painful condition, most commonly in the acute phase or postoperatively. The large-diameter, A-beta fibers are targeted with this treatment. The submotor stimulation is comfortable, providing excitation of large afferent (sensory) nerves. Pain reduction is attributed to the spinal gate mechanism. When the parameters of the stimulation are adjusted to target the large-diameter A-beta afferent nerve fibers, the release of enkephalins into the dorsal horn is triggered. Depolarization results in a tingling sensation. Avoiding muscle contraction is desirable because of the discomfort associated with prolonged muscle twitch and the potential for muscle contractions to stress damaged tissue and slow repair.

The pain relief generally lasts only as long as the stimulation. Any machine that allows stimulation of large-diameter sensory nerves can be used for this treatment. Sensory TENS is commonly used to reduce pain following an injury or after surgery in combination with ice, elevation, and compression.

To apply sensory TENS, the following parameters should be available on the unit: phase duration, pulse rate, and amplitude. The target nerve fiber is A-beta (sensory), which has a low capacitance and therefore does not require a very long phase duration. The phase duration should be low and generally is less than 100 μs. Longer phase durations increase the possibility of stimulating pain fibers, which should be avoided in sensory TENS. The pulse rate should be set high and generally is 60 to 120 pulses per second (pps). The pulse rate should be high enough so that the athlete cannot differentiate the individual pulses. The amplitude should create a strong sensory perception, but remain submotor. If the muscles begin to contract, lower the amplitude. There should not be a duty cycle with this type of treatment, and the stimulator should be set in the continuous mode.

The treatment time can theoretically last up to 24 h. However, the athlete can be instructed to use the device for intermittent 20- to 30-min treatments to see whether the pain is diminishing. If pain is not reduced, then electrode placement should be adjusted. The clinician should emphasize that TENS treatments do not replace rehabilitation progression. In the athletic training room, treatments generally are used in combination with ice or heat to reduce pain or spasm (figure 10.2). The treatment time for the TENS is consistent with the recommended time for thermotherapy, which ranges from 10 to 45 min depending on the depth of the target structure for the heat or cold therapy.

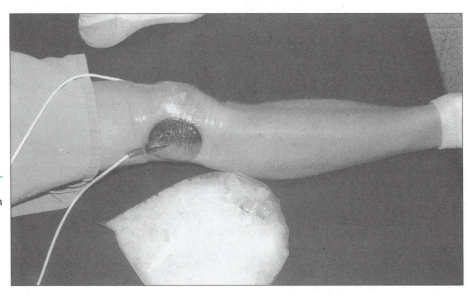

**Figure 10.2** Sensory transcutaneous electrical nerve stimulation is often used with ice as a pain management technique with acute injuries. So that effective cooling may take place, make sure the electrodes do not insulate the area.

Many TENS units allow the clinician to use a "modulation" mode to decrease accommodation to the stimulation. This is most often used with sensory TENS, since the large-diameter nerve fibers that are targeted with this type of stimulation accommodate quickly. Some manufacturers modulate the amplitude, the pulse rate, or the phase duration, usually by varying the parameter by 20% above and below the preset value. Different parameters may be modulated depending on the device (see figure 10.3). Some TENS units allow modulation of amplitude, phase duration, or pulse rate or "multimodulation," such that two or more parameters are modulated.

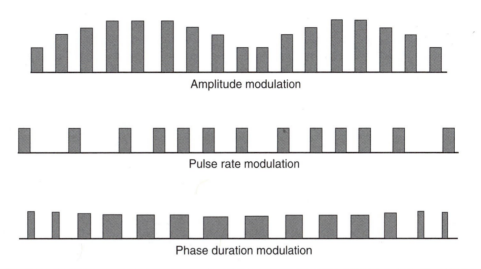

Amplitude modulation

Pulse rate modulation

Phase duration modulation

**Figure 10.3**  Modulation mode. Examples of modulation of the waveform include amplitude modulation, pulse rate modulation, and phase duration modulation. Modulation of the waveform helps to reduce accommodation.

## Motor TENS

Motor TENS may also be referred to as low-rate TENS and has been equated with acupuncture in its mechanism of pain relief. This mode of TENS incorporates the motor pain modulation theory. Motor TENS is more vigorous than sensory TENS and is used to treat subacute pain or trigger points. Motor TENS should not be used on acute injuries; in this situation, vigorous contractions may increase discomfort or cause bleeding.

Motor stimulation is theorized to release endogenous opiates from a descending inhibition of pain and may provide relief for a longer duration, lasting from 1 to 3 h after a 30-min treatment. Pain relief may be delayed compared to that with sensory TENS, but lasts longer, sometimes as long as 4 h.

To apply motor TENS, set the phase duration, pulse rate, and amplitude to the following specifications. The phase duration should be high, in a range of 200 to 300 μ, to target the A-delta (fast pain) nerve fiber. Because the motor nerve fibers are deep, elicitation of the A-delta fibers corresponds to a visible muscle contraction. The pulse rate should be low, with distinct, separate pulses in the range of 2 to 4 pps. The amplitude should cause the elicitation of strong, visible contractions but should not cause pain. A strong, tolerable muscle contraction indicates the stimulation of A-delta fibers. Treatment time generally lasts 20 to 30 min, although the pain relief may not occur for 30 to 120 min. A duty cycle is not necessary for motor TENS, and the continuous mode should be selected.

It is sometimes recommended that treatment be initiated with the sensory TENS technique to obtain the rapid onset of pain relief. As the pain subsides, the parameters can be adjusted to deliver motor TENS for prolonged pain relief. Again, this should be done only when the muscle contractions do not perpetuate the inflammatory response.

### Noxious TENS

A noxious stimulus is applied to elicit pain relief through the central biasing mechanism. This mode of TENS is commonly used with point stimulators because the amplitude should be the maximum tolerable level to trigger descending serotonergic tracts to inhibit pain. The small diameter of the probe creates a high current density to the target area without subjecting a broad area to the noxious stimulus. Units may incorporate an ohm meter to identify points of lower skin resistance that correlate highly with trigger and acupuncture points. Body charts may help locate appropriate points for optimal pain relief.

The key to appropriate noxious TENS is to use a machine that allows the stimulation of C fibers. Very few machines allow a phase duration long enough to elicit a response of C fibers, since long phase durations have the potential to apply a great deal of current. The Neuroprobe or a galvanic stimulator can be used (figure 10.4). The recommended phase duration is between 10 to 20 ms. This is in contrast to what is possible with most TENS units, which have a maximum of 250 $\mu$s (milli- = $10^{-3}$; micro- = $10^{-6}$).

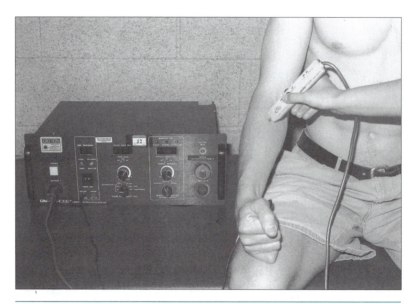

**Figure 10.4** Neuroprobe point stimulation. A monopolar electrode configuration is used with the active electrode in the remote and the dispersive electrode in the athlete's hand.

To apply noxious TENS, the parameters should be set to the following specifications. Again, the ability to stimulate C fibers may be prohibited in many stimulators to protect the athlete. The phase duration must be longer than 1 ms, 10-20 is recommended, and the amplitude should be as high as tolerable. The pulse rate may vary, but the clinician should choose either a high frequency or a low frequency. The high-frequency 100 to 150 pps prevents the discrimination of individual pulses and is classically used in noxious TENS. A low frequency of 2 to 7 pps, however, will elicit the benefits of motor TENS in conjunction with noxious TENS. If the stimulator parameters are capable of overcoming the capacitance of C fibers, then the A-delta fibers will be stimulated as well, providing an added benefit. Each point should be stimulated for 30 sec, and generally 8 to 10 points are treated in a session.

Do not expect good results for TENS treatments if the athlete is taking narcotic analgesics. The electrical stimulation produces natural opioids that compete for the receptor sites occupied by the medication.

The pain modulation parameters are summarized in table 10.1.

**Table 10.1  Transcutaneous Electrical Nerve Stimulation Parameters**

| Type of TENS | Phase duration | Pulse frequency | Amplitude | Target nerve fiber |
|---|---|---|---|---|
| Sensory | <100 μs | 60-120 pps | Sensory, submotor | A-beta |
| Motor | 200-300 μs | 2-4 pps | Strong muscle contraction | A-delta |
| Noxious | >1 ms | 2-4 pps or 100-150 pps | Tolerable | C fiber |

## Types of TENS Units

Various types of machines can be used to deliver TENS in a clinical setting. Understanding the type of stimulator and how the treatment can be varied makes the clinician much more versatile. Companies that manufacture stimulators try to simplify the treatments by requiring the clinician to push one button to select the parameters. Computer chips are programmed appropriately. Although these machines simplify the delivery of stimulation, a clinician may not appreciate the nuances of parameter selection.

The following section overviews different classes of electrical stimulators that are often used for TENS and pain modulation. These stimulators are biphasic low-voltage stimulators, portable TENS units, interferential units, and high-voltage stimulators.

### Low-Voltage Stimulators

Low-voltage stimulators are all TENS units that do not belong to a special class. Numerous manufacturers produce stimulators in this category. They can have either monophasic or biphasic current and have variable waveforms. Usually they have specific controls for phase duration, intensity, frequency, and duty cycles. Most of these units have limitations on the phase duration for safety reasons, so they are not effective as noxious pain stimulators.

### Portable TENS Units

Battery-operated portable TENS units allow a long duration of electrical stimulation (see figure 10.5). They can be lent or sold to an athlete or patient so that TENS can be used throughout the day or night for pain management. Portable TENS units are often used for electrical stimulation treatments during traveling with a team.

When using a portable TENS unit, complete a musculoskeletal evaluation to determine the source of pain and areas of associated pain. From the evaluation, determine sites for electrode placement, which may be around painful joints, on trigger or acupuncture points, at spinal nerve root levels or peripheral nerve trunks, or at a superficial point of the nerve supplying the painful area. Prepare the skin site by cleaning the area; electrodes should not be placed over abraded skin or open wounds. Secure electrodes at designated areas on the skin. Carbon-silicon-impregnated rubber electrodes require a conductive gel interface. Some pre-gelled electrodes contain an adherent. Thoroughly explain the treatment to the athlete.

Preset the phase duration and the pulse rate prior to application according to the type of TENS to be used. Gradually turn up the amplitude until the athlete feels a tingling sensation. Increase the amplitude until the stimulation is strong, but comfortable. Electrodes may have to be adjusted for better stimulation and pain relief. The athlete can be taught to adjust the amplitude independently but to keep the stimulation at the desired intensity (motor or submotor).

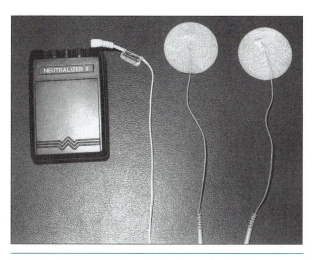

**Figure 10.5**  Portable transcutaneous electrical nerve stimulation units are available from many manufacturers. Most have two channels and allow the clinician to preadjust the rate, phase duration, and modulation.

During treatment, the amplitude may be adjusted to maximize pain relief and to account for accommodation. The fast response to sensory TENS allows rapid evaluation of electrode placement and effectiveness. If the athlete is responding well to sensory TENS, other modes may be utilized. After 20 to 30 min, reevaluate the athlete for pain and inspect electrode sites for **hyperemia.**

The athlete may be instructed in home use. Sensory TENS can be used throughout the day, but the athlete should be taught to turn the stimulation off periodically and to monitor the duration of pain relief.

## Interferential Stimulation Units

Interferential stimulation is another form of TENS used for pain relief, increased circulation, and muscle stimulation. We are categorizing interferential stimulation with TENS because it is primarily used for the modulation of pain. Interferential current simultaneously applies two medium-frequency currents to achieve deeper penetration of the stimulation. Medium- and high-frequency currents reduce the skin impedance that minimizes the penetration of low-frequency currents. Theoretically, a medium-frequency stimulation can be directed to a target tissue such as a joint. However, according to the pain modulation theories, sensory stimulation must evoke enkephalin intervention at the dorsal horn. Furthermore, because of bombardment of stimulation during the refractory period, medium-frequency currents must be modulated; otherwise there is minimal or no response in the tissues. Typical modulation techniques include the incorporation of an internal duty cycle as with Russian stimulation, or "interfering" the current to create a resultant "beat" frequency.

In order to modulate the medium frequency to a range that can create an action potential in the tissues, two slightly different medium-frequency (within the range of 1,000 to 10,000 Hz) sinusoidal wave currents are applied at the same time (figure 10.6). Typically interferential units use a carrier frequency of 4,000 or 5,000 Hz. This results in a phase duration of 125 μs or 100 μs (1 sec divided by 4,000 Hz = *pulse* duration). (Divide by 2 to get the *phase* duration). This phase duration is excellent for sensory pain modulation. The waveforms of the two carrier currents are superimposed on each other, which causes interference. Interference creates points of augmentation and attenuation of the phases where peaks and valleys are added together. The interference results in the modulation of a "beat" mode with a frequency that ranges from 1 to 100 beats per second, which is well within the conventional low-frequency range. The beat frequency is determined by the difference between the two carrier frequencies. For example, carrier frequencies of 4,000 and 4,150 have a beat frequency of 150 beats per second (bps); 2,500 and 2,550 have a beat frequency of 50 bps.

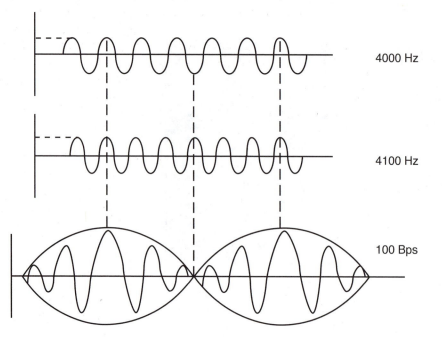

**Figure 10.6** Interferential stimulation. Two different medium-frequency currents are superimposed so that there is augmentation and attenuation of the currents. The resultant frequency is the beat frequency and is the difference between the two carrier frequencies.

4000 Hz

4100 Hz

100 Bps

The medium-frequency currents used with interferential units can cause a cutaneous nerve inhibition as with the action potential block mode of TENS. This action potential failure is known as Wedenski's inhibition and occurs as the stimulation is applied too fast in relation to the refractory period of the nerve. At a frequency of 5,000 Hz, the membrane is unable to stabilize, and the continuous function of the sodium-potassium pump causes an inhibitory effect. One can demonstrate Wedenski's inhibition by noting the anesthesia between the electrodes during medium-frequency stimulation. The patient should not be able to discriminate sharp or dull sensations between the electrodes during stimulation.

You can vary the frequency of the beats by changing one of the two carrier frequencies. The beat frequency, not the carrier frequencies, affects the tissues; and changes in this parameter alter the stimulation responses. The number of muscle twitches is greater as the beat frequency increases, until a tetanic contraction is attained. Some units have a feature that constantly changes the frequency of one of the carrier currents while the other remains constant. This mode is a "sweep frequency" that causes a rhythmic change throughout a range of frequencies. The purpose of the rhythmic mode is to reduce accommodation. Because the stimulation continuously changes, the body cannot adapt to it. The sweep frequency provides a more effective stimulation in this manner.

Some models include a rotating vector system that periodically changes the orientation of the electrical field 45° to further reduce accommodation. The efficacy of this modification has not been substantiated.

The beat frequency is selected according to the condition to be treated. A frequency of 60 to 100 bps is used for sensory TENS, 35 to 50 bps for muscle contraction, and 2 to 4 bps for motor TENS.

Four electrodes should be used for an interferential treatment, two for each carrier current in a quadripolar fashion. The electrodes of each current are placed diagonally over the treatment site (figure 10.7). The area to be treated should be surrounded by the electrodes if it is an extremity or joint. The electrodes should be placed all on one surface if the treatment area is large, such as the low back. Some interferential units also offer suction electrodes in which a mild vacuum is created under the electrode to allow it to stick to the body part. The electrodes are convenient to apply because they do not have to be strapped down and they stay in place throughout the treatment.

The passage of current through the tissues does not occur linearly between the electrodes but creates an electrical field. This field is purported to be shaped in a "cloverleaf" pattern

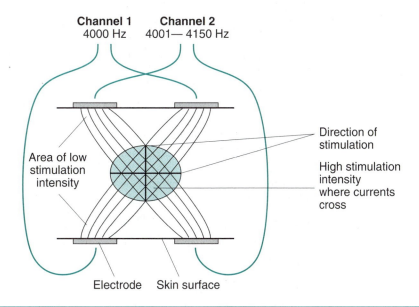

**Figure 10.7**   Stimulation produced with interferential current using four electrodes.

Reprinted by permission from Dynatronics Corporation.

situated three-dimensionally between the electrodes. If the conductivity of the tissues were uniform, this perfectly formed electrical field would occur with the maximal current concentration in the central region between the electrodes. However, differences in the tissue impedance affect the location of the electrical field and the degree of superposition of currents. Therefore, the concentration of current is not always centralized. To maximize the probability of properly placed electrodes and subsequent electrical fields, adjust the electrodes so that maximal intensity is perceived in the painful region.

Interferential stimulation can be used with other modalities. Although it is sometimes difficult with the suction electrodes, ice or heat can be used in conjunction with the stimulation. Treatment durations are dictated by the goal of treatment: pain relief, muscle reeducation, muscle spasm reduction, and so on. Interferential units have been shown to reduce pain and edema posttraumatically.

Contraindications to using interferential stimulators are the same as for any other form of TENS, but caution is necessary with the use of interferential machines in the proximity of diathermy units. The electrical field generated can cause power surges in the electrical modalities.

## Application

Turn the power for the interferential machine on prior to setting up electrodes. This prevents a power surge from transmitting to the patient during powering on. Select the interferential mode if the unit has multiple options of stimulation parameters. There may be an option of selecting the carrier frequency. Generally your decision will be determined by your treatment goal. For example, if there are options of 2,500 Hz and 5,000 Hz, remember that the higher the frequency, generally the better the depth of penetration (according to the formula that affects impedance). However, a 2,500-Hz current has a phase duration of 200 μs (1 / 2,000 = 400 μs biphasic; therefore each phase is 200 μs). A current with 5,000 Hz has only a 100-μs phase duration. Therefore if a longer phase duration is desired, which may be the case with use of **neuromuscular stimulation,** select the lower carrier frequency.

Select the treatment frequency. This also will be dictated by the treatment goal. Use the appropriate treatment frequencies for pain modulation or at tetany for neuromuscular stimulation. You may be able to select a frequency scan that modulates the frequency throughout a preset range to decrease accommodation. The treatment frequency is actually the difference between the two medium-frequency currents (e.g., 5,000 Hz and 5,100 Hz result in 100 bps).

Determine the duty cycle for the treatment. If the treatment is for pain, generally a continuous (no duty cycle) treatment is chosen. Neuromuscular treatments require a rest time, and both the "on" time and the "off" time should be selected as appropriate for the treatment.

Set up the electrodes. Moist sponges can be used to improve conductance. Two complete channels must be connected to the athlete. Ideally, the stimulation should cross between the electrodes. The electrodes should be firmly secured to the athlete.

Begin to increase the intensity of the stimulation, one circuit at a time. When the intensity of the second circuit is increased, the perception of stimulation may change. Increase each circuit a little at a time while getting feedback from the athlete about the location of maximal stimulation and the comfort level of the current. Amplitude should be adjusted only when the duty cycle is on rather than during the rest phase.

Some interferential units allow the clinician to "move" the current to allow better placement of the stimulation. This may be done with a joystick or a finger panel. This requires feedback from the athlete. Vector scan can be selected if the treatment site cannot be isolated. One circuit will intrinsically vary its amplitude, changing the location of maximal stimulation. This will reduce the time the treatment current is at the injury site, so a longer treatment duration is recommended. Check on the athlete for comfort during the treatment and make adjustments as necessary.

## Premodulated Interferential

Premodulated interferential stimulation is designed to make interferential stimulation easier to set up. The premise is that the two medium-frequency currents are crossed inside the machine so that only two electrodes or one channel is necessary for the treatment. However, the benefit of interferential stimulation is that with application of two medium-frequency currents to the skin, the beat frequency will be produced inside the body at the location of the pathology. By crossing the currents prior to applying them to the body, the treatment becomes very similar to time-modulated AC or burst mode TENS. The medium frequency is modified to a biologically active low frequency before it gets to the body. This method is still a very effective method of TENS application, since both sensory and motor pain modulation stimulation can be performed.

### Application of Premodulated Interferential

Determine your treatment goal—for example, sensory pain modulation, muscle spasm reduction by fatigue, or neuromuscular. Select "Pre-Mod" on the unit. Adjust the treatment frequency and duty cycle depending on the treatment goal.

Attach one channel (two electrodes) securely to the athlete and increase the intensity to the desired level depending on the treatment goal.

## *High-Voltage Stimulators*

High-voltage stimulators (HVS) are classified according to two distinct specifications: They must be able to transmit a voltage of at least 150 V and must use a twin-peaked monophasic current (see figure 10.8). The 150-V delineation is an arbitrarily set value that demarcates high- and low-voltage units. The major claims of this type of unit are that the high voltage allows deeper penetration of the energy and that the short phase duration of the twin peaks does not allow the capacitance of smaller sensory fibers (A-delta or C fibers) to be stimulated, resulting in greater comfort. Despite early concerns, these monophasic pulsatile waveforms do not cause ion flux. The phase duration is too short to drive the movement of charged particles. Therefore, TENS units with monophasic pulsatile waveforms do not cause skin irritation or the physiochemical responses seen with the application of DC current.

Since the stimulator is monophasic, there is a polarity difference in the electrodes, allowing the clinician to choose a positive or negative electrode for the treatment area. Again, since the phase duration is so short, there are minimal physiochemical changes under the electrodes. High-voltage units are used clinically for pain control, edema reduction, tissue healing, and muscle spasm reduction. Muscle reeducation or neuromuscular electrical stimulation (NMES) can be performed with high-voltage units if the stimulator allows a rest cycle.

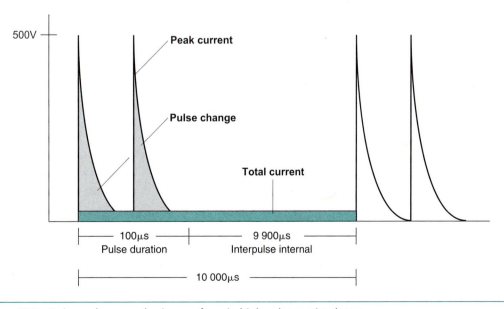

**Figure 10.8**  Twin-peak, monophasic waveform in high-voltage stimulators.

The voltage amplitude available with most high-voltage machines ranges from 0 to 500 V. The amplitude, as with most electrical stimulators, is determined by patient comfort and to meet the desired objective of the treatment (sensory or motor response). One of the features of the high-voltage machine is that although the voltage is high, there is a low average current. It is therefore a very safe modality. The twin-peaked waveform allows the high peak, but low average current. The decay of the pulse occurs almost immediately, and the second pulse begins before the first peak reaches the isoelectric line. The duration of both peaks together varies with each manufacturer, but is generally between 50 and 120 μs. The phase duration is not adjustable by the clinician, ensuring the safety of the unit.

Many claims have been made regarding the relevance of the polarity control of high-voltage units, although the low average current minimizes any ion flux or physiochemical response. However, during healing, the wound emits a charge potential depending on the stage of healing. It is believed that this potential is reinforced by application of the polarity of a like charge, either positive or negative, from the stimulator. This process promotes a stronger physiological response and has been associated with **chemotaxis** of leukocytes, which may enhance healing and edema reduction. However, the electrophoretic effect with this type of unit is negligible, especially with short treatment durations. The net ion flux across the membrane is minimal and is self-limiting. The short phase durations cause only a minor shift in ion migration, and with the interpulse interval the membrane can neutralize any change in the normal ion status. Iontophoresis cannot be performed with this unit because no net ion flux occurs. Several studies have addressed the possibility of edema reduction with high-voltage stimulation (Dolan et al. 2003; Goldman et al. 2003).

The frequency range offered by most high-voltage units is from 2 to 120 pps. The frequency adjustment allows the incorporation of either sensory or motor TENS principles when pain tolerance is the goal. The variation in frequencies also allows the clinician to optimize parameters for either muscle pumping or muscle reeducation. The phase duration cannot be changed and is so short that excitation of the smaller fibers for motor pain modulation or for a strong muscle contraction will be difficult to achieve.

Electrode placement for high voltage often utilizes the monopolar technique, although the bipolar can be used as well (see figure 10.9). The monopolar procedure uses one or more active electrodes and a larger dispersive electrode. The active electrodes are smaller in size and concentrate the current, and therefore the level of stimulation over the treatment site. As the name implies, the dispersive electrode spreads the same amount of current over a larger surface area, causing minimum, if any, sensory perception under the electrode. The active electrodes are placed over the treatment site, and the dispersive electrode is placed on a site distant to the treatment area. Since the distance between electrodes is increased with the monopolar method, there is potentially a deeper penetration of the current.

The bipolar technique, which uses equal-sized electrodes over the same treatment area, can also be used with high voltage. The larger electrode is replaced by a smaller one, although the cord must be plugged into the dispersive socket in the unit; otherwise the circuit is not complete.

A key feature of the high-voltage unit is its ability to be used with appendage submersion treatments. Submersion is a preferred method of treatment for acute ankle injuries because it provides circumferential cooling and sensory TENS for irregular surfaces. Even though the extremity is in a dependent position, the submersion method allows active range of motion during the treatment. The active electrodes are placed in the cold water bath (55° to 65° F), and a 20- to 30-min treatment is applied. The treatment is followed by other modalities and exercise as indicated for the condition. The treatment can be repeated several times throughout the day.

High-voltage stimulation with its monophasic current has the same applications as other TENS units—sensory and motor pain modulation and the effects on blood flow and edema reduction. High-voltage stimulation has the same contraindications as all other TENS and should not be used through the chest, whenever there is a cardiac pacemaker, or during pregnancy. It should not be used over the carotid sinus in the neck because of the proximity of the baroreceptors.

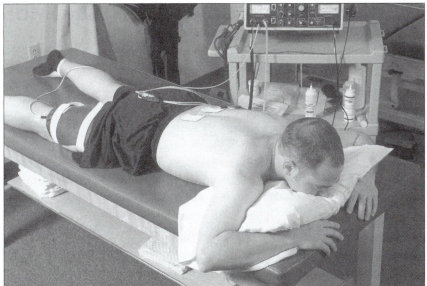

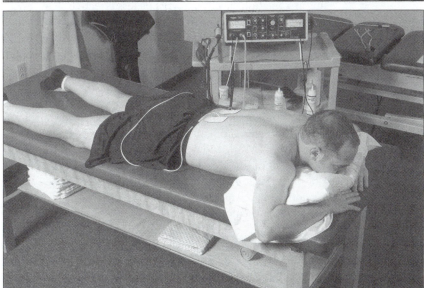

**Figure 10.9** Setups using a dispersive pad (monopolar) *(a)* and a small electrode (bipolar) *(b)*.

The evaluation should delineate the goal of the HVS. The high-voltage unit does not have an adjustable phase duration; therefore strong contraction as with motor TENS may not be possible. Check to see if your HVS has an adjustable duty cycle. If not, then the HVS cannot be used for NMES since there is no way to impose a rest time. The pulse frequency should be set depending on the goal of the treatment (sensory or motor TENS, muscle pumping or muscle contraction). If the HVS is to be used in a water bath, ensure that ground fault circuit interrupters are in good working order.

From the evaluation, determine whether a monopolar or bipolar electrode configuration is desired. Set up the electrodes using the respective technique. Make sure the dispersive pad is not causing trans-thoracic current.

Increase the amplitude to get the desired response (depending on the treatment goal—sensory or motor response). The HVS has a short phase duration, and the sensory nerves accommodate quickly to this stimulus. The amplitude may have to be increased periodically during the treatment. When the treatment time has ended, turn the amplitude back to zero and disconnect the electrodes. Evaluate the treatment response and inspect the skin. Return all electrodes and power down the stimulator.

# MUSCLE REEDUCATION: NEUROMUSCULAR ELECTRICAL STIMULATORS

Electrical stimulation can be used clinically to help to retrain the neuromuscular function that is lost from **arthrogenic muscle inhibition** following injury or surgery. The muscles "shut down" in order to protect the joint, but this inhibition must be overcome to allow controlled rehabilitation. One mechanism to help retrain the muscle function is with electrical muscle stimulation. The treatment is still TENS by definition, but the goal of the treatment is to elicit a strong muscle contraction through stimulation of the alpha motor nerve. The injured individual is taught to contract the muscle with the stimulation to overcome the natural inhibition. This use of electrical stimulation is termed neuromuscular electrical stimulation or NMES because the goal is to retrain the neuromuscular component to achieve an improved ability to produce muscle force.

Originally NMES was developed to increase the strength of muscles in trained athletes. Kots (1977) claimed that NMES combined with intense training resulted in greater strength gains than training alone. However, there is little evidence that NMES is any more beneficial than volitional isometric contractions in building strength. In fact, because isometric strength gains are position specific, NMES is less effective than resistance through the normal range of motion in a healthy individual.

NMES can also be applied to slow disuse atrophy in innervated muscle. At one time NMES was most commonly used to prevent disuse atrophy in postoperative care following anterior cruciate ligament reconstruction. When intra-articular graft placement procedures were developed, fixation of the graft was difficult, and patients were placed in plaster casts for up to 6 weeks following surgery. It was found that NMES limited disuse atrophy during cast immobilization. However, improved graft fixation now allows for range of motion and active quadriceps and hamstring contractions to be initiated soon after surgery, eliminating the need for NMES. Today, prolonged cast immobilization is reserved for unstable fractures. NMES is contraindicated in these cases, because active muscle contractions can alter alignment of the fracture site and delay healing.

Evidence-based medicine shows that NMES assists muscular function when neuromuscular inhibition is present following injury or surgery (Snyder-Mackler 1991, 1995; Robertson 2002; Lewek 2001; Currier 1993). Some data are inconclusive (Lieber 1996), and NMES is not as helpful when applied on normal subjects who are able to exercise independently.

## Muscle "Strengthening" Versus Force Capacity Enhancement

In order for a muscle to become stronger, a load must be placed on the muscle and adaptation must occur. Strength is measured by an increased ability to do work, usually by the ability to lift weights or produce more force. For strength to increase merely through utilization of electrical stimulation, the stimulation must be as great as a similar overload imposed in the form of exercise. Currier reports that a force equal to 40% to 60% of the maximal voluntary force must be imposed with electrical stimulation for "strengthening" to occur (Currier, Lehman, and Lightfoot 1979). For example, if the athlete is able to lift 20 lb with the biceps volitionally, to strengthen the muscle electrically the stimulation should be strong enough to lift 8 to 12 lb. This level of electrical stimulation is rarely tolerable, and in normal situations it is easier to exercise rather than use electrical stimulation for muscle strengthening.

In an injured population, electrical stimulation can assist neuromuscular function. If there is inhibition of a muscle from effusion or prolonged immobilization, electrical stimulation can be used to help teach the athlete to contract the muscle. In this manner, the force capacity or ability of the muscle to contract is enhanced, but the muscle is not truly "strengthened." Electrical muscle stimulation always occurs through the motor nerve rather than by depolarizing the muscle membrane directly whenever the peripheral nerve is intact. Therefore, although muscle contraction is the goal, the technique is termed *neuromuscular electrical stimulation* or NMES.

NMES can be used in sports medicine for muscle reeducation following injury or surgery, the reduction of disuse atrophy with immobilization, or augmentation of the function of an impaired muscle (functional electrical stimulation). For example, NMES may be used to assist dorsiflexion with foot-drop. Additionally, NMES may be used for focal stimulation of a weakness (e.g., stimulation of paraspinals on the convex side of scoliosis).

## Endogenous Versus Exogenous Muscle Contractions

The "all-or-nothing" principle affects the type of muscle contraction that is elicited with NMES (exogenous), and this creates a difference compared to physiological contractions (endogenous). According to the law of Dubois Reymond, if the amplitude of the stimulation exceeds threshold, the phase duration exceeds capacitance, and the rate of rise of the leading edge is fast enough to prevent accommodation, there will be an action potential. When electrical stimulation is applied to target alpha motor neurons, the entire motor unit associated with the stimulated nerve will respond. The large-diameter motor nerves are preferentially stimulated because they have a lower capacitance. Large-diameter motor nerves correspond to fast-twitch (glycolytic) fibers. These muscle fibers fatigue quickly because of the energy system utilized to produce a contraction. This is in contrast to a normal physiological contraction; in such contractions, slow-twitch fibers are recruited first, and if the task requires a greater force, the fast-twitch fibers will be called upon as needed.

Furthermore, because of the all-or-nothing principle, the contraction will be maintained as long as the stimulation is applied. There is no inhibition if the contraction becomes too strong; therefore the body cannot protect itself against an intense contraction. An electrically stimulated contraction is also synchronous, meaning that the individual motor units cannot "rest" as with an endogenous contraction. These factors contribute to the increased fatigue associated with NMES. The differences between physiologic and electrical muscle contractions are summarized in table 10.2.

## Fatigue and Neuromuscular Electrical Stimulation

Electrically produced contractions cause greater fatigue than physiological contractions, primarily because of the energy system used in the fast-twitch fibers. In order to reduce fatigue

### Table 10.2   Differences Between Physiological and Electrical Muscle Contractions

|  | Physiological | Electrical |
| --- | --- | --- |
| Order of recruitment | Slow-twitch fibers are excited first. Fast-twitch fibers are excited if increased force is required, preserving energy. | Larger-diameter, fast-twitch fibers are recruited first because they have a lower capacitance. Slow-twitch fibers are recruited if the stimulation is increased. |
| Synchrony of firing | There is asynchronous firing to promote a continuous contraction. This reduces the potential for fatigue of any one motor unit. | There is synchronous firing depending on the frequency of the stimulation. The contraction continues until the stimulation is off. |
| Inhibition | If the stimulation is strong, the Golgi tendon organ (GTO) will cause inhibition, which relaxes the muscle to prevent too strong a contraction. | The GTO is excited, but inhibition of the alpha motor neuron is overcome because of direct stimulation of the peripheral nerve. |
| Fatigue | There is minimal fatigue because of the order of recruitment and asynchrony of firing of motor units. | The muscle fatigues rapidly from the fast-twitch fiber recruitment, which uses the phosphocreatine energy system, and from the synchronous nature of the firing. |

with electrical stimulation, a duty cycle or *rest time* must be imposed. Generally, a 1:5 "on" to "off" time is required to allow enough time to regenerate the local energy utilized for the contraction. The phosphocreatine energy system is depleted rapidly (in 10-15 sec) and requires 30 sec to 1 min to replace. The rest time allows quality contractions to be produced throughout the treatment. With use of NMES for muscle reeducation or to promote quality muscle function, generally a 10-sec contraction is followed by a 45- to 50-sec rest time. As the athlete accommodates to the overload (after 1 to 2 weeks of training), the rest time can be reduced to 30 sec. Because of muscle fatigue, the duty cycle is probably the most important feature of a neuromuscular stimulator.

## Neuromuscular Electrical Stimulation Parameters

The electrical stimulator's parameters of phase duration, pulse frequency, amplitude, and duty cycle can be adjusted to optimize the NMES treatment.

The phase duration with NMES should be high enough to overcome the capacitance of motor nerve fibers. Although the capacitance of these motor fibers is low, these fibers are deep, and a high phase duration is recommended (250 to 300 $\mu$s) so that there is increased recruitment of many motor units.

The goal is to produce a tetanus contraction; therefore the pulse rate should be 35 to 50 pps. Usually 50 pps is used. Higher frequencies (over 100 pps) do not cause a stronger contraction and promote early fatigue.

The amplitude with NMES depends on the goal of the treatment. If the purpose is to teach the athlete to contract the muscle, then the intensity should produce a strong, tolerable contraction. The athlete should superimpose a voluntary contraction with the electrical contraction whenever possible to enhance the force production. If the goal is "strengthening" the muscle, then the amplitude should be 40% to 60% of the maximal volitional force.

As described previously, the duty cycle is probably the most important parameter in NMES treatment since the electrically produced contractions cause more fatigue than endogenous contractions. The duty cycle should be 1:5 (10 sec on and 50 sec off) in the initial treatments, and as the athlete adapts to the stimulation the duty cycle can be reduced to 1:3. The "on" time does not include the ramp time, so if a long ramp time is desired, increase the "on" time. For example, if the "on" time is 10 sec, but there is a 3-sec ramp, then the maximal intensity is on for only 7 sec. Increase the "on" time in this case to 13 sec so that there is a maximal contraction for the full 10 sec.

## Types of Neuromuscular Stimulators

Any machine can be used as long as there is a duty cycle control. Ideally, the unit should be able to produce a strong, tetanus contraction. Commonly the *Russian stimulator* is used; this machine has unique parameters that were popularized by Kots, a Russian researcher who presented impressive results on muscle strengthening with electrical stimulation in 1977. The Russian stimulation parameters are preset and cannot be adjusted to vary the treatment.

## Russian Stimulation Parameters (Time-Modulated Medium-Frequency AC Stimulation)

- Sinusoidal AC current with a carrier frequency of 2,500 Hz (200-$\mu$s phase duration)
- Bursted or "time-modulated AC" with a 10-ms "on" time and 10-ms "off" time, which ultimately results in a 50 burst per minute frequency
- Duty cycle preset at 10 sec on and 50 sec off (with a 2- to 3-sec ramp)

# Neuromuscular Stimulation Application

The following is an example of a stimulation protocol for the quadriceps muscle.

Explain the treatment protocol to the athlete, who is encouraged to increase the current intensity for as strong a contraction as can be tolerated. Also encourage the athlete to superimpose a volitional contraction in conjunction with the stimulation.

Place one electrode over the femoral nerve in the femoral triangle and the other over the distal quadriceps proximal to the patella. The athlete should be positioned in a device such as an Orthotron that adds isometric resistance to the contraction and limits the complete excursion of the limb. Terminal extension should be avoided to prevent joint "jamming" and soft tissue damage (figure 10.10). The optimal knee angle to obtain maximal quadriceps muscle force using NMES is at 60° of knee flexion.

Treatment parameters may vary according to the type of unit utilized. The phase duration is often preset; otherwise select 200 to 300 µs. The pulse frequency is also often preset, but if it is adjustable, select 40 to 50 Hz (30 to 40 Hz postoperatively) for tetany. The amplitude should be adjusted and increased to tolerance of a maximal contraction. Make sure that the amplitude is adjusted only when the stimulation is on rather than during the rest phase. The duty cycle should be set at 15 sec on and 50 sec off (this is preset on some units; otherwise use a 1:5 on:off ratio). Select the ramp time at 2 to 3 sec.

The treatment duration may vary according to the type of neuromuscular stimulator being used and the goal of the treatment. For example, the larger clinical models require only 10 to 15 contractions when maximally tolerated contractions are elicited. However, when the athlete is being "taught" to contract a muscle following a surgical procedure, a greater number of submaximal contractions can be performed. With use of home portable units, the treatment can be repeated up to three times a day for up to 1 h, although overfatigue of the muscle groups should be discouraged. Generally these units do not elicit a maximal contraction.

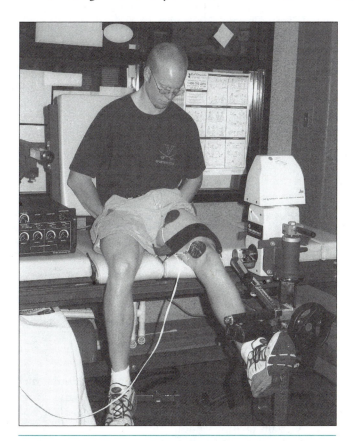

**Figure 10.10**   Neuromuscular electrical stimulation for force capacity enhancement. Block terminal extension to protect the joint. Use a concomitant maximal volitional contraction.

The athlete should be placed in a position to allow the best contraction of the muscle. If there is a deficit in the muscle function in part of the range, such as with an extension lag of the knee, then the muscle should be strengthened in the weak aspect of the range (figure 10.11).

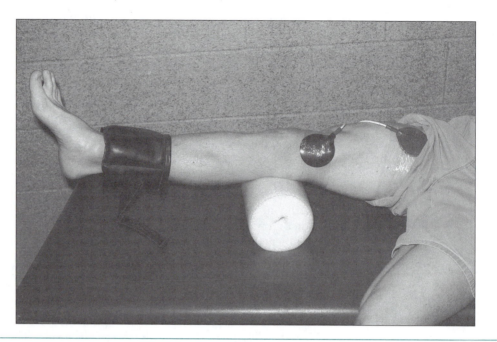

**Figure 10.11**  Neuromuscular electrical stimulation for muscle reeducation. Use the electrical stimulation to teach the athlete how to contract the muscle after an injury or surgery. Active exercise with the stimulation is encouraged.

If reciprocal stimulation of agonist–antagonist muscle groups is desired, then the joint should be positioned so that both muscle groups can benefit. This is generally in the mid-range of the joint motion.

When one is attempting to increase the force generated by the muscle with augmentation of electrical stimulation, the end range of the joint should be blocked. This position is necessary to minimize potential injury to the joint, since the inhibition caused normally by the Golgi tendon organ is unable to take place as long as the stimulation is on. Blocking terminal extension also prevents hyperextension of the joint.

## IONTOPHORESIS AND STIMULATION OF DENERVATED MUSCLE: DIRECT CURRENT STIMULATOR

As discussed in chapter 9, there are two major classifications of waveforms: monophasic and biphasic. Biphasic waveforms have no polarity effects. Monophasic waveforms are polar since one electrode is positive and the other is negative. If the phase duration is short, as with an HVS, the polar effects are minimal and there are no physiochemical effects under either electrode.

A galvanic current, with its long phase duration (at least 1 sec), has strong polar effects and is capable of changing the pH under the electrodes, creating a physiochemical effect. One electrode is always positive (the anode), and one electrode is always negative (cathode). Certain physiochemical effects occur in the tissues under each electrode (see figure 10.12 and table 10.3).

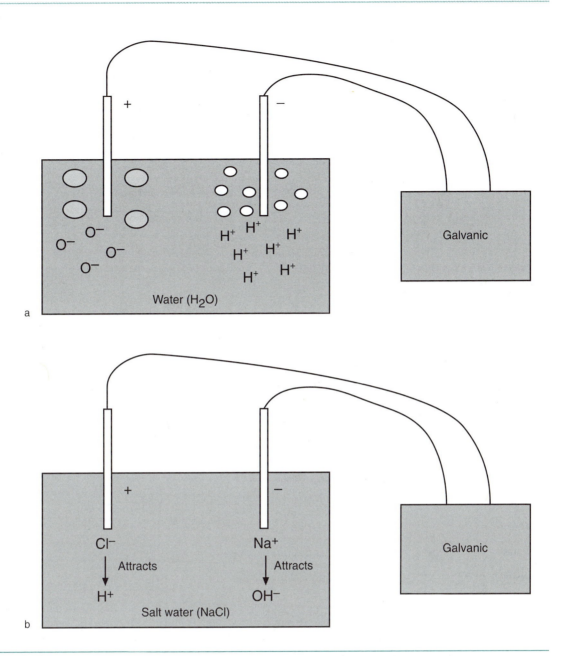

**Figure 10.12** *(a)* Place each level of a galvanic stimulator into a container of water. Turn on the current and note the development of many small bubbles at the *negative* electrode (hydrogen ions) and the development of a few larger bubbles at the *positive* electrode (oxygen ions). *(b)* Place each lead into a container of salt water. The salt water dissociates in water into $Na^+$ and $Cl^-$ ions. The $Cl^-$ is attracted to the positive electrode, which forms HCl acid. The $Na^+$ is attracted to the negative electrode, which forms NaOH, a strong base. This is similar to what happens in the body.

## Iontophoresis

**Iontophoresis** is the process in which ions in solution are transferred through the intact skin via an electrical potential. It is based on the electrical principle that "like" charges are repelled. Therefore, the ions in solution (of similar charge) migrate away from the electrical source into the body. Iontophoresis is a noninvasive method to introduce drugs locally (table 10.4). Iontophoresis has been shown to be effective in clinical trials (Gulick 2000), but there are numerous negative and inconclusive reports (Runeson 2002; Smutok 2002; Gudeman 1997). Furthermore, you should check state practice acts before administering iontophoresis. Some states, such as Virginia, consider iontophoresis the application of a prescription medication. Therefore only physicians can apply the device unless the treatment is delivered in an

**Table 10.3　Polarity Effects With Galvanic Stimulation**

| Positive | Negative |
| --- | --- |
| Attracts acids | Attracts alkali |
| Repels alkali | Repels acids |
| Hardens tissue | Softens tissue |
| Contracts tissue | Dilates tissue |
| Stops hemorrhage | Increases hemorrhage |
| Diminishes congestion | Increases congestion |
| Sedating | Stimulating |
| Relieves pain in acute conditions by reducing congestion | Reduces pain in chronic conditions because of softening effect |
| Scars formed are hard and firm | Scars are soft and pliable |

**Table 10.4　Pathology and Recommended Ions Used With Iontophoresis**

| Condition | Medication | Polarity |
| --- | --- | --- |
| Pain and inflammation | Salicylate | − |
|  | Hydrocortisone | + |
|  | Lidocaine | + |
|  | Dexamethasone | − |
| Calcium deposits | Acetic acid | − |
| Fungi | Copper | + |
| Adhesions | Chlorine | − |
| Edema | Magnesium sulfate | + |
| Spasms | Magnesium sulfate | + |

inpatient hospital setting. Pennsylvania requires a physician prescription for the medication, which the patient is responsible for obtaining. The treatment may be applied by an athletic trainer or physical therapist.

A DC generator is required for iontophoresis. Other monophasic stimulators have short phase durations, and the current does not flow long enough to cause physiochemical changes or a driving effect.

Commercially produced units make the application of iontophoresis very easy (figure 10.13). The medication is placed into a specially made electrode and applied at the treatment site. Some units have a feature to alter the duration of the treatment depending on the intensity of current used. The clinician sets the milliamp-minutes on this type of unit to keep dosage as consistent as possible.

The most common application of iontophoresis in sport rehabilitation is the use of dexamethasone to suppress inflammation, although there are no well-defined guidelines for such a treatment approach. The relationship between tissue repair and inflammation was emphasized in chapter 3, which pointed out that suppressing inflammation during tissue healing may be inappropriate.

However, small amounts of **necrotic** tissue or mechanical stimulation sometimes cause persistent pain that fails to respond to rest and other treatment interventions. With age, the vascularity of tendon declines, which may compromise the body's ability to phagocytize necrotic tissues. In these circumstances there is empirical evidence that an injectable or

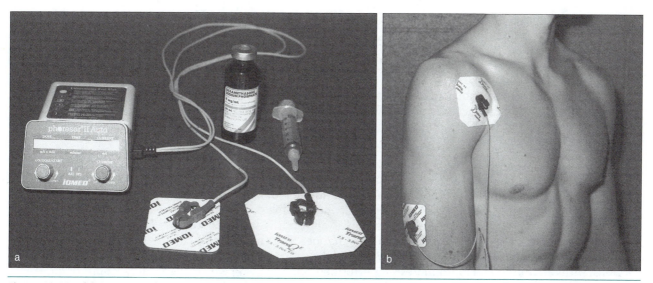

**Figure 10.13** *(a)* Commercial iontophoresis unit: small galvanic generator with one electrode that can be injected with the desired medication. The other electrode is dispersive. *(b)* Iontophoresis treatment. The active electrode on the anterior aspect of the shoulder contains the medication.

iontophoresed steroidal anti-inflammatory medication can break a cycle of irritation and pain. These treatments can relieve symptoms for months or even permanently.

Lidocaine can be used to anesthetize a small area of skin and underlying tissues. The injection of lidocaine or other anesthetics into trigger points can be effective in managing myofascial pain syndromes. Iontophoresis offers a means of delivering the medication without needles. However, the treatment of multiple trigger points with iontophoresis would be extremely time-consuming.

At one time it was common to mix lidocaine and dexamethasone for iontophoresis to buffer the solution and thus minimize skin irritation. Iontophoresis must be conducted with water-soluble medications, but a direct current passing through water causes hydrolysis, lowering the pH of the drug solution. When lidocaine is used to buffer the free hydrogen ions, less change in pH occurs. Unfortunately, this practice also diminishes the delivery of dexamethasone into the tissues (figure 10.14). The use of buffered electrodes, which were marketed in the 1990s, minimizes the risk of skin irritation. Thus, there is no longer a need to mix lidocaine and dexamethasone.

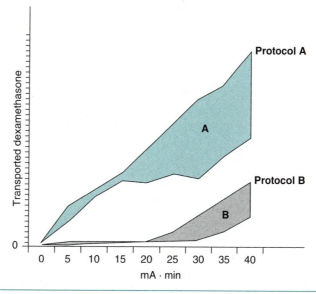

**Figure 10.14** Dexamethasone delivery is enhanced by using a buffered electrode (Protocol A) instead of a lidocaine-dexamethasone mixture (Protocol B).

## The Effects of pH Buffering on Drug Delivery During Iontophoresis

Iontophoresis must be conducted using water-soluble drugs. However, a direct current passing through an aqueous solution causes the hydrolysis of water, thus creating potentially harmful changes in the pH of the drug solution.

$OH^-$ raises pH.

$H^+$ lowers pH.

Because the most commonly used drug in iontophoresis is the negatively charged dexamethasone sodium phosphate, a potential problem is the accumulation of hydroxide ions, which are also negatively charged. If allowed to accumulate, they will be driven into the skin along with the drug ions. Depending on the length of the treatment, this can result in alkaline burns at the skin surface. Fortunately, there are ways to prevent these potentially dangerous pH changes. The method most frequently used in delivering dexamethasone sodium phosphate involves mixing the drug with lidocaine hydrochloride. When the two substances are mixed and iontophoresis is performed, the following electrochemical reactions occur:

$$DexPO_4^{-2} + 2Na^+ + OH^- + H^+ \ LidoH^+ + Cl^-$$

An additional consideration with iontophoresis, which parallels concerns raised for phonophoresis, is the inability to precisely quantify the amount of medication delivered into the tissues. Continued investigation of the techniques is needed to provide treatment protocols with demonstrated efficacy.

### Treatment Procedures

Since the purpose of application of iontophoresis is to introduce a medication, a physician should prescribe the treatment. Even topically applied steroids can have a systemic effect; therefore administration of pharmaceutical agents should be monitored by a physician.

The electrical stimulators used in athletic training for iontophoresis deliver DC. The substance to be driven into the tissue must carry an electrical charge in solution. The solution is placed in a treatment electrode that is buffered to minimize skin irritation (figure 10.15).

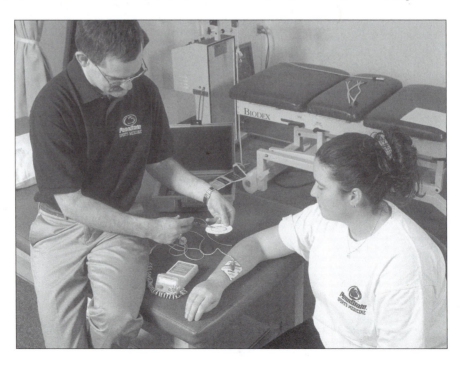

**Figure 10.15** Electrode preparation.

The maximum current delivered by the stimulator is 5 mA. Because DC is used, waveform duty cycle, frequency, phase duration, and ramp cannot be adjusted, and the only parameters of concern are polarity and dosage. The polarity of the treatment electrode should be the same as that of the ion to be driven into the tissue, because like charges repel. The unit of iontophoresis dosage is milliamperes per minute (mA/min). With buffered electrodes, the maximum dosage is 80 mA/min. The higher the dosage, the greater the amount of medication driven into the tissues. The dosage is determined by the amplitude of current that the recipient is able to tolerate multiplied by the length of the treatment. For example, if a 3-mA peak current is the most an individual can tolerate and the current is applied for 25 min, the dosage is 75 mA/min.

### Safety

Safe application of iontophoresis requires proper equipment and clinical judgment. Iontophoresis carries all of the cautions and contraindications of TENS. In addition, medications to which the individual is allergic contraindicate iontophoresis. Even with modern electrodes designed for iontophoresis, skin irritation and chemical burns are possible. Instruct the recipient to report any sensation of burning, and if the individual does so, interrupt the treatment and inspect the skin. Terminate treatment if you have any concern that burning may be occurring. Some individuals, especially fair-skinned people, are very sensitive and cannot be treated with iontophoresis.

Although homemade electrodes and DC generators have been used for iontophoresis, it is strongly recommended that you use commercial stimulators and electrodes designed specifically for iontophoresis, to protect the individual as well as yourself. Proper equipment reduces the risk of skin injury substantially.

## Direct Stimulation of Denervated Muscle

When the conduction of impulses to muscle by alpha motor neurons is disrupted, the individual loses control of the affected muscle. **Alpha motor neurons** conduct impulses from the spinal cord to the muscle and are also referred to as lower motor neurons, in contrast to the motor neurons of the spinal cord that are referred to as upper motor neurons. When the nerve to the muscle is not functioning, the muscle is denervated, or without innervation.

Denervation can be caused by injury or disease, but you will most likely encounter denervated muscle secondary to trauma. Severe knee sprains and dislocations can injure the peroneal nerve where it passes behind the head of the fibula, denervating muscles in the anterior tibial or lateral compartments of the leg. Injury to the brachial plexus can denervate the deltoid and other muscles of the arm.

Unlike upper motor neurons of the spinal cord, injury to which results in permanent paralysis, alpha motor neurons can regenerate and active control of the muscle can be restored. This reinnervation process is very slow and does not always occur.

However, because reinnervation is possible, clinicians have attempted to maintain the muscle through electrically stimulated contractions. The efficacy of electrical stimulation of denervated muscle has not been established. Electrical stimulation does not bring about reinnervation; however, a regularly stimulated muscle may recover force-generating capacity sooner if reinnervation occurs.

Although lower and upper motor neuron lesions are uncommon, it is important to understand the difference between these types of lesions. It is also important to understand that with lower motor neuron injury, the parameters of stimulation required for NMES will not elicit a contraction because the capacitance of muscle is much greater than that of the alpha motor neuron. Therefore, when NMES fails to elicit a contraction of the target muscle, one must suspect a lower motor neuron injury. If this diagnosis is confirmed, a low-frequency AC or DC current must be applied to overcome the capacitance of the muscle. The stimulation of denervated muscle carries the same contraindications as TENS.

The stimulation is uncomfortable because of the depolarization of small-diameter afferent nerves. Work closely with the directing physician in treating individuals with lower motor neuron lesions, and obtain the necessary equipment should stimulation of denervated muscle be requested.

# WOUND HEALING: MICROCURRENT ELECTRICAL NERVE STIMULATOR

Microcurrent is a form of electrotherapy in which the stimulus amplitude is in the micro-amperage (millionth of an ampere) range. Microcurrent stimulators have been referred to as microcurrent electrical nerve stimulators (MENS) and low-intensity stimulators (LIS). MENS is a poor name because the peak amplitude generated is usually below the rheobase of even A-beta afferent fibers. Thus, the electrical current does not result in nerve depolarization. Moreover, the theoretical basis underlying the application of microcurrent does not involve nerve fiber depolarization.

A substantial body of evidence shows that electrical stimulation has physiological effects that are not related to nerve fiber depolarization. Electrical stimulation has been shown to speed repair in slow-healing surface wounds such as decubitus ulcers in humans (Houghton et al. 2003; Barron, Jacobson, and Tidd 1985; Gentzkow et al. 1988; Kloth and Feeder 1988). Enhanced repair in deeper tissue has been reported in animal models with the use of indwelling electrodes (Akai et al. 1991; Nessler and Mass 1987; Tart and Dahners 1989; Litke and Dahners 1994; Owoeye et al. 1987). Exciting work on the effects of microcurrent on edema formation in the acute inflammatory phase is ongoing; however, this work is limited to animal models.

There is also great interest in the use of pulsed ultrasound and pulsed electromagnetic fields to facilitate healing of nonunion and slow-healing fractures. The effects of these stimulators will be discussed in the next chapter.

Although the effects and potential benefits of microcurrent stimulation warrant continued investigation, the work completed so far has limitations. There is no evidence that using electrical stimulation facilitates the normal repair response in healthy humans. Whether microcurrent has application in the treatment of musculoskeletal injuries sustained by physically active people has yet to be determined. There is some testimonial evidence of the benefits of microcurrent in the treatment of these injuries; however, controlled investigations using delayed-onset muscle soreness as a model for musculoskeletal injury suggest that microcurrent may relieve pain but does not speed recovery (Denegar et al. 1992). Some reports even question the pain-relieving effects of microcurrent (Lerner and Kirsch 1981; Weber, Servedino, and Woodall 1994). The subsensory effects of microcurrent may influence the peripheral mechanisms of the inflammatory and pain processes.

Where does the evidence leave the certified athletic trainer who must decide whether to apply microcurrent? At this time, the only application of microcurrent shown to be effective is in treatment of slow-healing skin lesions, a condition that a certified athletic trainer is not prepared to treat. The prospects for other uses of microcurrent will depend on future research findings. Clearly, electricity can alter tissue responses. However, research based on animal models and the use of indwelling electrodes does not provide answers about using surface electrode stimulation in humans to facilitate deep tissue repair or alter capillary membrane permeability to minimize swelling.

Microcurrent stimulation is safe, although the cautions identified for TENS should be observed. The major challenge is developing a theoretical basis and substantiating the clinical efficacy of microcurrent in the treatment of musculoskeletal injuries. Throughout your career you should continue to review the research literature and critically assess whether there is enough evidence to warrant the application of any modality, including microcurrent stimulation. Table 10.5 summarizes the indications and contraindications for the forms of electrotherapy discussed in this chapter.

## Table 10.5 Indications and Contraindications for Electrotherapy

| | Indications | Contraindications |
|---|---|---|
| TENS Neuromuscular stimulation | Pain control<br>Restore neuromuscular control<br>Retard atrophy | Electrode placement over carotid artery<br>Cardiac pacemaker (unless approved by MD; monitoring may be necessary)<br>Pregnancy |
| Iontophoresis | With dexamethasone: chronic inflammation<br>With lidocaine: local anesthesia | Electrode placement over carotid artery<br>Cardiac pacemaker (unless approved by MD; monitoring may be necessary)<br>Pregnancy<br>Medications to which individual is allergic or hypersensitive |
| Stimulation of denervated tissues | Lower motor neuron lesion | Same as for TENS |
| Microcurrent | Slow-healing wounds<br>Inflammatory conditions | Same as for TENS |

## SUMMARY

1. Understand the clinical uses for electrical stimulation in the rehabilitation process.

   Electrical stimulation has numerous clinical uses including pain modulation, neuromuscular facilitation, and wound healing. An athletic trainer can use various commercial stimulators to complement the rehabilitation process. Electrical stimulation helps to reduce pain, making therapeutic exercise and daily activities more comfortable. Additionally the stimulation can be modified to encourage muscle reeducation. When the muscle activity is facilitated, active exercise can be directed to assist the return to function.

2. Analyze the waveform of the available device and determine whether the treatment goal can be met using that stimulator.

   There are numerous stimulators on the market. Many new machines offer programmed treatment parameters, making treatment selection as easy as pushing a button. However, the athletic trainer should understand the intrinsics of the preprogrammed treatments with respect to waveform, amplitude, phase duration, and frequency. Understanding how the electrical configuration can be altered to target different tissue types is essential in understanding therapeutic modalities. The athletic trainer should be able to differentiate waveforms, types of stimulators, and methods of application used in electrical stimulation treatment.

3. Incorporate pain modulation theories with the electrical stimulation principles to determine the amplitude, phase duration, and pulse frequency necessary for a variety of clinical purposes.

   Pain modulation theories were reviewed in chapter 4. Electrical stimulation can be varied to target different nerve fiber types to maximize the analgesia addressed by each of the pain modulation theories: sensory, noxious, and motor. The phase duration, amplitude, and frequency can be adjusted to target the A-beta, C, and A-delta fibers to respectively utilize these theories clinically.

4. Describe the use of neuromuscular electrical stimulation, including Russian stimulation, for muscle reeducation.

   Muscle inhibition is common after injury or a surgical procedure. Electrical stimulation, specifically NMES, can be used to facilitate contraction of a muscle and thus assist the reeducation of the muscle. Neuromuscular electrical stimulation is most effective when used in combination with active exercise.

5. Describe the uses of a galvanic stimulator.

> Galvanic current is the same as direct current (DC). This unique current in physical medicine is a monophasic current with a phase duration of at least 1 sec. It has the highest phase charge or average current of any stimulator. Its primary uses are for iontophoresis to transcutaneously deliver medication and for stimulation of denervated muscles. Muscles that have lost the peripheral nerve can maintain some contractility while the nerve is regenerating. The stimulation does not promote nerve growth.

6. Understand the use of microcurrent electrical stimulation.

> Microcurrent electrical stimulation uses subsensory stimulation to promote wound healing. There are various suggestions regarding the waveforms, phase duration, frequency, and amplitude to maximize the results. Most researchers use a monophasic current to create an electrical field potential of a specific polarity around the injured site in order to enhance normal chemotactic effects of the inflammatory process.

7. Identify contraindications for the application of electrotherapy.

> Electrical stimulation should not be used in pregnancy, on a patient with a cardiac pacemaker, or over the carotid sinus in the neck. Caution should be exercised with the use of stimulators with high phase charges such as galvanic stimulators. Additionally, the electrical stimulation should not be placed so that it goes through the chest.

## CITED SOURCES

Abelson K, Langley GB, Sheppeard H, Vlieg M, Wigley RD: Transcutaneous electrical nerve stimulation in rheumatoid arthritis. *New Zealand Medical Journal* 96:156-8, 1983.

Akai M, Wadano Y, Yabuki T, Oda H, Sirasaki Y, Tateishi T: Effect of a direct current on modification of bone and ligament repair process: Experimental investigation of a rabbit model. *J Jpn Orthop Assoc* 65:196-206, 1991.

Ballegaard S, Christophersen SJ, Dawids SG, Hesse J, Olsen NV: Acupuncture and transcutaneous electric nerve stimulation in the treatment of pain associated with chronic pancreatitis. A randomized study. *Scandinavian Journal of Gastroenterology* 20:1249-54, 1985.

Barron JJ, Jacobson WE, Tidd G: Treatment of decubitus ulcers: A new approach. *Minn Med* 68:103-106, 1985.

Currier DP, Lehman J, Lightfoot P: Electrical stimulation in exercise of the quadriceps femoris muscle. *Phys Ther* 59:1508, 1979.

Currier DP, Ray JM, Nyland J, Rooney JG, Noteboom JT, Kellogg R: Effects of electrical and electromagnetic stimulation after anterior cruciate ligament reconstruction. *J Orthop Sports Phys Ther* Apr;17(4):177-84, 1993.

Denegar CR, Yoho AP, Corowicz AJ, Bifulco N: The effects of low volt, microamperage stimulation on delayed onset muscle soreness. *J Sport Rehab* 1:95-102, 192.

Dolan MG, Mychaskiw AM, Mattacola CG, Mendel FC: Effects of cool-water immersion and high-voltage electric stimulation for 3 continuous hours on acute edema in rats. *J Athl Train* Dec;38(4): 325-329, 2003.

Gentzkow GD: Electrical stimulation to heal dermal wounds. *J Dermatol Surg Oncol* Aug;19(8):753-8, 1993.

Goldman R, Brewley B, Zhou L, Golden M: Electrotherapy reverses inframalleolar ischemia: a retrospective, observational study. *Adv Skin Wound Care* Mar-Apr;16(2):79-89, 2003.

Grimmer K: A controlled double blind study comparing the effects of strong burst mode TENS and high rate TENS on painful osteoarthritic knees. *Australian Journal of Physiotherapy* 48:49-56, 1992.

Gudeman SD, Eisele SA, Heidt RS Jr, Colosimo AJ, Stroupe AL: Treatment of plantar fasciitis by iontophoresis of 0.4% dexamethasone. A randomized, double-blind, placebo-controlled study. *Am J Sports Med* May-Jun;25(3):312-6, 1997.

Gulick DT: Effects of acetic acid iontophoresis on heel spur reabsorption. *Phys Ther Case Rep* 3:64-70, 2000.

Houghton PE, Kincaid CB, Lovell M, Campbell KE, Keast DH, Woodbury MG, Harris KA: Effect of electrical stimulation on chronic leg ulcer size and appearance. *Phys Ther* Jan;83(1):17-28, 2003.

Hsueh T, Cheng P, Kuan T, Hong C: The immediate effectiveness of electrical nerve stimulation and electrical muscle stimulation on myofascial trigger points. *American Journal of Physical Medicine and Rehabilitation* 76:471-6, 1997.

Jensen H, Zesler R, Christensen T: Transcutaneous electrical nerve stimulation (TNS) for painful osteoarthrosis of the knee. *International Journal of Rehabilitation Research* 14:356-8, 1991.

Kloth LC, Feeder JA: Acceleration of wound healing with high voltage, monophasic, pulsed current. *Phys Ther* 68:503-508, 1988.

Kots YM: *Electrostimulation.* Paper presented at the Canadian-Soviet Exchange Symposium on Electrostimulation of Skeletal Muscles, Concordia University, Montreal, 1977.

Kumar D, Marshall HJ: Diabetic peripheral neuropathy: amelioration of pain with transcutaneous electrostimulation. *Diabetis Care* 20:1702-5, 1997.

Lerner FN, Kirsch DL: Micro-stimulation and placebo effect. *J Chiropractic* 15:101-106, 1981.

Lewek M, Stevens J, Snyder-Mackler L: The use of electrical stimulation to increase quadriceps femoris muscle force in an elderly patient following a total knee arthroplasty. *Phys Ther* Sep;81(9): 1565-71, 2002.

Lewis B, Lewis D, Cumming G: The comparative analgesic efficacy of transcutaneous electrical nerve stimulation and a non-steroidal anti-inflammatory drug for painful osteoarthritis. *British Journal of Rheumatology* 33:455-60, 1994.

Lewis D, Lewis B, Sturrock RD: Transcutaneous electrical nerve stimulation in osteoarthrosis: a therapeutic alternative? *Annals of Rheumatic Diseases* 43:47-9, 1984.

Lieber RL, Silva PD, Daniel DM: Equal effectiveness of electrical and volitional strength training for quadriceps femoris muscles after anterior cruciate ligament surgery. *J Orthop Res* Jan;14(1):131-8, 1996.

Litke DS, Dahners LE: Effects of different levels of direct current on early ligament healing in a rat model. *J Orthop Res* Sep;12(5):683-8, 1994.

Mannheimer C, Carlsson C: The analgesic effect of transcutaneous electrical nerve stimulation (TNS) in patients with rheumatoid arthritis. A comparative study of different pulse patterns. *Pain* 6:329-34, 1979.

Moore SR, Shurman J: Combined neuromuscular electrical nerve stimulation and transcutaneous electrical nerve stimulation for treatment of chronic back pain: a double-blind, repeated measures comparison. *Archives in Physical Medicine and Rehabilitation* 78:55-60, 1997.

Moystad A, Krogstad BS, Larheim TA: Transcutaneous nerve stimulation in a group of patients with rheumatic disease involving the temporomandibular joint. *Journal of Prosthetic Dentistry* 64:596-600, 1990.

Nash TP, Williams JD, Machin D: TENS: Does the type of stimulus really matter? *Pain Clinic* 3: 161-8, 1990.

Nessler JP, Mass DP: Direct-current electrical stimulation of tendon healing in vitro. *Clin Orthop* Apr;(217):303-12, 1987.

Owoeye I, Spielholz NI, Fetto J, Nelson AS: Low-intensity pulsed galvanic current and the healing of tenotomized rat Achilles tendon: Preliminary report using low load-to-breaking measurements. *Arch Phys Med Rehabil* 68:415-418, 1987.

Robertson VJ, Ward AR: Vastus medialis electrical stimulation to improve lower extremity function following a lateral patellar retinacular release. *J Orthop Sports Phys Ther* Sep;32(9):437-43, 2002.

Runeson L, Haker E: Iontophoresis with cortisone in the treatment of lateral epicondylalgia (tennis elbow)--a double-blind study. *Scand J Med Sci Sports* Jun;12(3):136-42, 2002.

Smith CR, Lewith GT, Machin D: Preliminary study to establish a controlled method of assessing transcutaneous nerve stimulation as treatment for the pain caused by osteo-arthritis of the knee. *Physiotherapy* 69:266-8, 1983.

Smutok MA, Mayo MF, Gabaree CL, Ferslew KE, Panus PC: Failure to detect dexamethasone phosphate in the local venous blood postcathodic lontophoresis in humans. *J Orthop Sports Phys Ther* Sep;32(9):461-8, 2002.

Snyder-Mackler L, Delitto A, Bailey SL, Stralka SW: Strength of the quadriceps femoris muscle and functional recovery after reconstruction of the anterior cruciate ligament. A prospective, randomized clinical trial of electrical stimulation. *J Bone Joint Surg* 77(8) 1166-1173, 1995.

Snyder-Mackler L, Ladin Z, Schepsis AA, Young JC: Electrical stimulation of the thigh muscles after reconstruction of the anterior cruciate ligament. Effects of electrically elicited contraction of the quadriceps femoris and hamstring muscles on gait and on strength of the thigh muscles. *J Bone Joint Surg* 73(7) 1025-1036, 1991.

Tart RP, Dahners LE: Effects of electrical stimulation on joint contracture in a rat model. *J Orthop Res* 7(4):538-42, 1989.

Taylor P, Hallett M, Flaherty L: Treatment of osteoarthritis of the knee with transcutaneous electrical nerve stimulation. *Pain* 11:233-40, 1981.

Thorsteinsson G, Stonnington HH, Stillwell GK, Elveback LR: The placebo effect of transcutaneous electrical stimulation. *Pain* 5:31-41, 1978.

Vinterberg H, Donde R, Andersen RB : Transcutaneous nerve stimulation for relief of pain in patients with rheumatoid arthritis. *Ugeskr Laeger* 140:1149-50, 1978.

Weber MD, Servedino FJ, Woodall WR: The effects of three modalities on delayed onset muscle soreness. *J Orthop Sports Phys Ther* 20:236-242, 1994.

## ADDITIONAL READINGS

Abram SE, Reynolds AC, Cusick JF: Failure of naloxone to reverse analgesia from transcutaneous electrical stimulation in patients with chronic pain. *Anesth Analg* 60:81-84, 1981.

Akai M, Oda H, Shirasaki Y, Teteishi T: Electrical stimulation of ligament healing: An experimental study of the patella ligament of rabbits. *Clin Orthop Rel Res* 235:296-301, 1988.

Clement-Jones V, Tomlin S, Rees LH, McLoughlin L, Besser GM, Wen HL: Increased beta-endorphin but not met-enkephalin levels in human cerebrospinal fluid after acupuncture for recurrent pain. *Lancet*: 946-948, 1980.

Denegar CR, Huff CB: High and low frequency TENS in the treatment of induced musculoskeletal pain. *J Athl Train* 23:235-237, 1988.

Denegar CR, Perrin DH: Effects of transcutaneous electrical nerve stimulation, cold and a combined treatment on pain, decreased range of motion and strength loss associated with delayed onset muscle soreness. *J Athl Train* 27:200-206, 1992.

Denegar CR, Perrin DH, Rogol AD, Rutt R: Influence of transcutaneous electrical nerve stimulation on pain, range of motion and serum cortisol concentration in females with induced delayed onset muscle soreness. *J Orthop Phys Ther* 11:100-103, 1989.

Deyo RA, Walsh NE, Martin DC, Schoenfeld LS, Ramamurthy S: A controlled trial of transcutaneous electrical nerve stimulation (TENS) and exercise for chronic low back pain. *N Engl J Med* 322: 1627-1634, 1990.

Gangarosa L, Payne L, Hayakawa K: Iontophoretic treatment of herpetic whitlow. *Arch Phys Med Rehabil* 70:336-340, 1989.

Gentzkow GD: Electrical stimulation to heal dermal wounds. *J Dermatol Surg Oncol* 19:753-758, 1993.

Gersh MR: *Electrotherapy in Rehabilitation.* Baltimore, Davis, 1992.

Grice K: Hyperhydrosis and its treatment by iontophoresis. *Physiotherapy* 66:43-44, 1980.

Grice K, Satter H, Baker H: Treatment of idiopathic hyperhydrosis with iontophoresis of tap water and poldine methylsulfate. *Br J Dermatol* 86:72-78, 1972.

Haggard H, Straus M, Greenburg L: Fungus infections of hands and feet treated with copper iontophoresis. *JAMA* 112:1229, 1939.

Kahn J: *Principles and Practices of Electrotherapy.* New York, Churchill Livingstone, 1987.

Kenney TG, Dahners LE: The effect of electrical stimulation on ligament healing in a rat model with a dosage study. *Trans Orthop Res Soc* 13:348, 1988.

Litke DS, Dahners LE: The effects of low level direct current electrical stimulation on ligament healing in a rat model: A dosage study. *Trans Orthop Res Soc* 17:669, 1992.

Melzack R: Prolonged relief of pain by intense transcutaneous somatic stimulation. *Pain* 1:357-373, 1975.

Nessler JP, Mass DP: Direct current electrical stimulation of tendon healing in vitro. *Clin Orthop* 217: 303-312, 1985.

Psaki C, Carroll J: Acetic acid ionization: A study to determine the absorptive effects upon calcific tendinitis of the shoulder. *Phys Ther Rev* 35:84-87, 1955.

Robinson AJ: Basic concepts in electricity and contemporary terminology in electrotherapy. In Robinson AJ, Snyder-Mackler L (Eds), *Clinical Electrotherapy,* 2nd ed. Baltimore, Williams & Wilkins, 1995.

Rosenburg M, Curtis L, Bourke DL: Transcutaneous electrical nerve stimulation for the relief of postoperative pain. *Pain* 5:129-133, 1978.

Shrivastera S, Singh G: Tap water iontophoresis for palmar hyperhydrosis. *Br J Dermatol* 96:189-195, 1977.

Sloan J, Sotani K: Iontophoresis in dermatology. *J Am Acad Dermatol* 15:671-684, 1986.

Wolcott LE, Wheeler PC, Hardwicke HM, Rowley BA: Accelerated healing of skin ulcers by electrotherapy: Preliminary clinical results. *South Med J* 62:795-801, 1969.

Wood JM, Evans III PE, Schallreuter KU, Jacobson WE, Sufit R, Newman J, White C, Jacoboo M: A multicenter study on the use of pulsed low intensity direct current for healing chronic stage II and III decubitus ulcers. *Arch Dermatol* 129:999-1009, 1993.

# Ultrasound, Diathermy, and Electromagnetic Fields

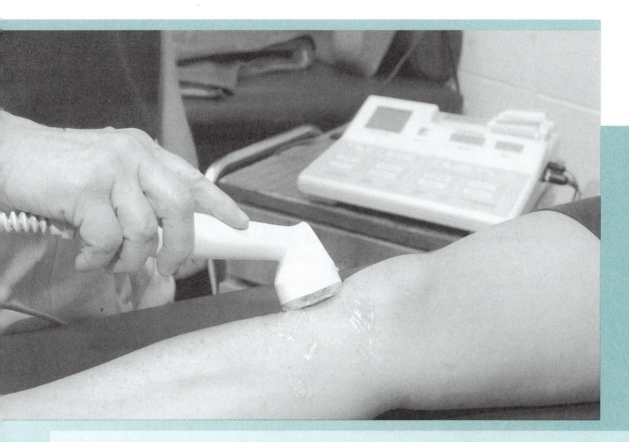

## *Objectives*

After reading this chapter, the student will be able to

1. describe how therapeutic ultrasound is generated by the treatment unit;

2. define beam nonuniformity ratio (BNR) and effective radiating area (ERA);

3. identify and describe the use of effective conducting media for ultrasound treatments;

4. define dose, duty cycle, treatment duration, and frequency as parameters of therapeutic ultrasound;

5. describe the thermal effects of therapeutic ultrasound;

6. describe the treatment parameters and physiological effects of pulsed ultrasound;

7. discuss the technique and efficacy of phonophoresis;

8. identify contraindications and precautions for treatment with therapeutic ultrasound;

9. identify indications for treatment with therapeutic ultrasound;

10. describe the differences between therapeutic ultrasound and diathermy;

11. identify the two mechanisms through which diathermy can be used to heat deep tissues;

12. identify the contraindications and precautions for the application of diathermy; and

13. describe the potential uses of diathermy and pulsed electromagnetic field therapy in athletic training and other allied medical fields.

**T**wo individuals are awaiting treatment. The first is a 22-year-old track athlete who sustained a strain of the biceps femoris 3 weeks ago. The second is a 36-year-old tennis player diagnosed with calcific tendinitis of the long head of the biceps brachii. Is treatment with ultrasound or diathermy indicated in the treatment of either athlete? What parameters should be selected with use of the modalities? How is the energy transmitted into the tissues? This chapter examines current uses and the evidence of efficacy of ultrasound and diathermy and pulsed electromagnetic fields.

This chapter focuses on therapeutic ultrasound and, to a lesser extent, the therapeutic use of electromagnetic fields. Ultrasound is commonly used by certified athletic trainers and physical therapists. With appropriate parameter adjustment, ultrasound can be applied to heat deeper tissues including muscles, tendons, ligaments, joint capsules, and scar tissue. Unlike the superficial heating modalities discussed in chapter 8, ultrasound energy penetrates through the skin and subcutaneous fat. Thus, ultrasound can be considered a deep-heating modality.

Not all of the purported benefits of ultrasound are attributable to thermal effects. When ultrasound is pulsed, less heating occurs than when treatment time remains the same. Responses to pulsed ultrasound are believed to be due to the effect of the sound energy at the cellular level as opposed to tissue heating.

Sound energy also has been used to drive medication through the skin. This process, known as **phonophoresis,** has been used commonly in athletic training and physical therapy despite very little evidence of efficacy. These issues are explored in greater detail later in this chapter.

Electromagnetic fields **(diathermy)** also can be applied to heat deeper tissues. At one time diathermy was a popular deep-heating modality. Because diathermy is more cumbersome to apply and has more contraindications than ultrasound, diathermy is less commonly used by certified athletic trainers. However, new diathermy devices have come on the market, and diathermy is available in more facilities than it was a few years ago. Diathermy allows for heating of larger areas of tissue. The discussion of diathermy also provides an introduction to treatments with pulsed electromagnetic fields.

Pulsed electromagnetic field and specially designed pulsed ultrasound devices have been developed to facilitate bone healing, and the use of these modalities in treating physically active individuals has increased. Therefore, diathermy and treatment with pulsed electromagnetic fields are discussed in this chapter to provide background on what is known and yet to be answered regarding the impact of these modalities on tissue healing.

## APPLICATION OF ACOUSTIC ENERGY: ULTRASOUND

**Ultrasound** differs from the modalities discussed in the previous three chapters in that it transmits energy that falls within the acoustic, rather than electromagnetic, spectrum. Ultrasound is used in medicine for imaging and for loosening joint replacements requiring revision, as well as for therapeutic benefits. Different frequencies of ultrasound are used for each application. The ultrasound units used in athletic training and physical therapy emit sound energy at frequencies between 800 KHz (800,000 Hz) and 3 MHz (3,000,000 Hz). Modern high-quality ultrasound units can transmit sound waves at frequencies of 1 and 3 MHz. Some units are adjustable to 1, 2, and 3 MHz (figure 11.1). The importance of frequency and the applications of ultrasound at various frequencies will be discussed in detail. Initially, it is important to understand that therapeutic ultrasound uses acoustic energy, delivered at very specific high frequencies, for therapeutic purposes.

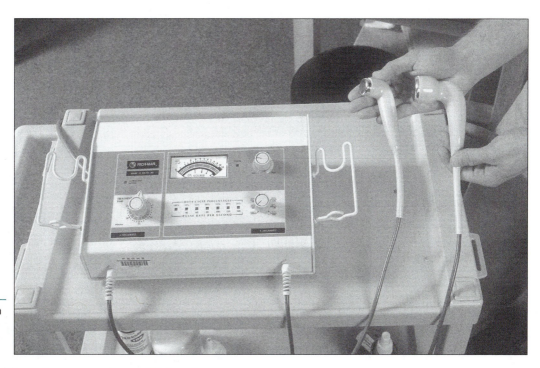

**Figure 11.1** Modern ultrasound unit with multiple frequencies and sound heads.

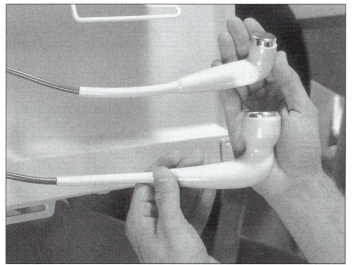

**Figure 11.2** Components of an ultrasound unit.

Ultrasound machines use electrical current to create a mechanical vibration in a crystalline material housed in the "head" of the unit. Vibration of the crystalline material produces a wave of acoustic energy (ultrasound) (figure 11.2). The crystalline material is usually lead zirconate titanate, although natural crystals and other synthetics have been used. The sound energy emitted from the ultrasound head travels through tissues and is absorbed.

Ultrasound is now used extensively for diagnostic imaging. Ultrasound of 1 MHz to 10 MHz is used to image deep structures such as the abdomen and superficial structures such as the eye, respectively. Ultrasound is also routinely used for prenatal examination. Through ultrasound, some correctable birth defects can be identified and the sex of the fetus can also be determined. The sound energy used for imaging differs in amplitude and pulse characteristics from that used for therapeutic purposes.

## Crystal Quality and Size: Beam Nonuniformity Ratio and Effective Radiating Area

Two terms describe the size and quality of an ultrasound crystal found in therapeutic ultrasound devices. **Effective radiating area (ERA)** is the area that receives at least 5% of the peak sound energy. This is essentially the size of the area to which sound energy is conducted when the head of the ultrasound unit contacts the skin. The ERA is somewhat smaller than the surface area of the sound head.

The beam of sound energy emitted from a crystal is not uniform but rather is characterized by areas of high intensity and lower intensity (figure 11.3). **Beam nonuniformity ratio (BNR)** is the ratio between the average intensity of the ultrasound beam across the ERA divided by the peak intensity of the ultrasound beam; the lower the BNR, the more uniform the intensity of the sound wave.

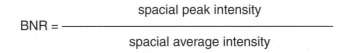

$$BNR = \frac{\text{spacial peak intensity}}{\text{spacial average intensity}}$$

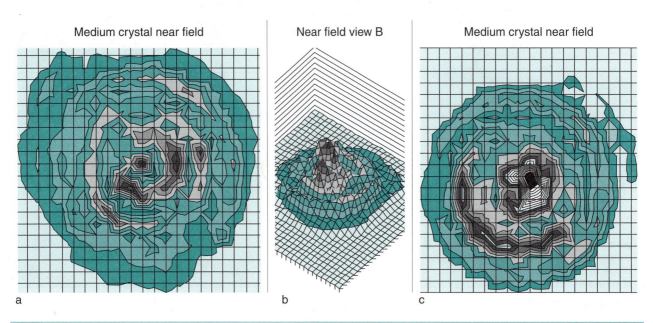

Medium crystal near field       Near field view B       Medium crystal near field

a                               b                       c

Figure 11.3   Beam scan of a crystal with a beam nonuniformity ratio (BNR) of 2.32, top view *(a)* and side view *(b)*. When tested on 40 subjects, the ultrasound transducer housing this crystal produced a very comfortable treatment at 1.5 to 2.0 W/cm². Beam scan of a crystal with a BNR of 7.75, top view *(c)*. When this was tested on 40 subjects, the ultrasound transducer housing the crystal produced an uncomfortable treatment at 1.5 W/cm², and was not tolerated at 2.0 W/cm².

Courtesy of Brigham Young University Sports Injury Research Center.

A low BNR minimizes the risk of developing "hot spots" and allows the certified athletic trainer to deliver higher doses of ultrasound without causing pain and discomfort. The BNR must be listed by the manufacturer on all units. Ideally, the BNR would be 1; however, this is impossible, and the acceptable range is between 2 and 6. Investigate the BNR before purchasing an ultrasound unit. A unit with a low BNR may be more expensive but will allow for greater comfort and safety and maximum delivery of sound energy.

Unfortunately, BNR and ERA may not adequately define how an ultrasound unit will function. Holcomb and Joyce (2003) reported that there were significant differences in the change in tissue temperature between two ultrasound units with a BNR of 3.7 and 2.3 and an ERA of 4.9 and 4.6 cm, respectively. These authors speculated that the area of peak intensity or peak area of the maximum beam nonuniformity ratio (PAMBNR) as described by Draper (1999) might explain why two ultrasound units differ in performance. Certainly a small spike of peak amplitude as illustrated in figure 11.4 will deliver less energy and therefore have less thermal effect than that provided by a larger area of peak amplitude. The issue of equipment performance and parameters is likely to be a central issue in the future study of the efficacy of treatment with ultrasound.

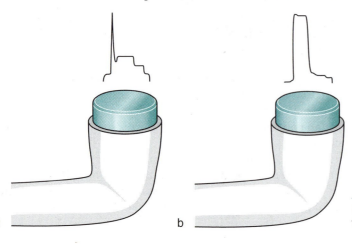

a       b

Figure 11.4   The area of peak intensity may affect the performance of ultrasound devices.

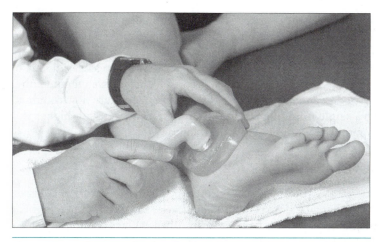

**Figure 11.5**  Ultrasound gel and gel pads.

## Conducting Media

Air is a poor conductor of ultrasound energy. To maximize delivery of sound energy to the tissues, a conducting medium must be used. Several substances have been used to conduct ultrasound, including ultrasound gel, gel pads, mineral oil, lotions, and water. The amount of sound energy conducted varies substantially between conducting media. Commercial ultrasound gel (Draper 1996; Draper et al. 1993; Klucinec et al. 2000) and gel pads (Klucinec et al. 2000; Klucinec 1996) (figure 11.5) are superior conducting media. Water is not a good conducting medium (Draper 1996; Draper et al. 1993; Klucinec et al. 2000; Klucinec 1996; Forrest and Rosen 1989, 1992), attenuating as much as 65% of the sound energy (Klucinec et al. 2000), and should not be used to administer therapeutic ultrasound. The conducting capacities of most gels and creams have not been established. However, some have been shown to be very poor conductors of sound energy (Draper 1996; Draper et al. 1993; Klucinec et al. 2000; Klucinec 1996; Forrest and Rosen 1989, 1992; Cameron and Monroe 1992). When applying ultrasound, use gels and gel pads known to be effective conductors.

## Parameters of Treatment With Ultrasound

As with electrotherapy, you can alter the treatment parameters of ultrasound depending on the desired effect. Fortunately, the number of adjustable parameters is smaller. You can control the amplitude of the sound waves and therefore the amount of sound energy being emitted from the sound head. The sound energy emitted by the crystal is measured in watts (W). The dose of sound energy delivered is based on the amount of energy being emitted divided by the radiating area of the crystal measured in square centimeters ($cm^2$). Thus, ultrasound dose is measured in W/cm2. You can also adjust the duty cycle, duration of treatment, and frequency.

Duty cycle refers to the process of interrupting delivery of the sound wave so that periods of sound wave emission are interspersed with periods of interruption. Figure 11.6 depicts pulsed and continuous ultrasound.

Often you can select between several duty cycles. Duty cycle is calculated by dividing the time during which sound is delivered by the total time the sound head is applied. For example, if ultrasound is transmitted for 150 ms out of every second of treatment, then the duty cycle is 150/1,000, or 15%. When the emission of sound energy is not interrupted, the duty cycle equals 100% and the ultrasound is referred to as continuous ultrasound.

Much has been learned regarding the treatment duration needed to elevate tissue temperatures to beneficial

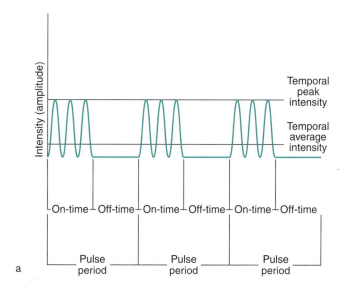

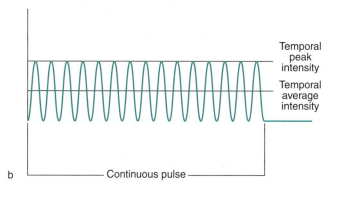

**Figure 11.6**  In pulsed ultrasound, energy is generated only during the "on" time *(a)*. Duty cycle is determined by the ratio of "on" time to pulse, in this case 50%. Continuous ultrasound is shown in *(b)*.

levels. An interaction among the frequency, dose, and treatment duration has also been found. Findings indicate that recipes for duration and intensities of ultrasound treatments used in the past do not increase tissue temperature sufficiently.

The frequency of the sound waves affects the depth at which the greatest amount of ultrasound energy is absorbed, as well as the time required to increase tissue temperature. Ultrasound units that allow for treatment with more than one frequency are now common, but some older units have a single fixed frequency of 1 MHz. Treatments with higher frequencies are often more appropriate for musculoskeletal injuries.

## Sound Energy Absorption in Tissues

The amount of acoustic energy absorbed by tissues is influenced by many factors. The tissue characteristics, as well as the frequency, dose (W/cm²), duty cycle, and duration of treatment with ultrasound, affect the amount of acoustic energy absorbed. When continuous ultrasound is delivered, the greater the energy absorption, the greater the tissue heating. Tissues with greater protein density have a higher rate of absorption, whereas tissues with a higher water content have lower absorption rates. Thus, tendon, ligament, and muscle tissue absorb more sound energy than skin and adipose tissue. Superficial bones and nerves absorb the most energy.

Ultrasound at a higher frequency (3 MHz) is absorbed more rapidly than that at a lower frequency (1 MHz) (figure 11.7). Therefore, ultrasound at higher frequencies affects tissues that are more superficial, whereas at a lower frequency less energy is absorbed superficially and more is available to penetrate into deeper tissues. Thus, if the goal of treatment is to heat the capsular tissue at a joint such as the elbow with ultrasound, you should use a 3-MHz frequency. Temperature increases of up to 8° have been reported with 3-MHz ultrasound at 1 W/cm² in 4 min in superficial tissues such as the patella tendon (Chan et al. 1998). If the target tissue is deeper, for example over the gastrocnemius-soleus complex, a lower frequency (1 MHz) is necessary; 10 min of continuous 1-MHz ultrasound at 2.0 will elevate temperature about 4° at a depth of 2.5 cm (Draper, Castel, and Castel 1995). The interactions between ultrasound parameters and thermal response are discussed further shortly.

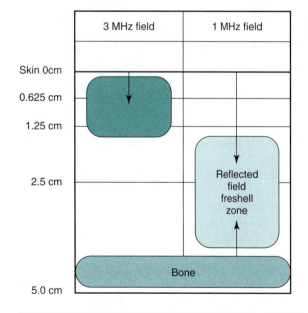

**Tissue penetration at 1 and 3 MHz based on actual measurement in human subjects**

**Figure 11.7**   Frequency and depth relationship.
Reprinted courtesy of Chris Castel.

## Thermal Effects of Ultrasound

Many of the benefits of ultrasound have been attributed to tissue heating. This section examines the effects of parameter adjustments on the thermal response to ultrasound. Draper (1996) suggested that an increase of 1° C (mild heating) increases metabolic activity; a 2° to 3° C increase reduces muscle spasm, increases blood flow, and reduces chronic inflammation; and a 4° C increase alters the viscoelastic properties of collagen.

An increase in temperature increases metabolic activity in deeper tissues. When these tissues are more active, the demand for oxygen is increased, which, in turn, increases local blood flow. Thus, one of the potential benefits of ultrasound is to increase local blood flow. The issues of tissue repair and treatment efficacy with ultrasound are discussed later in this chapter.

The analgesic and antispasmotic responses to ultrasound are not as great as those following cryotherapy, superficial heating, and transcutaneous electrical nerve stimulation (TENS) application. The primary effects of continuous ultrasound are increases in collagen elasticity in response to increased tissue temperature. By properly selecting treatment parameters you can increase temperature more than 4° in the target tissue.

### Duty Cycle and Tissue Heating

Continuous ultrasound results in therapeutically beneficial amounts of tissue heating. Pulsed ultrasound may have therapeutic benefits in certain circumstances (see "Efficacy of Ultrasound Therapy for Musculoskeletal Conditions" later in the chapter), but these effects are nonthermal. Certainly the sound energy delivered with a pulsed ultrasound treatment is absorbed into the tissues at depths determined by the frequency of the sound wave. However, the total energy delivered during pulsed ultrasound is less than with continuous ultrasound at the same intensity and duration. Thus, less local tissue heating occurs.

### Dose and Tissue Heating

The greater the dose of sound energy, the greater the amount of energy delivered to the tissues. Thus, with continuous ultrasound, a higher dose results in greater tissue heating in less time. Many clinicians administer ultrasound at a low dose, often 1.5 W/cm$^2$, because they were instructed in school to do so. This practice may have come about because older units caused discomfort at higher doses due to the characteristics of the crystal. Although higher doses of ultrasound, greater than 2.5 to 3.0 W/cm$^2$, can damage tissue, you should not limit the dose to 1.5 W/cm$^2$.

### Treatment Time and Tissue Heating

There is an interaction among frequency, dose, and the time required to increase tissue temperature. At a frequency of 3 MHz, 4 to 5 min is sufficient to achieve a 4° increase in local tissue temperature at a dose of 1.5 W/cm$^2$. However, when a 1-MHz frequency is applied, a 10-min treatment at a dose of 2.0 W/cm$^2$ is required to achieve the same increase in tissue temperature (Draper 1996; Draper, Castel, and Castel 1995). Although no minimum dose has been established for obtaining specific levels of heating, longer applications are needed when lower intensities of ultrasound are used. For example, a 1-MHz-frequency continuous ultrasound treatment at 1.5 W/cm$^2$ requires 12 min to increase tissue temperature 4° C as opposed to the 10 min needed at 2 W/cm$^2$ (Draper 1996) .

### Treatment Area, Sound Head Movement, and Tissue Heating

The parameters outlined in the previous sections to heat deeper tissues are predicated on treatment over an area no greater than three times the ERA of the crystal and a slow, controlled movement of the ultrasound head (figure 11.8). When larger areas are treated, the amount of acoustic energy reaching any single area is decreased. In addition, heat buildup is allowed to dissipate from the target tissue. Thus, there is less temperature increase during treatment and therefore less change in tissue elasticity and local blood flow during and after treatment.

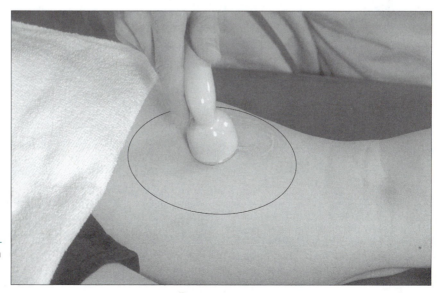

**Figure 11.8** Treating an area two to three times the effective radiating area.

Treating larger areas such as the lower back has little or no effect on the tissues, although there may be a placebo effect. Thus, ultrasound should not be applied over large areas. Currently, the best recommendation for treatment technique suggests covering a treatment area two to three times the area of the ERA with the sound head covering less than 2 in./sec.

Moving the sound head slowly prevents hot spots from developing in areas of peak amplitude and helps you maintain good contact with the skin or gel pad surface. With higher-quality, lower BNR rating crystals, the sound head can be moved more slowly, resulting in a more uniform heating and greater patient comfort. Rapid, sloppy movement of the sound head with frequent breaks in contact between the skin or gel pad decreases the thermal response to treatment.

### Tissue Cooling

Tissue temperatures fall fairly rapidly following ultrasound therapy. Draper and Ricard (1995) reported that when 3-MHz ultrasound was used to heat muscle tissue at the depth of 1.2 cm to an average of 5.3°, the tissue cooled 2° within the first 3.5 min. Rose et al. (1996) reported that tissues at 2.5 and 5 cm deep heating 4° by 1-MHz continuous ultrasound cooled 2° in less than 7 min. From these studies it is apparent that the thermal response to ultrasound is short-lived and that superficial tissues cool more rapidly than deeper ones. Thus, any stretching or manual therapies should be performed immediately following treatment, or even initiated in the last few minutes of treatment when possible, if the benefits of heating from ultrasound are to be realized.

## Nonthermal Effects of Ultrasound

When ultrasound is pulsed, very little heating occurs. However, pulsed ultrasound has been shown to affect tissue healing in some circumstances and alter cellular activity in vitro. From this work it can be concluded that some of the responses to ultrasound cannot be attributed to a thermal response. This section discusses the nonthermal effects of ultrasound and reviews the demonstrated clinical benefits of pulsed ultrasound.

### Acoustical Streaming and Stable Cavitation

The literature related to the nonthermal benefits of ultrasound attributes most of the effects to acoustical streaming and **stable** cavitation (figure 11.9). Acoustical streaming is the movement of fluids along cell membranes due to the mechanical pressure exerted by the sound waves. The movement occurs only in the direction of the sound wave. Acoustical streaming facilitates fluid movement and increases cell membrane permeability.

**Cavitation** is the formation of gas-filled bubbles. Ultrasound produces pressure changes in tissue fluids that create the bubbles and cause them to expand and contract. Stable cavitation refers to a rhythmic cycle of expansion and contraction during repeated pressure changes over many acoustic cycles. Unstable cavitation refers to a collapse of the gas bubbles. Unstable cavitation, which is most associated with low-frequency, high-intensity sound waves, is believed to damage tissues. Stable cavitation, which occurs with therapeutic ultrasound, is thought to facilitate fluid movement and membrane transport.

The increased movement of fluid and dissolved nutrients to and across cell membranes is believed to be the mechanism by which pulsed ultrasound facilitates tissue repair. Certainly acoustical streaming and stable cavitation also occur during continuous ultrasound. Continuous ultrasound, as noted previously, is usually applied to heat tissues prior to stretching or manual therapy.

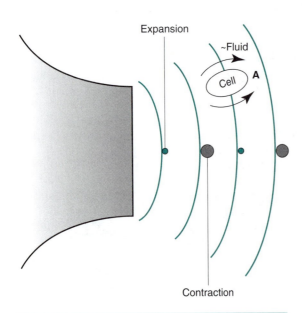

**Figure 11.9** Acoustical streaming and cavitation. Acoustical streaming is the movement of fluids around cells by sound waves. Cavitation is the expansion and contraction of air bubbles because of pressure changes in surrounding fluid due to acoustic energy.

### *Acute Injury and Tissue Healing*

Research on the impact of ultrasound in acute injury and tissue repair has been limited to animal models. The application of pulsed ultrasound has been studied following silver nitrate-induced inflammation in animal models. Pulsed ultrasound treatments of 2 to 4 min at low doses may transiently decrease capillary leakage (Fyfe and Chahl 1980). However, greater leakage of plasma over 24 h followed by a more rapid resolution of effusion has also been reported by the same investigators (Fyfe and Chahl 1985). The mechanism by which pulsed ultrasound affects swelling has not been fully explained, and much more study of mechanism and dose response is needed before pulsed ultrasound is routinely used following acute soft tissue injury.

In animal studies, investigators have found that after treatments with pulsed ultrasound, tissue repair is expedited (Dyson and Pond 1970) and tensile strength of healing tissues increased (Dyson and Pond 1970; Enwemeka, Rodriquez, and Mendosa 1989; Friedar 1988; da Cunha, Parizotto, and Vidal Bde 2001). Takakura et al. (2002) reported that pulsed ultrasound enhanced early repair of medial collateral ligament injuries in rats but did not result in improved load to failure, stiffness, or energy absorption at 3 weeks into the healing process. Saini, Roy, and Singh (2002), however, reported that 10 min of 0.5 W/cm$^2$ of continuous ultrasound on the third postoperative day and continuing for 10 days resulted in differences in repair of severed Achilles tendons in a small sample of dogs until 120 days postoperatively. Treated animals also subjectively recovered from lameness more rapidly. None of the findings from these reports have been replicated in humans. Thus, at this time the optimal treatment parameters and cost benefit of ultrasound treatments following acute musculoskeletal injuries are unknown.

Further investigation of these issues is clearly warranted. Low doses of ultrasound may promote mast cell degranulation and speed the completion of acute inflammation, limit capillary leakiness, and promote collagen synthesis during the repair phase. Excessive exposure may result in tissue breakdown and prolong the acute inflammatory response. In closed wounds, sprains, strains, and fractures, the precise amount of sound energy reaching the damaged tissues is not known. However, when using pulsed ultrasound to treat acute injuries, proceed with caution. Too little is better than too much sound energy.

### *Chronic, Slow-to-Heal Skin Ulcers*

The treatment of chronic, slow-to-heal, and nonhealing ulcers is frustrating and expensive. In the past 10 to 20 years, clinicians have found that low doses of sound, electrical energy, and light energy appear to speed healing in many cases. Reports on the use of pulsed ultrasound in treating human patients with chronic ulcers suggest that pulsed ultrasound has a physiological impact (Callam, Harper, and Dale 1987; Dyson and Suckling 1978; Erikson, Lundeberg, and Malm 1991). However, the subjects of these studies differ from healthy athletes in many respects, and we must use caution in generalizing these results to the treatment of musculoskeletal injuries.

## Contraindications to Ultrasound

Ultrasound is a relatively safe, easy-to-use therapeutic modality with few contraindications. Of greatest concern is the use of ultrasound in individuals with cancer and the impact of ultrasound on fetal development. Ultrasound has been reported to promote growth (Sicard-Rosenbaum et al. 1995), and perhaps metastasis, of malignant cells in laboratory animals and should not be used near tumors. The impact of therapeutic ultrasound on fetal development in humans is not fully known. Thus, therapeutic ultrasound should not be applied near the abdomen during pregnancy or to women of childbearing age who could be pregnant. The energy delivered to the tissues with therapeutic ultrasound is much greater than with diagnostic ultrasound, a common practice during pregnancy. Ultrasound also should not be applied over an infection.

Despite considerable confusion in the literature over the years, ultrasound can be applied safely over metal implants such as plates and screws. Gersten (1958) and Lehman, Delateur, and Silverman (1966) concluded that it is safe to apply ultrasound over joint replacements that contain metal and synthetics such as polyethelene and are held in place by methyl methacrylate cement. However, because low-frequency ultrasound is used to loosen prostheses for removal and revision, and because the long-term impact of ultrasound on joint replacements is not fully known, it should not be used over joint replacements.

Ultrasound should not be applied over the heart or in the area of a cardiac pacemaker. Ultrasound should also not be applied over the eyes or genitalia. The use of ultrasound directly over open epiphyses should be minimized, because the impact of such exposure is not fully known and may involve accelerated closure of epiphyses. However, adolescents and children rarely experience problems for which ultrasound is indicated. Ultrasound is often used to treat back conditions. The use of ultrasound should be restricted to an area no more than three to four times the ERA to increase tissue temperature to therapeutic levels. Exposure of the spinal cord to ultrasound should be minimized. In patients who have had a laminectomy, do not apply ultrasound directly over the area of the cord that is no longer protected by bone. Although these precautions and contraindications should be observed, they rarely affect the selection of ultrasound as a therapeutic modality.

## Phonophoresis

Phonophoresis is similar to iontophoresis, discussed in the previous chapters, in that a modality is applied to drive medications into the tissues. Phonophoresis utilizes sound energy, as opposed to electromagnetic energy, to drive the medication; thus, the medications driven into the tissues do not possess an electrical charge in solution.

Hydrocortisone is one of the medications administered with phonophoresis by certified athletic trainers and other health care providers. The medication is often mixed in a cream. Unfortunately, many of the creams, gels, and ointments used to administer hydrocortisone with phonophoresis are poor conductors of ultrasound energy (Cameron and Monroe 1992). If you choose to use phonophoresis, use only commercial preparations in which hydrocortisone or other active ingredient is mixed in a gel that is known to be a good conductor of acoustic energy. Cagnie et al. (2003), for example, found that phonophoresis enhanced delivery of ketoprofen (a nonsteroidal anti-inflammatory medication) into synovial tissues when mixed in Fastum gel (Industrie Farmaceutiche Riunite srl, Florence, Italy). These investigators found higher levels of ketoprofen following ultrasound at a frequency of 1 MHz at 1.5 W/cm$^2$ at a 20% duty cycle for 5 min than with continuous ultrasound. Ketoprofen levels were higher in synovial than in adipose tissues, and little change in plasma concentrations was observed within 120 min of application.

Perhaps the greatest similarity between phonophoresis and iontophoresis is the lack of evidence concerning efficacy. Very little research evidence supports the practice of phonophoresis. The work of Griffin et al. (1967; Griffin and Touchstone 1972) is perhaps most commonly cited as evidence of the efficacy of phonophoresis in treating musculoskeletal conditions. However, the benefits of phonophoresis observed by Griffin may have been due to placebo, because more recent studies have questioned the bioavailability of phoresed medications and the efficacy of phonophoresis (Darrow et al. 1999; Cicone, Leggin, and Callamaro 1991; Oziomek, Perrin, and Harrold 1991) and shown that phonophoresis (pulsed) did not affect responses to therapy consisting of cryotherapy and exercise in the treatment of tendinopathy (Penderghest, Kimura, and Gulick 1998). As noted by Cagnie et al. (2003), "Changes in tissue levels of drugs used in phonophoresis do not necessarily indicate that a particular drug will have a therapeutic effect."

As with iontophoresis, the exact amount of medication reaching target tissues following phonophoresis is often unknown. Thus, the clinician does not know whether a pharmacologically effective dose of medication has been administered. The concerns regarding the pathophysiology of the tissue raised in the discussion of iontophoresis also should be considered in connection with the use of phonophoresis.

Iontophoresis and phonophoresis have potential as medication delivery mechanisms in several areas of health care. However, much more work must be done to identify conditions that may respond to treatments. Additionally the optimal parameters needed for delivery of particular medications must be established. Finally, the efficacy of treatments must be investigated through clinical trials before continued use of these treatments by certified athletic trainers is warranted.

# EFFICACY OF ULTRASOUND THERAPY FOR MUSCULOSKELETAL CONDITIONS

The use of ultrasound in the treatment of musculoskeletal conditions has been studied through clinical trials, allowing for the preparation of several systematic reviews. Several more will likely be available once this edition is printed. A search of the Physiotherapy Evidence Database using the search term "ultrasound" revealed more than 10 systematic reviews or meta-analysis reports related to ultrasound in the treatment of arthritic and soft tissue conditions. Numerous clinical trials are also referenced.

It is not possible to review all of these reports in this chapter. To summarize, as of this writing there is a lack of evidence to support the use of ultrasound in the treatment of several musculoskeletal conditions. Systematic reviews have concluded that there is a lack of evidence to support the use of ultrasound in the treatment of patellofemoral pain syndrome (Brosseau 2001), osteoarthritis of the knee (Welch et al. 2001), acute ankle sprain (Van der Windt 2002), or plantar heel pain (plantar fasciitis) (Crawford, Atkins, and Edwards 2000). Randomized controlled clinical trials have shown a lack of benefit from ultrasound therapy for lateral epicondylalgia (tennis elbow) (Hacker and Lundeberg 1991), generalized shoulder pain (pulsed ultrasound) (Nykanen 1995), acute lateral ligament sprains of the ankle (Nyanzi et al. 1999), and subacromial bursitis (Downing and Weinstein 1986).

From a broader perspective, reports by Gam and Johannsen (1995), Van der Windt et al. (1999), and Robertson and Baker ( 2001) concluded that there is a lack of evidence to substantiate the use of ultrasound in treating musculoskeletal disorders. Robertson and Baker summarized the issue well when they wrote, "There is little evidence that active therapeutic ultrasound is more effective than placebo ultrasound for treating people with pain or a range of musculoskeletal disorders or for promoting soft tissue healing."

Does this lack of evidence mean that the reader should disregard all of the information in the earlier sections of this chapter? Draper (2002), in a letter to the editor in response to the paper by Robertson and Baker (2001), pointed out that the investigators in several studies included in this review employed inappropriate treatment parameters. In fact, two well-controlled clinical trials have shown that pulsed ultrasound improves treatment outcome for patients with calcific tendinitis of the shoulder and carpal tunnel syndrome. Ebenbichler et al. (1999) used ultrasound at 0.89 MHz, 20% duty cycle, at 2.5 $W/cm^2$ for 15 min, five times per week for 3 weeks and then three times per week for 3 weeks in patients with calcific tendinitis. At 9-month follow-up, resolution of the calcific lesion was found in 42% of patients treated with active ultrasound and in only 8% treated with placebo. Reduction in the calcific mass was found in a further 23% of the treated patients as compared to 12% of the placebo-treated group. Ebenbichler et al. (1999) applied 1-MHz ultrasound at 1 $W/cm^2$, 20% duty cycle, for 15 min five times per week for 2 weeks and then twice per week for 5 weeks in patients with carpal tunnel syndrome. Those receiving ultrasound had less pain and more normal electrodiagnostic studies at 6-month follow-up.

Furthermore, there is little evidence on which to make decisions regarding the use of ultrasound prior to tissue mobilization or stretching when range of motion is restricted. Draper et al. (1998) reported greater gains in dorsiflexion range of motion immediately following treatment in subjects receiving continuous ultrasound prior to stretching. However, after 10 treatments distributed over 5 days there were no differences between subjects treated with ultrasound and those who just performed stretching. Draper (personal communication 2003) has reported success in improving long-standing motion restrictions at the elbow when ultrasound or diathermy (discussed later in this chapter) is applied prior to joint mobilization. These results are important because (1) previous interventions had failed to reverse substantial limitations in functional range of motion; and (2) once restored, the motion gains were maintained. These results strongly suggest that ultrasound may be a beneficial adjunct to stretching and manual therapy in patients with motion restriction. Thus, the issue with the application of ultrasound and diathermy, as well as other modalities, is appropriate patient selection. Future clinical trials and case series reports will better guide decisions regarding ultrasound administration.

In summary, ultrasound should not be abandoned completely as a therapeutic modality. However, the liberal use of ultrasound in the management of a multitude of conditions without replicating parameters shown to produce results cannot continue either. Further research is clearly warranted to identify how this modality can be used to effectively treat athletes and others with musculoskeletal injuries.

# APPLICATION OF ELECTROMAGNETIC ENERGY: DIATHERMY AND PULSED ELECTROMAGNETIC FIELDS

Electromagnetic fields are found in two applications in the treatment of musculoskeletal injuries: diathermy and pulsed electromagnetic fields (PEMFs). The same principles apply to each application. The difference is that diathermy involves heating of tissues and PEMFs result in no tissue heating. The next two sections describe how heat is generated when diathermy is applied as well as explain why PEMFs do not cause heating.

## Diathermy

Diathermy is the therapeutic generation of local heating by high-frequency electromagnetic waves. Most diathermy units are classified as short-wave diathermy and generate an alternating current at 27.12 MHz. When the body is placed in an electric field, known as the capacitance technique, heating occurs due to the rapid rotation of **dipoles** (structures with positive and negative poles) (figure 11.10). As the current alternates between positive and negative, the dipoles rotate to align with the electric field. The mechanical friction and the movement of electrons result in local heating. Tissues with large numbers of dipoles, such as skin and muscle, have a greater capacitance to store an electrical charge. Thus, more current must be generated to cause dipole motion in these tissues. The greatest heating occurs in tissues with fewer dipoles, particularly fatty tissues. Thus, capacitance technique diathermy heats the subcutaneous fat more than the underlying muscle.

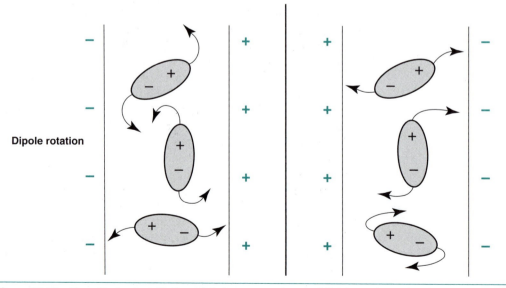

**Figure 11.10**    The effects of oscillating high-frequency electrical fields on the molecules and ions of the tissues. This figure shows dipole rotation; polar molecules rotate as the electrical field oscillates.

Reprinted by permission from Low and Reed.

Heating of tissue in a magnetic field, also known as the inductance technique, differs in that the body is not placed in an electrical field. Instead, magnetic waves are generated as an electrical current is driven through a coiled wire (figure 11.11). The magnetic field creates small currents in the tissues. The greatest heating occurs in tissue with low impedance, especially muscle. Thus, inductance technique is preferable for heating deeper tissues.

Like ultrasound, diathermy is effective for heating deeper tissues, but it can heat larger areas. Unlike ultrasound, pulsed diathermy can heat the deep tissues 3° to 4° C (Draper et al. 1999), although intra-articular temperatures rise to a lesser extent (Oosterveld et al. 1992). However, diathermy units are expensive and can be used on only one person at a time. In addition, diathermy carries a number of precautions and contraindications. All metal should be removed from the patient. In the past, metal implants and cardiac pacemakers were considered absolute contraindications for treatment with diathermy. Draper (personal communication 2003) has reported no adverse effects following the use of pulse diathermy (800 pulses per second [pps], 40-μs pulses) over metallic fixation of fractures around the elbow. Thus, the presence of metal should not be considered an absolute contraindication to the use of diathermy, but caution is advised until the range of safe parameters is better established. Diathermy must not be used near the uterus of a pregnant woman or near the abdomen or back of a woman of childbearing age who could be pregnant. Finally, diathermy should not be used on individuals with infections; acute inflammation; moist, open wounds; malignant tumors; or large joint effusions (table 11.1).

## Pulsed Electromagnetic Fields

Although diathermy is used on a limited basis in athletic training, the underlying technology has been used to promote tissue healing. Like ultrasound, diathermy can be pulsed to decrease the total energy transmitted to the tissues. Pulsed short-wave diathermy can be adjusted to provide a thermal response or to produce no tissue heating. When short-wave diathermy is adjusted to a low frequency (less than 600 pps) with a short phase duration (65 μs) into the nonthermal range, it is often classified as pulsed electromagnetic field (PEMF) or pulsed radio frequency energy (PRFE). This reclassification is important because diathermy implies heating, whereas the labels PEMF and PRFE imply a nonthermal therapy.

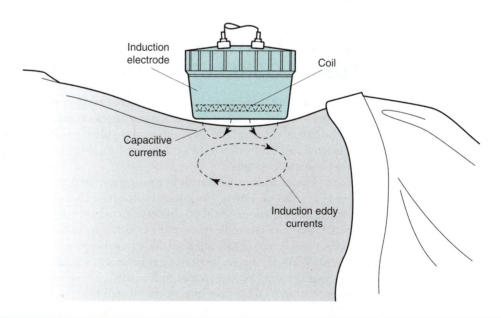

**Figure 11.11** With magnetic field diathermy applicators, eddy currents are induced in the tissues having highest conductivity.

**Table 11.1   Indications and Contraindications for Ultrasound and Diathermy**

| | Indications | Contraindications |
|---|---|---|
| **Ultrasound** | | |
| Continuous | Heat protein-rich, deeper tissue<br><br>Increase blood flow in deep tissues | Application over cardiac pacemaker, eyes, genitalia, joint replacements<br><br>Pregnancy<br><br>Cancer<br><br>Infection<br><br>Acute inflammation<br><br>Minimize exposure over open epiphyses and spinal cord |
| Pulsed | May speed repair in slow-to-heal wounds, including nonunion fractures and tendinopathy | Application over cardiac pacemaker, eyes, genitalia, joint replacements<br><br>Pregnancy<br><br>Cancer<br><br>Infection<br><br>Minimize exposure over open epiphyses and spinal cord |
| **Diathermy** | | |
| Continuous and pulsed | Heat large area of deeper tissue<br><br>Increase blood flow in deep tissues<br><br>Decrease pain and muscle spasm | Application over cardiac pacemaker, eyes, genitalia, joint replacements, and metal implants<br><br>Pregnancy<br><br>Open wounds<br><br>Cancer<br><br>Infection<br><br>Acute inflammation and joint effusion |

# EFFICACY OF DIATHERMY AND PEMF THERAPY FOR MUSCULOSKELETAL CONDITIONS

There are far fewer clinical trials and systematic reviews related to the application of diathermy than of ultrasound. No systematic reviews on diathermy were located in a search of the Cochrane database and Physiotherapy Evidence Database. Belanger's text identified reports from five controlled trials of diathermy on osteoarthritis (OA), three on neck pain, and three on ankle sprains.

None of the trials showed benefit in treating sprained ankles with diathermy (Pasila 1978; Barker 1985; McGill 1998). The conclusions of the studies on patients with OA were contradictory, although none of the studies conducted after 1970 (Clarke 1974; Svarcova 1990; Moffett 1996) were favorable to the use of diathermy in the treatment of OA.

McCray and Patton (1984) reported decreased trigger point sensitivity following diathermy treatment. While the longevity of this improvement was not addressed, a decrease in trigger point sensitivity may allow patients with myofascial pain to complete therapeutic exercise regimens central to their plan of care that would otherwise be painful. Foley-Nolan et al. (1990, 1992) reported less pain and greater cervical range of motion in patients with chronic (>8 weeks) neck pain and whiplash. These patients were treated, however, with nonthermal levels of PEMF. Thus, there is little evidence that diathermy enhances treatment outcomes in patients with musculoskeletal conditions. As noted in the discussion of ultrasound, this is not a reason to abandon all consideration of diathermy but rather indicates the need for clinical trials to identify situations in which treatment with diathermy will enhance care.

Draper et al. (2004) reported substantially greater gains in hamstring flexibility following 15-min treatments with 27.12-MHz diathermy pulsed at 800 bursts per second with 400-μs burst duration. Subjects received treatments for 5 days and retained substantially more flexibility at 3 days after the final treatment than subjects who completed the same stretching protocol without diathermy treatment. These results suggest that diathermy enhances treatments directed at soft tissue stretching.

Pulsed electromagnetic field therapy has been investigated with regard to tissue healing, with some studies suggesting that PEMF may speed wound healing (Brown and Baker 1987; Goldon et al. 1981; Itoh et al. 1991) and fracture healing. However, not all reports agree, and the use of PEMF in treating soft tissue injuries warrants further investigation. At present there is not enough information to recommend PEMF in the treatment of soft tissue injuries sustained by athletes.

## STIMULATION OF FRACTURE HEALING

In the past several years, the use of PEMF and pulsed ultrasound to treat nonunion and acute fractures has increased. Although more research is needed, there is evidence that these modalities can promote healing of nonunion fractures (Bassett 1984; Heckman, Ryaby, and McCabe 1994; Holmes 1994; Sharrard 1990), and the use of these treatments in sports medicine has increased. You should understand the physical properties of these units and stay up to date as the technology evolves, in case a "bone stimulator" (figure 11.12) is prescribed for your client.

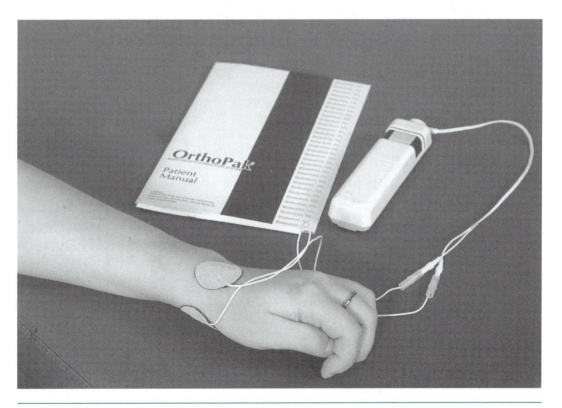

**Figure 11.12** Bone-stimulating unit.

## SUMMARY

1. Describe how therapeutic ultrasound is generated by the treatment unit.

   Ultrasound is generated through vibration of a crystal in an electrical circuit with alternating current. The rapid vibration of the crystal generates the emission of sound waves that are directed into tissues to achieve therapeutic effects.

2. Define BNR and ERA.

   BNR and ERA stand for beam nonuniformity ratio and effective radiating area, respectively. Because the crystals used in ultrasound equipment are not perfectly uniform, some parts of a crystal emit more sound energy than others. BNR is a ratio of the peak sound energy emitted from an ultrasound head divided by the average intensity emitted over the entire radiating area. ERA is simply the area of the crystal that emits at least 5% of the peak sound energy produced by the crystal.

3. Identify and describe the use of effective conducting media for ultrasound treatments.

   Because air is a poor conductor of ultrasound energy, a conducting medium must be used between the ultrasound head and the skin. Commercial ultrasound gels are designed to transmit ultrasound energy. Ultrasound gel is inexpensive and clearly the best transmitter of sound energy. Other conducting media, such as mineral oil, have been used but are substantially less efficient. A water bath has been recommended for ultrasound treatment over uneven surfaces such as the knuckles of the hand. Water, however, is also a poor conductor of high-frequency sound energy. Uneven surfaces are best treated with a gel pad, with ultrasound gel placed between the sound head and the pad and between the pad and the skin.

4. Define dose, duty cycle, treatment duration, and frequency as parameters of therapeutic ultrasound.

   Ultrasound dose is measured in watts of energy over the ERA, or $W/cm^2$. The frequency of therapeutic ultrasound ranges from 0.8 to 3 MHz, with higher frequency (3 MHz) used to treat more superficial tissues. When pulsed ultrasound is used, the duty cycle refers to the amount of time ultrasound is transmitted in relation to total treatment time. For example, a 20-ms burst of ultrasound followed by an 80-ms interruption would create a 20% duty cycle. Treatment duration is simply the length of time an ultrasound treatment is applied. To achieve optimal increases in tissue temperature, a longer (8-10 min) treatment of continuous (no duty cycle) ultrasound is required at 1 MHz than at 3 MHz (4-5 min).

5. Describe the thermal effects of therapeutic ultrasound.

   When 8 to 10 min of continuous 1-MHz ultrasound is delivered, temperature increases 4° in deeper (2.5-5 cm) tissues. A similar increase in temperature can be achieved at 1 to 2.5 cm with 4 to 5 min of continuous 3-MHz ultrasound.

6. Describe the treatment parameters and physiological effects of pulsed ultrasound.

   The primary parameter of pulsed ultrasound is duty cycle, which may vary from 10% to 90%. Pulsed ultrasound has been shown to increase the metabolic activity of fibroblasts in vitro and to speed healing of slow-to-heal skin lesions such as decubitus ulcers.

7. Discuss the technique and efficacy of phonophoresis.

   Phonophoresis is the use of ultrasound energy to drive medications through the skin. Although some studies have reported that medication can be driven through the skin, it is unknown whether pharmacologically effective doses can be delivered. There is little evidence that phonophoresis is clinically effective in treating musculoskeletal conditions.

8. Identify contraindications and precautions for treatment with therapeutic ultrasound.

> Ultrasound is contraindicated in individuals with cancer, infection, or acute inflammation or in those who are pregnant. Ultrasound should not be applied over the eyes, the genitalia, joint replacements, or cardiac pacemakers. Exposure over the spinal cord and epiphyses should be minimized.

9. Identify indications of treatment with therapeutic ultrasound.

> Continuous ultrasound is indicated when the certified athletic trainer wants to heat deep tissues. Heating will increase blood flow to the tissues and make them more elastic and less viscous. Thus, ultrasound is commonly used before manual therapies and stretching. Pulsed ultrasound may be used to treat slow-to-heal skin wounds and with special devices in the treatment of nonunion fractures.

10. Describe the differences between therapeutic ultrasound and diathermy.

> Diathermy heats deep tissues with electromagnetic energy as opposed to acoustic energy. Modern diathermy units are considerably more expensive than ultrasound but have similar heating effects and can heat larger areas of tissue.

11. Identify the two mechanisms through which diathermy can be used to heat deep tissues.

> Diathermy can heat tissues via a capacitance technique in which the individual becomes part of an alternating-current electrical field. The continuous reversal of the position of dipoles (structures with positive and negative poles) creates friction and therefore heat. Diathermy can also heat tissue via an inductance technique. When an electrical current is passed through a wire, magnetic or eddy currents are generated. This technique brings about the greatest heating in tissues with low impedance, such as muscle.

12. Identify the contraindications and precautions for the application of diathermy.

> In general, diathermy has the same contraindications as ultrasound. In addition, diathermy cannot be used over metal implants or open wounds.

13. Describe the potential uses of pulsed electromagnetic field therapy in athletic training and other allied medical fields.

> Pulsed electromagnetic fields (PEMF) are used to treat nonunion and acute fractures; PEMF may also speed healing following injury or surgery to tendons and ligaments and may relieve persistent pain. More study is needed to determine the best use of PEMF in treating musculoskeletal injuries.

## CITED SOURCES

Barker AT, Barlow PS, Porter J, Smith ME, Clifton S, Andrews L, O'Dowd WJ: A double-blind clinical trial of low-power pulsed short wave therapy in the treatment of a soft tissue injury. *Physiotherapy* 71:500-504, 1985.

Bassett CA: The development and application of pulsed electromagnetic fields (PEMFs) for ununited fractures and arthrodeses. *Orthop Clin North Am* 15:61-87, 1984.

Belanger AY: Evidence-based Guide to Therapeutic Physical Agents. Philadelphia, PA. Lippincott Williams & Wilkins, 175-176, 2002.

Brosseau L, Casimiro L, Robinson V, Milne S, Shea B, Judd M, Wells G, Tugwell P: Therapeutic ultrasound for treating patellofemoral pain. *The Cochrane Library* 4, 2001.

Brown M, Baker RD: Effect of pulsed shortwave diathermy on skeletal muscle injury in rabbits. *Phys Ther* 67:208-214, 1987.

Cagnie B, Vinck E, Rimbaut S, Vanderstraeten G: Phonophoresis versus topical applications of ketoprofen: Comparison between tissue and plasma levels. *Phys Ther* 83:707-712, 2003.

Callam MJ, Harper DR, Dale JJ: A controlled trial of weekly ultrasound therapy in chronic leg ulceration. *Lancet* 2:204-206, 1987.

Cameron MH, Monroe LG: Relative transmission of ultrasound by media customarily used by phonophoresis. *Phys Ther* 72:142-148, 1992.

Chan AK, Myrer JW, Measom GJ, Draper DO: Temperature changes in human patella tendon in response to therapeutic ultrasound. *J Athl Train* 33:130-135, 1998.

Cicone CD, Leggin BG, Callamaro JJ: The effects of ultrasound on trolamine salicylate phonophoresis on delayed onset muscle soreness. *Phys Ther* 71:666-675, 1991.

Clark GR, Willis LA, Stenners L, Nichols PJ. Evaluation of physiotherapu in the treatment of osteoarthritis of the knee. *Rheumatol Rehabil* 13:190-197, 1974.

Crawford F, Atkins D, Edwards J: Interventions for treating plantar heel pain. *The Cochrane Library* 3, 2000.

da Cunha A, Parizotto NA, Vidal Bde C: The effect of therapeutic ultrasound on repair of the achilles tendon (tendo achilles) of the rat. *Ultrasound Med Biol* 27:1691-1696, 2001.

Darrow H, Schulthies S, Draper D, Ricard M, Measom GJ: Serum dexamethasone levels after Decadron phonophoresis. *J Athl Train* 34:338-341, 1999.

Downing DS, Weinstein A: Ultrasound therapy of subacromial bursitis. A double blind trial. *Phys Ther* 66:194-199, 1986.

Draper DO: Ten mistakes commonly made with ultrasound use: Current research sheds lights on myths. *Athl Train Sports Health Care Persp* 2:95-107, 1996.

Draper DO: *A breakthrough on comfortable ultrasound treatments: Beam non-uniformity ratio is only half the equation.* Paper presented at Annual Meeting and Clinical Symposium of the National Athletic Trainers' Association, Kansas City, MO, June 18, 1999.

Draper DO, Anderson C, Schulthies SS, Richard MC. Immediate and residual changes in dorsiflexion range of motion using an ultrasound heat and stretch routine. *J Athl Train* 33;141-144, 1998.

Draper DO: Don't disregard ultrasound yet—the jury is still out. *Phys Ther* 82:190, 2002.

Draper DO, Castel JC, Castel D: Rates of temperature increase in human muscle during 1 MHz and 3 MHz continuous ultrasound. *J Orthop Sports Phys Ther* 22:142-150, 1995.

Draper DO, Castro JL, Feland B, Schulties S, Eggett D: Shortwave diathermy and prolonged stretching increase hamstring flexibility more than prolonged stretching alone. *J Orthop Sports Phys Ther* 34:13-20, 2004.

Draper DO, Knight KK, Fujiwara T, Castel JC: Temperature change in human muscle during and after pulsed short-wave diathermy. *J Orthop Sports Phys Ther* 29:13-22, 1999.

Draper DO, Ricard MD: Rate of temperature decay following 3 MHz ultrasound: The stretching window. *J Athl Train* 30:304-307, 1995.

Draper DO, Sunderland S, Kirkendall DT, Richard M: A comparison of temperature rise in human calf muscles following applications of underwater and topical gel ultrasound. *J Orthop Sports Phys Ther* 23:247-251, 1993.

Dyson M, Pond JB: The effect of pulsed ultrasound on tissue regeneration. *Physiotherapy* 64:105-108, 1970.

Dyson M, Suckling J: Stimulation of tissue repair by ultrasound: A survey of mechanisms involved. *Physiotherapy* 64:105-108, 1978.

Ebenbichler GR, Erdogmus CB, Resch KL, Funovics MA, Kainberger F, Barisani G, Aringer M, Nicolakis P, Weisinger GF, Baghestanian M, Preisinger E, Fialka-Moser V: Ultrasound therapy for calcific tendinitis of the shoulder. *N Engl J Med* 340:1533-1538, 1999.

Ebenbichler GR, Resch KL, Nicolakis P, Weisinger GF, Uhl F, Ghanem AH, Fialka V: Ultrasound treatment for treating the carpal tunnel syndrome: Randomized "sham" controlled study. *BMJ* 316: 731-735, 1998.

Enwemeka CS, Rodriquez O, Mendosa S: The effects of therapeutic ultrasound on tendon healing. *Am J Phys Med Rehabil* 6:283-287, 1989.

Erikson SV, Lundeberg T, Malm M: A placebo controlled trial of ultrasound in chronic leg ulceration. *Scand J Rehabil Med* 3:211-213, 1991.

Foley-Nolan D, Barry C, Coughlan RJ, O'Conner P, Rodeo D: Pulsed high frequency (27 MHz) electromagnetic therapy for persistent neck pain: A double blind, placebo controlled study of 20 patients. *Orthopedics* 13:445-451, 1990.

Foley-Nolan D, Moore K, Codd M, Barry C, O'Connor P, Coughlan RS. Low energy pulsed electromagmetic therapy for acute whiplash injuries. A double blind randomized controlled study. *Scand J Rehabil Med* 24:51-59,1992.

Forrest G, Rosen K: Ultrasound: Effectiveness of treatments given under water. *Arch Phys Med Rehabil* 70:28-29, 1989.

Forrest G, Rosen K: Ultrasound treatments in degassed water. *J Sport Rehab* 1:284-289, 1992.

Friedar S: A pilot study: The therapeutic effect of ultrasound following partial rupture of Achilles tendons in rats. *J Orthop Sports Phys Ther* 10:39-45, 1988.

Fyfe MC, Chahl LA: The effect of therapeutic ultrasound on experimental oedema in rats. *Ultrasound Med Biol* 6:107-111, 1980.

Fyfe MC, Chahl LA: The effect of single or repeated applications of "therapeutic" ultrasound on plasma extravasation during silver nitrate induced inflammation of the rat hindpaw ankle joint in vivo. *Ultrasound Med Biol* 11:273-283, 1985.

Gam AN, Johannsen F: Ultrasound therapy in musculoskeletal disorders: A meta-analysis. *Pain* 63: 85-91, 1995.

Gersten J: Effect of metallic objects on temperature rises produced in tissue by ultrasound. *Am J Phys Med* 37:75-82, 1958.

Goldon JH, Broadbent NRG, Nancarrow JD, Marshall T: The effects of Diapulse on the healing of wounds: A double blind randomized controlled trial in man. *Br J Plast Surg* 34:267-270, 1981.

Griffin JE, Echternach JL, Price RE, Touchstone JC: Patients treated with ultrasonic driven cortisone and with ultrasound alone. *Phys Ther* 44:20-27, 1967.

Griffin JE, Touchstone JC: Effects of ultrasonic frequency on phonophoresis of cortisol in swine tissue. *Am J Phys Med* 51:62-78, 1972.

Hacker E, Lundeberg T: Pulsed ultrasound treatment in lateral epicondylalgia. *Scand J Rehabil Med* 23:115-118, 1991.

Heckman J, Ryaby JP, McCabe R: Acceleration of tibial fracture-healing by noninvasive low-intensity pulsed ultrasound. *J Bone Joint Surg* 76:26-34, 1994.

Holcomb WR, Joyce CJ: A comparison of temperature increases produced by 2 commonly used ultrasound units. *J Athl Train* 38:24-27, 2003.

Holmes GB Jr. Treatment of delayed unions and nonunions of the proximal fifth metatarsal with pulsed elecromagnetic fields. *Foot Ankel Int* 15:552-556, 1994.

Itoh M, Montemayor Jr. JS, Matsumoto E, Eason A, Lee MH, Folk FS: Accelerated wound healing of pressure ulcers by pulsed high peak power electromagnetic energy (Diapulse). *Decubitus* 4:24-30, 1991.

Klucinec B: The effectiveness of the aquaflex gel pad in the transmission of acoustic energy. *J Athl Train* 31:313-317, 1996.

Klucinec B, Scheidler M, Denegar C, Domholt E, Burgess S: Transmissivity of common coupling agents used to deliver ultrasound through indirect methods. *J Orthop Sports Phys Ther* 30:263-269, 2000.

Kristiansen TK, Ryaby JP, McCabe J, Frey JJ, Roe LR: Accelerated healing of distal radial fractures with the use of specific, low-intensity ultrasound. A multicenter, prospective, randomized, double-blind, placebo-controlled study. *J Bone Joint Surg Am* 79:961-73, 1997.

Lehmann JF, Delateur B, Silverman DR: Selective heating effects of ultrasound in human beings. *Arch Phys Med Rehabil* 47:331-338, 1966.

Low J, Reed A. *Electrotherapy Explained*. Oxford, Butterworth- Heinemann Ltd. 1992, pg. 230.

McCray RE, Patton NJ. Pain relief at trigger points: A comparison of moist heat and shortwave diathermy. *J Orthop Sport Phys Ther* 5:175-178, 1984.

McGill SN: The effect of pulsed shortwave therapy on lateral ligament sprain of the ankle. *NZJ Physiother* 10:21-24, 1988.

Moffett JA, Richardson PH, Prost H, Osborn A. A placebo-controlled double blind trial to calculate the effectiveness of pulsed shortwave diathermy for osteoarthritic hip and knee pain. *Pain* 67:121-127, 1996.

Nyanzi CS, Langridge J, Heyworth JRC, Mani R: Randomized controlled study of ultrasound therapy in the management of acute lateral ligament sprains of the ankle joint. *Clin Rehabil* 31: 16-22, 1999.

Nykanen M: Pulsed ultrasound treatment of the painful shoulder: A randomized, double blind, placebo-controlled study. *Scand J Rehabil Med* 27:105-108, 1995.

Oosterveld FG, Rasker JJ, Jacobs JW, Overmars HJ: The effect of local heat and cold on the intraarticular and skin surfaces of the knee. *Arthritis Rheum* 35:146-151, 1992.

Oziomek RS, Perrin DH, Harrold DA, Denegar CR: Effect of ultrasound intensity and mode on serum salicylate levels following phonophoresis. *Med Sci Sports Exerc* 23:397-401, 1991.

Pasila M, Visuri T, Sundholm A: Pulsating shortwave diathermy: Value in treatment of recent ankle and foot sprains. *Arch Phys Med Rehab* 59:383-386, 1978.

Penderghest CE, Kimura IF, Gulick DT: Double-blind clinical efficacy study of pulsed phonophoresis on perceived pain associated with symptomatic tendinitis. *J Sport Rehab* 7:9-19, 1998.

Peppard A: Personal communication. Brockport, NY, 1977.

Robertson VJ, Baker KG: A review of therapeutic ultrasound: Effectiveness studies. *Phys Ther* 81: 1339-1350, 2001.

Rose S, Draper DO, Schulthies SS, Durant E: The stretching window part two: Rate of thermal decay in deep muscles following 1 MHz ultrasound. *J Athl Train* 31:139-143, 1996.

Saini NS, Roy KS, Bansal PS, Singh B, Simran PS: A preliminary study on the effect of ultrasound therapy on the healing of severed achilles tendons in five dogs. *J Vet Med A Physiol Pathol Clin Med* 49:321-328, 2002.

Sharrard WJW: A double blind trial of pulsed electromagnetic fields for delayed healing of tibial fractures. *J Bone Joint Surg* 72B:347-355, 1990.

Sicard-Rosenbaum L, Lord D, Danoff JV, Thom AK, Eckhaus MA: Effects of continuous therapeutic ultrasound on growth and metastasis of subcutaneous murine tumors. *Phys Ther* 75:3-11, 1995.

Svarcova J, Trnausky K, Zvarova J. The influence of ultrasound galvanic currents and shorwave diathermy on pain intensity in patients with osteoarthritis. *Scand J Reumatol Suppl* 67:83-85, 1987.

Takakura Y, Matsui N, Yoshiya S, Fujioka H, Muratsu H, Tsunoda M, Kurosaka M: Low-intensity pulsed ultrasound enhances early healing of medial collateral ligament injuries in rats. *J Ultrasound Med* 21:283-288, 2002.

Van der Windt DAWM, van der Heijden GJMG, van den Berg SGM, ter Riet G, de Winter AF, Bouter LM: Ultrasound therapy for musculoskeletal disorders: A systematic review. *Pain* 81:257-271, 1999.

Van der Windt DAWM, van der Heijden GJMG, van den Berg SGM, ter Riet G, de Winter AF, Bouter LM: Ultrasound therapy for acute ankle sprains. *The Cochrane Library* 1, 2002.

Welch V, Brosseau L, Peterson J, Shea B, Tugwell P, Wells G: Therapeutic ultrasound for osteoarthritis of the knee. *The Cochrane Library* 3, 2001.

## ADDITIONAL READINGS

Michlovitz SL: *Thermal Agents in Rehabilitation*, 3rd ed. Philadelphia, Davis, 1993.

Prentice WE: *Therapeutic Modalities for Allied Health Professionals*. New York, McGraw-Hill, 1998.

# CHAPTER 12

# Low-Level Laser Therapy

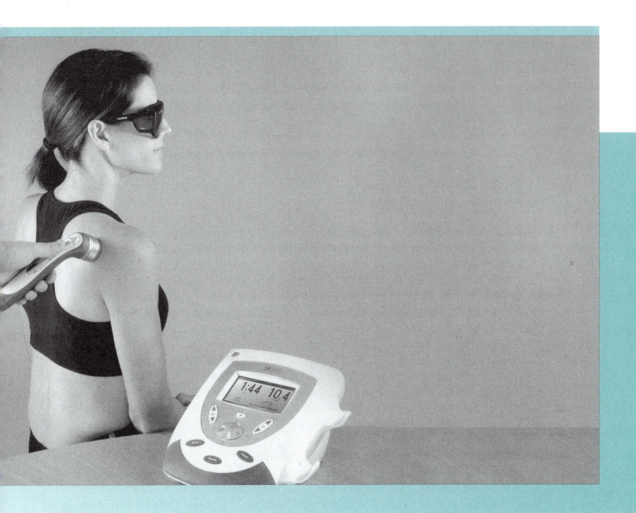

## Objectives

After reading this chapter, the student will be able to

1. understand the evolution of light therapy;
2. describe the unique characteristics of laser energy;
3. discuss the types of lasers available for soft tissue treatment and compare their energy outputs with respect to power, dosage modifications, wavelength, and pulse frequency;
4. perform a laser treatment using a commercially available device;
5. understand the biological effects of low-level laser therapy; and
6. describe the safety considerations and contraindications of low-level laser therapy.

A 60-year-old golfer is referred to the sports medicine clinic by an orthopedic surgeon for treatment of carpal tunnel syndrome. The surgeon has prescribed laser therapy in addition to therapeutic exercise. What is laser, how does it work, and when should it be used? These are the topics addressed in this chapter.

The recognition and application of light energy for healing are not new. Light has been associated with worship, superstitions, and healing powers throughout the ages since prehistoric times. The Phoenicians, early Hebrews, and Greeks had their sun god worship, and their reliance on the sun for health and healing (actinotherapy and heliotherapy) is well documented. When we think of light energy on biological tissues we can quickly appreciate the impact the sun has on photosynthesis and vision. These are two examples of biological processes that are dependent on the application and absorption of electromagnetic energy. Light energy has had numerous applications in health care throughout history, but as technological advancements occurred in medicine, its application diminished. Lasers are the most refined form of light energy and are now used extensively for medical and scientific purposes.

The use of lasers for soft tissue healing was discovered by accident. A Hungarian physician, Endre Mester, was researching the ability of ruby laser energy to destroy tumors in rats in the early 1960s (Mester et al. 1967). His laser was not nearly as powerful as he had originally thought; and as he applied this light energy, he noticed that the superficial surgical wounds he had imposed were healing faster than in the nontreated animals. Thus began the extensive investigation of using low-power lasers to heal soft tissue injury.

LASER is an acronym for light amplification of stimulated emission of radiation. Einstein conceptualized the laser in 1917, but the first working laser was not built until 1960 (Van Pelt et al. 1970). Lasers are commonplace now and are used in a variety of applications in fields such as communication, industry, and medicine. Therapeutic lasers used for wound healing and pain management have been called many things, including soft lasers, cold lasers, low-power lasers, low-intensity lasers, and biostimulators, to list a few. Presently, the most commonly utilized label to describe this type of therapy is low-level laser therapy (LLLT). The principal factor required to label this type of laser energy is that it does not raise the treated tissues above 36.5° C.

Low-level lasers have been used extensively in physical medicine throughout Europe and Canada for many years. Lasers were excluded in the first edition of this text because the Food and Drug Administration (FDA) had not approved the use of these devices for the treatment of musculoskeletal disorders in the United States. In 1999, however, the FDA started to evaluate Premarket Notifications 510(k) for these medical devices. The 510(k) approval is required for anyone who wants to market Class I, II, and some Class III devices intended for human use in the United States. The 510(k) must be submitted to the FDA at least 90 days before marketing unless the device is exempt from 510(k) requirements. A 510(k) is a premarketing submission made to the FDA to demonstrate that the device to be marketed is as safe and effective as, that is, substantially equivalent (SE) to, a legally marketed device that is not subject to premarket approval (PMA) (FDA 2002). The 510(k) allows a specific laser device to be used for specific conditions. Approval means that the approved laser can be sold, but that the only claim the manufacturer can make is for the indication described in the 510(k).

As of January of 2002, the FDA had granted the premarket notification for the application of LLLT for two clinical applications.

1. The "adjunctive use in providing temporary relief of minor chronic neck and shoulder pain of musculoskeletal origin." The laser is a 630-nanometer (nm) diode laser with a 10-mW output.

2. The "adjunctive use in the temporary relief of hand and wrist pain associated with Carpal Tunnel Syndrome." The approved device was a low-energy infrared laser containing a cluster of three 30-mW, 830-nm laser diodes.

In addition to those specific treatment parameters, several other laser companies have received premarket notification approvals for their devices for the same applications. One should be sure when purchasing a device that the company has obtained FDA approval for the product. Claims beyond those listed on the approval should not be marketed. Clinical data will most likely be generated and submitted to the FDA for approval that will further expand the application of LLLT. This assumption is based on the extensive research and clinical application of LLLT devices in other countries.

The FDA approvals offer certified athletic trainers and other health care providers another modality for the treatment of patients they serve. This was, to our knowledge, the first time that a therapeutic modality was approved only for the treatment of specific conditions. Although extensive applications of this modality for other maladies are described in the international literature, any use of a therapeutic laser of the management of other conditions is considered "off-label" application. We will review some of this literature later in the chapter. American clinicians should not bill for any application of LLLT other than those specifically approved, and the clinician bears full responsibility for any adverse effects.

Lasers come in many types and forms with differing applications. To understand the unique attributes of laser energy, some understanding of the electromagnetic spectrum and atomic theory is necessary. The acronym LASER provides considerable insight into its production: Light energy, or **photons,** are amplified and then stimulated and emitted as radiant energy. Thus, as ultrasound involves acoustic energy, laser delivers light energy that is absorbed in the tissues.

## ELECTROMAGNETIC ENERGY

Energy is the ability to do work. The electromagnetic spectrum is the total range of energy expressed in relation to the wavelength and frequency of this energy. Electromagnetic energy consists of photons that travel at the speed of light: 300,000,000 m/sec. This spectrum ranges from long wavelengths such as radio waves that are measured in meters to the opposite end of the spectrum with gamma rays that are measured in femtometers ($10^{-15}$). Photons of different wavelengths have different energy levels (figure 12.1). Photon energy is proportional to its frequency—the higher the frequency, the higher the photon energy. The high-energy photons are in the gamma, x-ray, and ultraviolet end of the spectrum and are capable of causing atom or molecular ionization.

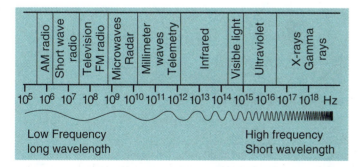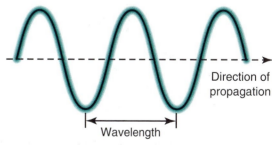

**Figure 12.1** The electromagnetic spectrum is a continuum of energies that are categorized by their wavelength and frequencies, which are inversely proportional. As the frequency increases, the wavelength shortens, and when there is a low frequency, the wavelength is long. The visible spectrum is within the electromagnetic spectrum and has wavelengths between 400 and 760 nm.

Reprinted by permission from Georgia State University Department of Physics and Astronomy.

The electromagnetic energy emitted from the sun is transmitted to earth. The earth's atmosphere absorbs the high-energy photons except for a portion of the ultraviolet range (UVB and UVC).

Photons are either produced naturally or man-made, but the two types have the same energy level and consequences. At wavelengths of 320 nm or shorter, the energy becomes ionizing, therefore dangerous for human exposure. Sunlight and light used for conventional illumination have a wide spectrum of electromagnetic energies. Neon lights are narrow-band lights that result in a predominant color. Light-emitting diodes (LEDs) use a relatively narrow band of electromagnetic energy that can result in a distinct color (red, yellow, green, or blue) or may also emit infrared frequencies that are invisible to the human eye. In contrast to the LEDs that have a narrow band of electromagnetic wavelengths, laser light is very wavelength specific and therefore energy specific. Light-emitting diodes should not be confused with laser light, although the two terms are often used interchangeably.

# LASER PRODUCTION

An atom has a nucleus consisting of protons and neutrons with electrons orbiting about in designated shells or valence levels. When energy is applied to an atom, the energy may be absorbed, causing one of the electrons to move and orbit in a higher shell. An atom in this state is labeled as "excited" and is unstable. The electron will return to a normal level of orbit (called **ground state**) as soon as possible. When this occurs, the energy that caused the excited state is released as a photon (packet of light). In a normal state, electrons are absorbing energy and releasing photons continuously as the atoms attempt to remain in their most stable form **(spontaneous emissions;** see figure 12.2).

How is the light amplified? When a quantity of atoms is retained in a chamber **(lasing chamber)** and excited by the application of energy, photons are released in this confined area. As a photon strikes another excited atom, it stimulates the release of an additional photon as the electron returns to its resting orbit. As this occurs, the original photon is unaffected and continues to influence other atoms. Thus, as more and more photons are generated, increasing amounts of light energy are produced **(amplification).** A lasing chamber is constructed with a semipermeable (also referred to as semireflective) mirror at one end. When the ability of the mirror to reflect light is exceeded, some laser light escapes from the chamber through the mirror (figure 12.3).

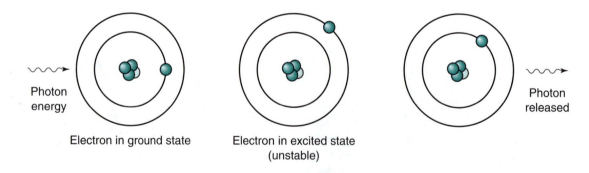

Photon energy

Electron in ground state

Electron in excited state (unstable)

Photon released

**Figure 12.2** Energy (photon) causes an atom to become excited, and an electron moves to a higher valence level. All matter seeks its most stable form and requires energy to be in an excited state. The matter releases an equal amount of energy (photon) as the atom goes back into its ground state. This process occurs naturally (spontaneous emission).

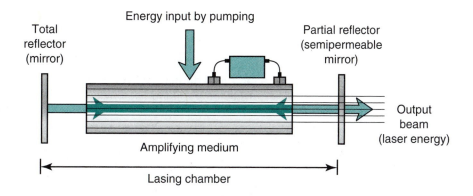

**Figure 12.3** Basic production of a laser. Energy is applied to a closed chamber to allow amplification of photons. The energy is released at one end in the form of a laser.

# Laser Components

There are thousands of types of lasers that are categorized by the way they are made. The four categories of lasers include gas (helium-neon), solid (ruby), liquid (dye), and semiconductor (diode).

The typical anatomy of a laser includes the following:

- Lasing medium: gas, semiconductor, liquid
- Power supply: energy source
- Resonating cavity: mirrored chamber

The lasing medium contains specific elements that will discharge photons of a specific wavelength and, therefore, energy. The power source applies energy into the lasing medium. The lasing medium stores the energy by raising the atom's outer electrons into a higher-valance orbit. This creates an environment where the majority of atoms are in their excited state, a condition that is called population inversion. When a photon of a specific energy identical to that being stored collides with an excited atom, an identical photon is produced. This photon, along with the incident photon, is released; the release is termed stimulated emission (figure 12.4). These photons further stimulate adjacent excited atoms, resulting in more photons being released. Depending on the elements of the lasing medium, the stimulated emission produces photons of a specific wavelength (monochromic) that are in a fixed phase relationship (coherent). The resonating chamber is composed of a chamber (gas), channel (diode), or rod (solid state) that further concentrates the production of the photons by the use of mirrors. The mirrors are placed at each end of the chamber. One mirror is totally reflective and the other mirror is partially reflective. As the photon concentration increases, the photons are emitted through the partially reflective end.

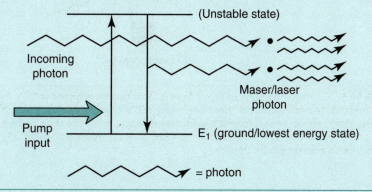

**Figure 12.4** When energy is applied (pumping source), the atoms are in their excited state. When a photon strikes this atom, another photon is released in addition to the original photon. The additional photon causes more photons to be released when they strike additional excited atoms. This is termed stimulated emissions.

# PROPERTIES OF LASER LIGHT

What is unique about laser light? Laser light has three related properties: **monochromaticity, coherence,** and **collimation.** "Monochromic" means that the light is of one color or one wavelength that is specific to the energy level of the photon. The wavelengths of light energy range from 100 to 10,000 nm (billionths of meters). If the wavelength is less than 400 nm, the light falls into the ultraviolet spectrum. Visible light has wavelengths of 400 to 700 nm. The infrared spectrum lies between 700 and 10,000 nm. Two points can be drawn from this information. First, not all lasers emit light in the visible spectrum; secondly, when the light of a laser is visible, the light is of a single color since it is monochromic.

"Coherent" means that all of the waves of light energy are of the same length and are traveling in a similar phase relationship. This characteristic increases the wave amplitude characteristic (constructive interference). Furthermore, all of the energy is traveling in the same direction. This leads to the third characteristic of lasers, which is collimation.

"Collimation" refers to the degree to which the beam remains parallel with distance. A perfectly collimated beam would have parallel sides and would never expand at all. A laser beam does diverge somewhat and even obeys the inverse square law as the distance from the laser source is increased. The divergence of laser is minimal and varies with the type of laser (gas vs. diode), and can be modified with the use of lenses. The collimation of the laser is a safety concern for both the patient and practitioner as the energy is concentrated to a thin beam. When the energy is focused on a small part of the retina, damage can result whether the laser is visible or not. Properties of laser and white light are compared in figure 12.5.

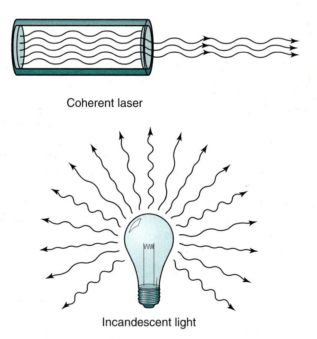

Coherent laser

Incandescent light

**Figure 12.5** Contrast the light emitted from a laser to that emitted from a light bulb. White light contains many different colors and therefore many wavelengths of light. Since the waves are of different lengths, they cannot remain in phase and they diverge. Thus, the light from a single bulb can illuminate a large area. The light emitted from a laser does not readily diverge, allowing travel over long distances and greater penetration.

# LASER CLASSIFICATION

Scientists have established safe exposure limits for different types of laser energy and developed a system of laser hazard classifications (American National Standards Institute [ANSI Z136.1-2000]). There are five levels in the classification system: 1, 2, 3a, 3b, and 4. Categories 1, 2, and 3a are considered safe; 3b has certain risks; and 4 has the chance for serious risk. Standardized safety measures must be utilized to reduce the chance of adverse responses to laser exposure. Laser manufacturers are required to certify and label their devices in the appropriate category.

- **Class 1 lasers.** A Class 1 laser is considered to be incapable of producing damaging radiation levels and is therefore determined to be eye safe. These lasers are exempt from most control measures. Many lasers in this class are lasers that are embedded in an enclosure that prohibits or limits access to the laser radiation. Laser printers and CD players are examples of a Class 1 laser.

- **Class 2: low-power visible lasers.** Class 2 lasers are low-power lasers that also emit visible radiation (400- to 700-nm wavelength). These lasers can exceed the Class 1 accessible emissions level (AEL) but do not exceed 1 mW. For this laser class, the normal human aversion response of 0.25 sec to bright radiant sources naturally protects the eye if the beam is viewed directly. The potential for an eye hazard exists if this normal reflex motion is overcome and the exposure times are greater than 0.25 sec.

- **Class 3: medium-power lasers.** Class 3 lasers are medium-power lasers or laser systems that require control measures to prevent viewing of the direct beam. Control measures emphasize preventing exposure of the eye to the primary or reflected beam.

- **Class 3a lasers.** Class 3a lasers have an output power up to 5 mW. Viewing of the direct beam is normally not hazardous if it occurs for only momentary periods with the unaided eye. These lasers may present a hazard if viewed using collecting optics, which is any type of lens including glasses.

- **Class 3b lasers.** Class 3b lasers are medium-power lasers that have an output power of 5 mW to 500 mW. Viewing these lasers under direct beam and specular reflection conditions is hazardous. The diffuse reflection is usually not a hazard except for higher-power Class 3b lasers. The Class 3b laser is not normally a fire hazard. Many of the LLLT devices are classified as 3b lasers.

- **Class 4: high-power lasers.** Class 4 lasers are high-power lasers that exceed 500 mW. Direct beam, specular reflections, and diffuse reflections from these lasers present a hazard to both the eye and skin. A Class 4 laser can also present a fire hazard (radiant power > 2 W/cm² is an ignition hazard). In addition, these lasers can create hazardous airborne contaminants and have a potentially lethal high-voltage power supply. The entire beam path must be enclosed to reduce the potential hazards.

Lasers must be labeled appropriately to alert the user of potential hazards. Figure 12.6 demonstrates some standard labels for Class 2, 3, and 4 lasers.

# LASER PARAMETER SELECTION

Parameter selection is perhaps the most difficult aspect of LLLT since there are so many variables that must be considered. When one is determining the best-fit laser for therapeutic treatment, the following patient and laser parameters should be evaluated. Patient considerations include the type and condition of the tissue and acute or chronic condition; and even pigmentation may have an impact on the laser treatment outcome. Laser parameters that must be considered include wavelength, output power, average power, power density (intensity), and energy density (dosage). These factors are summarized in "Considerations for the Proper Selection of LLLT Treatment Parameters and Devices" on page 204. It is important to understand these parameters to effectively operate different systems or to obtain comparable clinical outcomes. Many of the LLLT therapy devices marketed are menu driven, so selecting the tissue type and chronicity of the injury provides a specific treatment dosage.

Class 2 and Class 3a laser signs

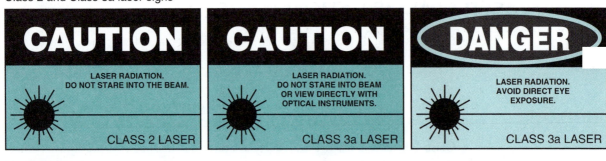

Class 3b laser signs

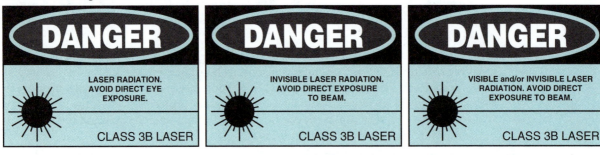

Class 4 laser signs

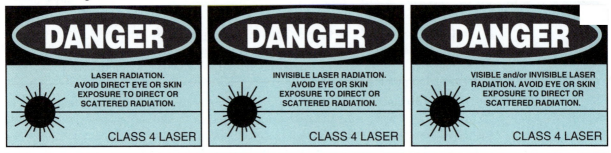

**Figure 12.6** Lasers must be identified and marked according to their classification. The required labels need to be placed near the aperture to alert the user of potential hazards.

# Considerations for the Proper Selection of LLLT Treatment Parameters and Devices

The clinician should take into consideration both patient factors and the types of clinical lasers available. These factors are used to determine the best outcomes.

## Patient Parameters

- Medical history and proper diagnosis: Diabetes or other medical conditions may alter clinical efficacy.
- Stage of the injury: Acute and chronic conditions require different dosages.
- Medications: Some medications may make the patient photosensitive (e.g., antibiotics).
- Pigmentation of the tissues: Dark skin absorbs light energy more than light skin.

## Laser Parameters

- Wavelength
- Output power
- Average power
- Intensity
- Dosage

One of the major problems with determining the efficacy of LLLT is that laser treatment is often poorly documented in the literature. Different laser types were used and dosages were varied or not reported. Therefore outcomes cannot be evaluated in a methodical manner. The equipment being marketed today is not well described, so the clinician may not know exactly what treatment parameters were delivered in a given study. It is important for the clinician to be aware of equipment features so that consistent energy levels can be delivered for a given condition.

## Wavelength and Types of Lasers Used in Low-Level Laser Therapy

A basic premise of electromagnetic energy is that the longer the wavelength (lower frequency), the greater the penetration. When determining the best-fit wavelength for laser application, the depth of the target tissue is an important consideration. Therefore, the HeNe laser with a wavelength to 632 nm is more appropriate for dermatological (more superficial) conditions, and the GaAs with a wavelength of 904 nm is better for deeper structures. The ideal wavelength for specific problems has not been fully determined. Penetration is also affected by the power delivered (figure 12.7). Since energy can be absorbed while being transmitted, enough energy must be present at the target tissue to evoke a response.

Different types of lasers are available that allow the application of varied photon energy and depth of penetration. The various elements used in the laser production result in the different photon energy levels emitted. The elements themselves are not introduced into the body. The types of lasers with LLLT have evolved to make the treatment application easier—the entire laser production can be housed in a handheld unit. When you are choosing a laser, factors to consider are the wavelength (which affects the depth of penetration), the ease of application, and the intensity or power density. Devices with multiple lasers in their surfaces make treating larger areas much more time efficient, but this feature adds to the expense.

### Helium-Neon (HeNe)

The helium-neon laser was one of the first therapeutic lasers developed in the 1970s. It was initially a gas laser that emitted a red visible light with a wavelength of 632 nm. It is presently

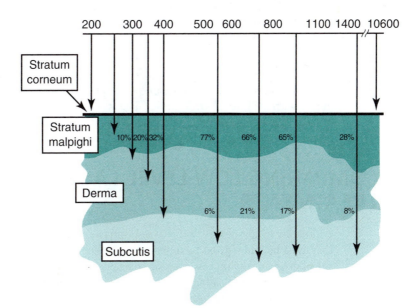

**Figure 12.7**  Depth of penetration. Wavelength of the laser is associated with the color (infrared, red, etc.) and the depth of penetration. Some laser energy is absorbed in the superficial, subcutaneous area, which decreases its ability to penetrate to deeper tissues.

Image courtesy of the Lawrence Berkeley National Library.

available also as a semiconductor laser that eliminates the need for the gas chamber and fiber optics. Initially the typical power output was from 1 to 2 milliwatts (mW) and was delivered by a fiber optic probe. Currently HeNe lasers are being produced with higher outputs, up to 25 mW. The depth of penetration with this wavelength is from 6 to 10 mm. The HeNe is commonly used in superficial wound care.

### Indium-Gallium-Aluminum-Phosphide (InGaAlP or GaAlInP)

This type of laser is a semiconductor that emits a wavelength between 630 to 700 nm. It is gradually replacing the HeNe lasers in some applications because it does not require fiber optics. Semiconductor lasers have less coherence than gas lasers, so the treatment times need to be longer given the same output power. These lasers are commonly used in superficial wound care.

### Gallium-Arsenide (GaAs)

This is a semiconductor laser that utilizes an infrared wavelength of 904 nm, which is invisible to humans. It was first developed in the early 1980s and had an output power that ranged from 1-mW to 5-mW maximum output. The early GaAs lasers were pulsed and with the low output power provided minimal energy dosages. Presently, the output is up to 100 mW and can be superpulsed. Therefore, there is a short **pulse-train** (burst) duration (100-200 ns) that is repeated up to 1,000 bursts per second. The depth of penetration has been reported to be 30 to 50 mm. This type of laser is being applied on deeper tissues such as tendons and ligaments.

### Gallium-Aluminum-Arsenide (GaAlAs)

This is also a semiconductor laser in the infrared region with wavelengths that range from 780 to 890 nm but are most commonly between 800 and 830 nm. They are delivered in a continuous wave mode. This type of laser became more popular in the 1990s. The output power of these laser devices ranges from 30 to 100 mW, but the device has been manufactured with an output of up to 1,000 mW.

Typically the gallium-aluminum-arsenide (GaAlAs) lasers are used for deeper ligament and tendon injuries, and the indium-gallium-aluminum-phosphide (InGaAlP or GaAlInP) or HeNe lasers are used for superficial and dermatological problems. Higher output of the laser allows for shorter treatment times.

### Combination Probes

Probes are produced that contain a grouping of several single-wavelength laser diodes in one probe. Cluster probes may combine LEDs with a single laser or may contain multiple laser diodes with a single LED. A single LED is often intended to be a visible signal when infrared (invisible) laser energy is being applied. The LED is often reported to be therapeutic, but this light is not a laser and cannot be compared to any LLLT reported in the literature.

## COMPARING LOW-LEVEL LASER THERAPY TREATMENTS

Ultimately the tissues are going to respond to energy. There are several operational definitions that must be understood to appreciate how energy is varied with laser application. Although the photon energy that is intrinsic to a specific type of laser will not vary, the output power of the laser unit may affect the outcome. Descriptions of the power and how it is delivered to the patient must be consistent if one is to compare treatments. The dosage of the laser is determined by the intensity of the laser and the time of application. However, the number of application points and how close each irradiated site is to the next must also be consistent. The beam diameter varies with the type of laser (semiconductor vs. gas) as well as the equipment quality (fiber optics). Most LLLT equipment has narrow beam diameters, but the treatment is delivered per square centimeter. The rationale is that once the laser energy penetrates the skin, there will be absorption, reflection, refraction, and transmission of the energy. The narrow beam might be irradiating a larger diameter within the tissues. Furthermore, this generalization to a 1-cm treatment area makes the application easily reproducible.

The dosage of laser therapy is determined by the total amount of energy applied to the tissues. Microchip technology has simplified the calculations that the clinician must make so that the only variable is the time per irradiated area. The computations in the next section seem complex, but you will see that determining the dosage involves minimal math skill. Generally the higher the power of the laser, the shorter the time required to deliver the same dosage. The following definitions provide the basis for making laser treatments more consistent so that treatment outcomes can be compared when different types of lasers are used.

## Output Power

The power of laser energy is measured in watts (W) or milliwatts (mW = $10^{-3}$W). The output power is important in categorizing the laser for safety and should be clearly described with each device. The output power is not adjustable by the clinician.

The laser equipment you own will change with age; the stated output of the laser does not stay consistent over time. You should use a power meter to determine the output power of your device to make dosage application correct. This factor is determined by the calibration of the therapeutic device.

## Power Density

The power density of the laser is much like the power output or average power, but this parameter takes into consideration the actual beam diameter. Power density is also termed "intensity," which is the average power per unit area in square centimeters (watts or milliwatts per $cm^2$ [$mW/cm^2$]).

$$power\ density = intensity = power\ (W)\ /\ beam\ diameter\ in\ cm^2 = W/cm^2$$

If the light is spread over a larger area, this will result in a lower power density (intensity) than if it were concentrated on a smaller area. The beam diameter determines the power density; therefore, it is affected by the degree of collimation the beam contains. Gas lasers have less divergence than semiconductor lasers. However, the use of fiber optics will increase the degree of divergence. The power density is usually programmed in the laser unit and reported simply as watts per $cm^2$ or mwatts per $cm^2$.

## Average Power

Laser energy can be applied in a continuous or pulse-train (burst) frequency mode (figure 12.8). Knowing the average power is important in determining dosage when you are utilizing a pulsed laser. If the laser is delivered in a continuous (cw) mode, then the average power is equal to the peak output power of the device. If the laser is pulsed (burst), then the average power is equal to the peak output power multiplied by the duty cycle. Therefore, if the peak power output of a laser is 5 mW (0.005 W) with a 25% duty cycle, then the average output is 1.25 mW (0.00125 W).

Different methods are used to create the pulsing of a laser, but with low-level lasers the most common method is by creating a duty cycle. However, low-level lasers may have a single pulse.

If a laser delivered output power of 50 mW in a continuous mode, it would take 20 sec to deliver 1 joule (J) [(50 mW = 0.050 W) × 20 sec = 1 J]. If the laser were pulsed to a 25% duty cycle, then it would take 80 sec to deliver 1 J (0.050 W × 0.25 = 0.0125 mW × 80 sec = 1 J). A longer time is needed to obtain the same dosage when the laser is pulsed. Pulse-train frequencies should not be confused with the carrier frequency of the laser, which is wavelength dependent.

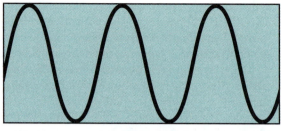

Continuous wave

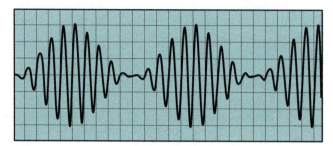

Pulse train

**Figure 12.8**    Continuous wave versus pulse train.

If the desired treatment dosage were 2 J, then the treatment time would be peak output power × duty cycle.

> 0.005 W × 0.25 = 0.00125 W average power
> dosage = joules (watts per second) / cm²
> joules / average power = treatment time per cm² of treatment area

For example, 2 J / 0.00125 W = 1,600 sec (26.67 min/cm²). If the laser device was not pulsed, for example, 2 J / 0.005 W = 400 sec (6.67 min/cm²).

## Energy Density or Dosage

Energy density is the most important treatment parameter, describing the amount of energy applied per unit area. Dosage is measured in joules (a joule is equal to 1 watt per second). Therefore if the wattage or power is known, then the number of joules is affected by the treatment time per irradiated area. Treatment outcomes are dosage dependent, so this parameter must be consistently determined.

The difference between power density and energy density (dosage) is the time component.

> intensity = watts / beam area in cm²
> dosage = intensity × irradiation time (seconds) = joules / cm²

The grid technique of irradiating each square centimeter of affected tissue is typically used. Therefore the total treatment time is affected by the intensity of the laser and the size of the treatment area. For example, if the laser is applied over a small area such as the transverse carpal ligament, then the treatment time will be significantly less than in treating the paraspinal musculature.

## Recommended Dosage Range

The Arndt-Shultz principle is highly applicable with this type of modality. This principle suggests that some energy may elicit a small response in biological tissues. While more energy could have improved the result, too much energy negates the beneficial effect of the treatment.

The range of laser dosage that has elicited a reported therapeutic response is between 0.001 $J/cm^2$ and 10 $J/cm^2$. There is believed to be a minimal "window threshold" of energy needed to elicit a response. This explains why supermarket cashiers can get carpal tunnel syndrome despite the scanners! An excessive dose may result in a suppressive effect. It has been recommended that dosage between 0.5 and 1.0 $J/cm^2$ be used for open wounds and between 2.0 and 4.0 $J/cm^2$ with intact skin (table 12.1) (Tume and Tume 1994).

## Pulsing Frequencies

Although there are different methods of pulsing lasers that will vary the power output, there is some interest in the impact that pulsing frequencies have on the outcome of laser treatments. Research is under way to determine if this parameter may affect therapeutic outcomes. Questions exist about whether the pulsing frequencies interfere with the resonating frequencies inherent in the tissue or whether the depth of penetration of the energy may be altered. Further research is needed to determine the relevance of this parameter.

## Treatment Frequency

There is considerable variation in responses to laser therapy, so treatments should be individualized to the patient. The general recommendation is to use the least amount of energy that elicits the most benefit. Generally, laser treatments delivered three to four times a week with moderate doses are more effective than higher doses fewer times per week. Acute conditions should be treated more frequently than chronic conditions, but not more than once daily. Laser energy has a cumulative effect, so small doses spaced farther apart have elicited more effective outcomes.

## Application Techniques

There are different methods of applying laser energy during the treatment. The classical considerations should be maintained with respect to targeting the treatment area. The various techniques are described next, and combinations of the techniques may be used when indicated clinically.

### Point Application

Point application is used in treating acupuncture or trigger points; the laser is applied directly over a point, and the dosage is delivered. Power density considerations make the cosine law

## Table 12.1   Treatment Dosages Recommended in the Literature

| Clinical condition | Dosage (joules) |
| --- | --- |
| Wound healing | 0.5-4 |
| Revascularization | 2-3 |
| Pain relief | 1-4 |
| Muscle spasms | 2 |
| Circulation | 1-3 |
| Nerve stimulation | 0.1-0.5 |
| Nerve cell regeneration | 2 |
| Inflammatory condition | 1-3 |
| Chronic conditions | 3-6 |

and the inverse square law (especially with highly diverging laser beams) very relevant with laser application. The laser application should be positioned in firm contact with the skin when appropriate or as close to the skin surface as possible. The applicator should also be positioned so it is perpendicular to the treatment surface. This will reduce energy loss due to diffusion or reflection.

There can be a considerable variation in the beam characteristics between lasers, but in application of point stimulation the point is generally considered to be in a 1-cm$^2$ area. Although the beam may have a spot contact of a 2-mm diameter, there will be a spread effect of up to 1 cm within the tissues. To treat trigger points or acupuncture points, the treatment is applied to individual points and then moved to the next point. When a surface area is being covered, two methods can be utilized to apply the laser energy—scanning and grid technique.

### Scanning

With scanning technique, the laser head is held close to the tissue surface and moved in a slow and steady manner over the treatment area. The scanning lines are approximately 1 cm apart, and the treatment is continued until the dosage is completed. There are expensive commercially produced laser devices that apply a scanning technique. The patient lies under the lasing head, which mechanically moves over the treatment area.

### Grid

With the grid technique, the treatment area is determined and a grid matrix in 1-cm squares is imaged over this area. Point application is used for a specified amount of dosage per square centimeter, which will ultimately distribute the total dosage over the treatment area in the treatment grid. This technique is considered to be more accurate than the scanning technique. Firm contact should be made with the skin unless there is an open wound; in this case a 1- to 2-mm distance is maintained.

## Tips for Effective Treatment Application

The following suggestions should be considered when one is administering laser treatment to ensure the most effective and consistent outcomes.

- The laser should be maintained so that it is perpendicular to the treatment surface.
- Firm contact should be maintained with the treatment site unless an open wound is present. If contact is not appropriate, then the laser should be held as close to the surface as possible.
- Determine the appropriate treatment dosage for the individual points as well as the total treatment dose, that is, 1 J/cm$^2$ for a total of 20 J.
- Treatment should be minimal at first, and the dosage and treatment frequency should gradually increase as tolerated to obtain the optimal outcomes.
- Treatment application can use one of several techniques:
  - "Surround the dragon:" This technique utilizes point application around the perimeter of the pain site or lesion.
  - Grid technique: Fill in the pain area or lesion using point application in an imaginary 1-cm$^2$ grid.
  - Acupuncture point: Use an acupuncture chart to locate appropriate points at which to treat involved structures or pain syndromes.
- Ask the patient for any sensations or changes in his or her condition during treatment.
- Establish pre- and posttreatment changes in pain, edema, or functional capacity.
- Ask the patient prior to the next treatment about reaction to the previous treatment.
- Adjust the dosage according to the response elicited from the previous treatment:
  - Decrease the dosage if undesirable outcomes occurred.
  - Increase the dosage if there were no results.

# BIOLOGICAL EFFECTS OF LASER

Low-level laser therapy has been studied for over 40 years, with mixed outcomes reported. The applications have been extensive, involving dermatology, respiratory conditions, arthritic conditions, soft tissue and bone healing, pain, and nerve lesions, to name a few. Conclusions on efficacy are difficult to ascertain because many of the reported outcomes are in non-peer-reviewed literature, anecdotal reports, uncontrolled studies, or published abstracts; or controlled studies have poorly described methodology or show contradictory outcomes. The FDA relies on clinical data to allow an expansion in the application of LLLT. Ideal studies are from multiclinical sites and are randomized, blinded, placebo-controlled studies that verify safety and efficacy. As far as the FDA is concerned, the safety considerations have been largely satisfied but further research is needed to determine efficacy with medical conditions other than carpal tunnel syndrome and neck pain.

Of the methodological flaws noted, dosage has been and remains a significant pitfall in research. Frequently, studies used very low doses of laser. The treatment parameters that should be documented to allow consistency in further research include the following:

- Laser model
- Laser type and wavelength
- Probe description (single/cluster)
- Output power
- Pulsing/Pulsing duration
- Pulse frequency
- Dosage
- Power density (intensity)
- Treatment technique (distance)
- Treatment time
- Treatment frequency

The potential use of LLLT in sports medicine would be to enhance wound healing and pain management following injury. It would be helpful to find a modality that could be applied acutely and one that would expedite the return of an athlete to competition by providing these outcomes. Low-level laser therapy has been reported to expedite the inflammatory process, decrease pain, and promote tissue healing. Studies have suggested that lasers promote fibroblast proliferation, promote the synthesis of Type I and III procollagen mRNA (Abergel et al. 1984), hasten bone healing (Ozawa et al. 1995), and help in the revascularization of wounds (Kovacs, Mester, and Gorog 1974).

The proposed mechanism of action of laser therapy is associated with the ability of the cell to absorb the photon and transform the energy into adenosine triphosphate (ATP). The ATP is a form of energy that the cell uses to function. The cell must absorb the light energy for this process to occur. We know that certain cells have the capacity to absorb light energy, as in the skin reacting to sunlight. These light-absorbing components of the cells are termed chromophores or photoacceptors and are contained within the mitochondria and cell membrane. Cell components such as cytochrome c, porphyrins, and flavins also have a light absorbing capability (Karu 1987).

Production of ATP is essential to cell function. Normally ATP is produced by the mitochondria, using oxygen as the primary fuel. Laser stimulation has been shown to enhance the production of ATP by forming singlet oxygen, reactive oxygen species (ROS), or nitric oxide, all of which influence the normal formation of ATP (Derr and Fine 1965; Lubart et al. 1990). The increased ATP prompts homeostatic function of the cells to resume. Furthermore, the ATP energy may drive the messenger RNA to foster cell mitosis and proliferation.

The proposal that laser energy merely promotes normal cellular function rather than changing cell function explains why injured tissues respond to laser therapy while there is little effect on noninjured cells. This is in contrast to the application of high levels of laser energy or excessive doses that cause damage to cells. Again, the effect of the laser is dependent on the intensity of the energy, the exposure time, and the irradiated area. The wavelength of the laser affects the depth of penetration of the energy.

## Inflammation

The effect of LLLT on inflammation has been reported to be pro-inflammatory rather than anti-inflammatory (Kana et al. 1981). Laser has been shown to enhance the degranulation of mast cells that results in histamine production. Histamine, a powerful chemical mediator, tends to accelerate the inflammatory cascade. As the inflammatory process progresses more rapidly, the proliferative phase of healing begins sooner, subsequently enhancing the wound healing process. The effect of laser on inflammation suggests that LLLT may begin early in the injury process and may be combined with RICE (rest, ice, compression, elevation) as an initial intervention.

## Pain

The FDA is allowing the marketing of approved LLLT devices for the treatment of symptoms associated with carpal tunnel syndrome and for adjunctive use in providing temporary relief of minor chronic neck and shoulder pain of musculoskeletal origin. The effect on other painful conditions has been reported, but the effectiveness is equivocal. Numerous studies have shown that LLLT is effective in reducing pain, but the exact mechanisms are still to be determined. The production of endogenous opioids, nitric oxide, serotonin, and acetycholine has been reported to be a source of analgesic effects elicited from laser radiation (Laakso et al. 1994; Choi, Srikantha, and Wu 1986). These mechanisms need further study. Another proposed mechanism for pain reduction is a direct effect on nerve conduction velocity and somatosensory evoked potentials. These changes have been measured after the application of LLLT, but their ability to influence pain is not well understood.

## Wound Healing

Wound healing has been enhanced with the application of laser energy (Woodruff et al. 2004; Enwemeka et al. 2004). The most promising investigations have involved using laser to promote the healing of ulcers and other injuries to the skin. Research outcomes have varied for different reasons, including the use of different wavelengths and dosages and the use of healthy animal models.

Laser radiation results in **biomodulation,** meaning that it can stimulate or inhibit. This is analogized to sunlight and tanning. Some energy is effective in stimulating melatonin, but excessive light results in damage (suntan vs. sunburn). Low-dosage laser would be ineffective, while excessive energy may inhibit rather than stimulate healing. Acute injuries can be treated more frequently (daily) than chronic wounds, which should be treated only two to three times per week. Chronic wounds do not respond to aggressive interventions.

Laser energy is more effective in treating pathological states; therefore, when healthy subjects are used, the outcomes may be subdued. Although tissue healing is accelerated, no hyperplastic effects have been reported (Bosatra, Jucca, and Olliaro 1984). During the course of healing, lased wounds had more collagen and had a higher tensile strength than the controls, but by day 14 the wounds were similar (Abergel et al. 1987; Kana et al. 1981; Surinchak et al. 1983). This shows that laser energy catalyzes normalization rather than creating a supernormal effect.

Systemic effects from laser therapy have been reported (Mester et al. 1971; Kana et al. 1981). This is why research using laser treatments on one body part and using another site on the same subject or animal as the control may give misleading results. These systemic effects are not always observed in the research but should be considered.

## Adjunctive Therapy

Other modalities in addition to LLLT can be beneficial, although thermal devices should be used after the laser treatment. Blood, specifically the hemoglobin, absorbs laser energy, so any modality that increases blood flow could make LLLT less effective. Generally it is recommended that tissues be cooled prior to laser treatment and heated afterward if these therapies are indicated. When combining laser treatment with ultrasound, it was felt that the individual therapies obtained the best outcomes and the clinician should choose the most appropriate modality rather than combining them (Gum et al. 1997).

Medications may have an effect on laser efficacy, although more research on this issue is needed. Medications such as nonsteroidal anti-inflammatory drugs, steroids, and calcium channel blockers, to list a few, are thought to block membrane channels and pigment receptors (Meersman 1999), which are important for laser actions, and therefore reduce laser effectiveness. Other medications such as procaine, certain antibiotics, and copper-based local substances may enhance the effectiveness of laser energy by enhancing the receptor sites. Researchers should be sensitive to the presence of medications with subject selection when designing laser studies.

# SAFETY CONSIDERATIONS

It is important to ensure a proper diagnosis, as with the application of any modality. Make sure you are aware of what condition you are treating.

- **Eye safety.** Never look into the aperture of the laser. The cornea transmits light energy and the eye focuses the light on the retina. Wavelengths over 700 nm are invisible; therefore, the light reflex response will be absent. This could result in retinal damage. Eye protection should be provided for both the clinician and the patient depending on whether the classification of the laser is 3b or higher. Laser warning signs should be present. It is also recommended that the laser probe be kept in contact with the skin whenever possible. Safety keys are provided with many laser units to help avoid indiscriminant activation of the laser.

- **Cell proliferation.** There was a decrease in mitotic activity with very high doses of laser energy, but a proliferation with low doses, of 0.5 to 1.5 J/cm² in open wounds and up to 4 J/cm² in closed wounds. These energy levels will also vary with different types of lasers (lower doses were more effective with the GaAs lasers; higher energies were needed with the HeNe) (Mester, Mester, and Mester 1985). Adult doses should not exceed 50 J, and the maximum dosage for children under 14 years of age is 25 J (Tume and Tume 1994).

- **Fatigue reactions.** Fatigue has been reported after laser treatments (Tuner and Hode 2002). This was short-term and was more common in chronic pain conditions.

- **Pain response.** The patient may complain of a pain response the day after treatment. This is believed to be due to an activation of tissue healing mechanisms that had become dormant (Tuner and Hode 2002). This should be a positive response sign, especially in a chronic injury condition.

# CONTRAINDICATIONS AND PRECAUTIONS

Because low-level laser therapy can inhibit cell function when applied in high doses, laser therapy should be applied at appropriate dosages. A number of contraindications warrant special considerations.

- **Pregnancy.** No published research is present that addresses the effect of laser therapy on the unborn child. As a precautionary measure, laser therapy should be avoided in pregnant women, especially with application to certain acupuncture points and over the lower abdomen.

- **Cancer.** No mutagenic effects have been reported with the use of LLLT. Cancerous cells in vitro have been stimulated to grow, but in vivo studies resulted in a reduction in tumor size that was attributed to an enhanced immunological system (Wohlgemuth et al. 2001). Only oncologists should treat cancer patients.

- **Thyroid gland.** Thyroid gland activity has been modified by laser energy; therefore treating over this area should be avoided (Hernandez, Santisteban, and del Valle-Soto 1989).

- **Children.** No studies have identified any impact on open growth plates. Since there are limited studies on the use of LLLT in children, the treatment should not be done unless the benefits clearly outweigh the potential for risk when there are open growth plates. Generally the maximum dosage for children is recommended to be less than 25 J (Tume and Tume 1994).

Low-level laser therapy is still under scrutiny using evidence-based research standards. Laser therapy is making gains as research is more controlled and as multicenter studies and contemporary diagnostic measures are being utilized. Low-level laser therapy has been utilized for treatment of many neuromusculoskeletal conditions in many countries, and no adverse effects have been reported in over 1,700 publications. Additional research is required to obtain data concerning success rates in treating specific conditions, length of exposure, frequency of treatments, and related therapeutic protocols.

## SUMMARY

1. Understand the evolution of light therapy.

   Clinicians throughout the ages have used actinotherapy or light therapy to heal wounds and sicknesses without understanding the physiological impact of the application of light. Modern-day uses of light therapy include ultraviolet light and laser therapy. Laser applies the most refined photon or light energy.

2. Describe the unique characteristics of laser energy.

   Laser energy is composed of photons with all of the same energy and will subsequently be only one color (monochromatic). These photons all have the same wavelength and frequency and travel in parallel with each other, making them collimated. Additionally, the photons are in phase with one another or coherent. These factors—monochromaticity, coherence, and collimation—are unique characteristics of laser light.

3. Discuss the types of lasers available for soft tissue treatment and compare their energy outputs with respect to power, dosage modifications, wavelength, and pulse frequency.

   There are different types of lasers that are made from a variety of elements, each producing a laser with a certain wavelength. Some types of lasers are more powerful than others, and some must be pulsed to be categorized for LLLT. Considering the variables in production, it is important for the clinician to understand how to compare clinical outcomes using the available parameters. The power is used to categorize the laser and is not adjustable by the clinician. The dosage takes into consideration the total amount of energy delivered and is calculated as the power (intensity) × treatment time. Dosage is measured in joules per square centimeter since most LLLT applications apply the energy over a 1-cm² area. Wavelength and pulse frequency are also parameters that are not controlled by the clinician but affect the depth of penetration and the amount of energy delivered.

4. Perform a laser treatment using a commercially available device.

   The most consistent method for applying LLLT is use of the grid technique. The laser is applied with the device perpendicular to the target tissue, and direct, light pressure is maintained using the applicator. The laser is applied for the designated duration in each square centimeter of an imaginary grid that covers the treatment area. The dosage is determined by the time during which each area is treated.

5. Understand the biological effects of LLLT.

The physiological effects of LLLT are the result of the ability of the body to absorb energy from the photon application. Specifically, the application of low levels of light energy causes an increase in the production of ATP. Cell proliferation is enhanced when a stimulus exists, as in an inflammatory state. Low-level laser therapy can be used in sports medicine to promote tissue healing and for pain.

6. Describe the safety considerations and contraindications of LLLT.

Low-level laser therapy can inhibit cell function when applied in high doses; therefore laser therapy should be applied at appropriate dosages. This form of therapy should not be used in pregnancy, over open epiphyseal plates, in cancer patients, or over the thyroid gland. The clinician should exercise caution when treating around the eyes, since some lasers used in LLLT are invisible and prolonged exposure can damage the retina.

## CITED SOURCES

Abergel RP, Lyons R, Castel J: Biostimulation of wound healing by lasers: Experimental approaches in animal models and fibroblast cultures. *J Dermatol Surg Oncol* 13:127-133, 1987.

Abergel RP, Meeker CA, Lam TS, Dwyer RM, Lesavoy MA, Uitto J: Control of connective tissue metabolism by lasers: Recent developments and future prospects. *Am J Acad Dermatol* 11:1142-1150, 1984.

Bosatra M, Jucca A, Olliaro P: In vitro fibroblast and dermis fibroblast activation by laser irradiation at low energy. *Dermatologica* 168:157-162, 1984.

Choi JJ, Srikantha K, Wu WH: A comparison of electroacupuncture, transcutaneous electrical nerve stimulation and laser photobiostimulation on pain relief and glucocorticoid excretion. *Int J Acupunct Electrother Res* 11:45-51, 1986.

Derr VE, Fine S: Free radical occurrence in some laser-irradiated biologic materials. *Fed Proc* 24(1 Suppl 14):99-103, 1965.

Enwemeka CS, Parker J, Dowdy D, Harkness E, Sanford LE, Woodruff LD: The effects of laser therapy on tissue repair and pain control. A meta analysis of the literature. *Photomed Laser Surg* Aug 1;22(4):323-329, 2004.

Gum SL, Reddy GK, Stehno-Bittel L, Enwemeka CS: Combined ultrasound, electrical stimulation, and laser promote collagen synthesis with moderate changes in tendon biomechanics. *Am J Phys Med Rehabil* 76(4):288-296, 1997.

Hernandez LC, Santisteban P, del Valle-Soto ME: Changes in mRNA of thyroglobin, cytoskeleton of thyroid cell and thyroid hormone levels induced by IR-laser radiation. *Laser Ther* 1(4):203-208, 1989.

Kana JS, Hutschenreiter G, Haina D, Waidelich W: Effect of low-power density laser radiation on healing of open skin wounds in rats. *Arch Surg* 115:293-296, 1981.

Karu T: Photobiological fundamentals of low power laser therapy. *IEEE J Quantum Elect* 23(10):1703-1717, 1987.

Kovacs IB, Mester E, Gorog P: Laser-induced stimulation of the vascularization of the healing wound. *Separatum Experientia* 30:341-343, 1974.

Laakso E, Cramond T, Richardson C, Galligan J: Plasma ACTH and B-endorphin levels in response to low level laser therapy (LLLT) for myofascial trigger points. *Laser Ther* 6(3): 133-142, 1994.

Lubart R, Malik Z, Rochkind S, Fisher T: A possible mechanism of low level laser-living cell interaction. *Laser Ther* 2(2):65-68, 1990.

Meersman P: Laser pharmacology and Achilles tendinopathy. *Laser Ther* 11(3):144-150, 1999.

Mester E, Mester A, Mester A: The biomedical effect of laser application. *Lasers Surg Med* 5:31-39, 1985.

Mester E, Szende B, Tota JG: Effect of laser on hair growth of mice [in Hungarian]. *Kiserl Orvostud* 19:628-631, 1967.

Mester E, Spiry T, Szende B, Tota JG: The effect of laser rays on wound healing. *Am J Surg* 122(4): 532-535, 1971.

Ozawa Y, Shimizu N, Mishima H, Kariya G, Yamaguchi M, Takiguchi H, Iwasawa T, Abiko Y: Stimulatory effects of low-power laser irradiation on bone formation in vitro. *Proc SPIE* 1984: 281-288, 1995.

Surinchak JS, Alago ML, Bellamy RF, Stuck BE, Belkin M: Effects of low-level energy lasers on the healing of full-thickness skin defects. *Lasers Surg Med* 2(3): 267-274, 1983.

Tume KG, Tume S: *A Practitioner's Guide to Laser Therapy and Musculoskeletal Injuries.* Southern Pain Control Centre, South Australia, 1994, 16.

Tuner J, Hode L: *Laser Therapy. Clinical Practice and Scientific Background.* Prima Books, Talinn Estonia, 2002, 103.

U.S. Food and Drug Administration. CDRH Consumer Information: Laser Facts. 2002. http://www.fda.gov/cdrh/consumer/laserfacts.html

Van Pelt W, Stewart H, Peterson R: *Laser Fundamentals and Experiments.* U.S. Department of Health, Education, and Welfare, Rockville, MD, 1970.

Wohlgemuth WA, Warner G, Reiss T, Wagner T, Bohndorf K: In vivo laser-induced interstitial thermotherapy of pig liver with a temperature-controlled diode laser and MRI correlation. *Lasers Surg Med* (29(4): 374-378, 2001.

Woodruff LD, Bounkeo JM, Brannon WM, Dawes Jr. KS, Barham CD, Waddell DL, Enwemeka CS: The efficacy of laser therapy in the treatment of wounds: A meta-analysis of the literature. *Photomed Laser Surg* June 1;22(3):241-247, 2004.

# Mechanical Energy

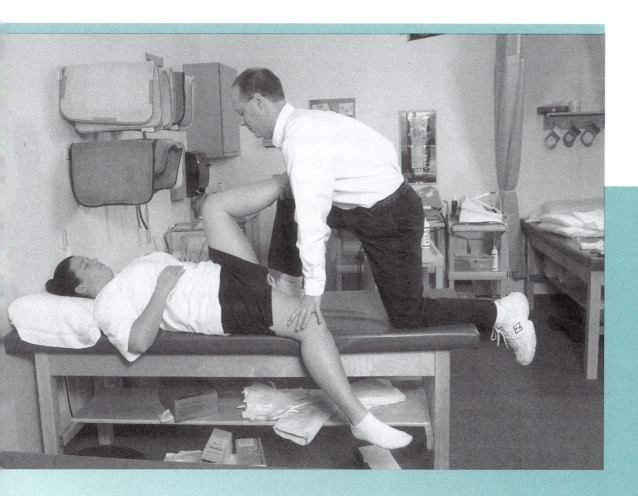

## *Objectives*

After reading this chapter, the student will be able to

1. discuss the potential benefits of using manual therapy techniques in rehabilitation;

2. describe massage, myofascial release, strain–counterstrain, muscle energy, and joint mobilization;

3. describe the afferent and efferent innervation of intrafusal and extrafusal muscle fibers and the relationship between the gamma and alpha motor neurons;

4. apply the "convex–concave rule" in performing joint mobilization;

5. describe the manual and mechanical traction techniques used to treat cervical spine dysfunction;

6. identify contraindications for manual therapies and mechanical traction;

7. describe the mechanical traction techniques used to treat lumbar spine dysfunction; and

8. describe the application of, and contraindications for, intermittent compression therapy.

A field hockey player is referred for care of her injured right wrist. She states that she injured the wrist 2 months ago when she fell on her outstretched hand. She was diagnosed as having a carpal sprain, and her arm was placed in a cast for 3 weeks due to concerns over a possible fracture of the scaphoid. Recent x-rays did not reveal a fracture. However, she complains of pain after activities and of stiffness in the wrist. Whirlpool treatments and stretching of the wrist flexors and extensors have not provided any benefits. Evaluation of the wrist reveals restrictions in wrist extension and decreased anterior glide of the radial carpal and midcarpal joints. The certified athletic trainer performs grade II, III, and finally IV joint mobilization at each articulation twice in a three day period. After three treatments over 6 days, range of the wrist is nearly normal, and the athlete is experiencing much less pain after activity. How did the new treatment make a difference? Joint mobilization and other manual therapy techniques can speed recovery from a variety of musculoskeletal injuries. This chapter introduces manual therapies and other modality applications that deliver mechanical energy to the body.

Some therapeutic modalities, such as mechanical traction and intermittent compression, are beneficial because they exert mechanical forces on the body. However, the most common "devices" used in athletic training to impart a mechanical force on the body are the hands of the athletic trainer, which are powerful assessment and treatment tools. In past years, many certified athletic trainers abandoned manual therapy because of demands on their time and infatuation with devices such as transcutaneous electrical nerve stimulation (TENS) and isokinetic dynamometers. Now, manual therapy techniques, which have largely been developed in osteopathic medicine, chiropractic medicine, and physical therapy, are increasingly being practiced by certified athletic trainers.

This chapter covers the topics of mechanical traction, intermittent compression, and manual therapy. Much of the chapter is devoted to introducing several manual therapy approaches. However, this chapter is intended only to introduce manual therapy. Detailed discussion of manual therapy techniques has been reserved for another of the texts in the Athletic Training Education Series: *Therapeutic Exercise for Musculoskeletal Injuries, Second Edition* (Houglum 2005). Issues of treatment efficacy are, however, discussed as in the previous three chapters.

Much of this text is devoted to understanding how therapeutic modalities affect the nervous system and connective tissues. Although manual therapies can be thought of as procedures as opposed to applications, the certified athletic trainer's hands affect the connective tissues and alter neural input. Some clinicians shun the use of therapeutic modalities such as ultrasound and TENS for newer manual techniques, whereas others view manual therapies as a subspecialty separate from contemporary athletic training practice. A treatment that combines modalities like ultrasound or TENS and manual techniques may provide the greatest relief of symptoms. For example, when treating an individual with myofascial pain, you may find TENS, superficial heat, or occasionally cold combined with massage, strain–counterstrain, or release techniques to be effective. All alter neural activity at the spinal level and relieve pain and muscle spasm. Also, because heated tissues are more pliable, ultrasound may be useful before treatments such as joint mobilization in which the goal is to stretch connective tissues and restore normal joint function.

Unlike cold therapy or TENS, manual treatment cannot be learned from a book but must be learned through laboratory instruction and hands-on practice. Students, as well as experienced clinicians, will continually refine their manual therapy skills and add variations and new techniques. Over the years, proprioceptive neuromuscular facilitation, joint mobilization, myofascial release, and strain–counterstrain techniques have been used to treat physically active individuals. These skills have largely been developed from clinical observation and passed from teacher to student. In many cases various techniques are recommended for treating the same condition. For example, patients with neck pain may respond to myofascial release, joint mobilization, or strain–counterstrain. No single manual therapy approach has been shown to be universally superior to another. Controlled clinical trials are needed to assess the efficacy of many applications of manual therapy. Developing skill in the manual therapy techniques offers you a greater number of options when you are developing a plan of care and improves the clinician's ability to evaluate the musculoskeletal system. Manual therapy techniques can be applied in any setting; these skills require time and practice rather than a large budget and athletic training room. Practice, experience, and attention to the clinical literature will guide your development of manual therapy skills and your ability to integrate traditional therapeutic modalities with manual therapy. This chapter will provide a foundation on which you can build your skills and will inspire you to pursue further training in manual therapy.

# MANUAL THERAPIES

Unfortunately, the scientific foundation for manual therapy has evolved more slowly than the art. There is relatively little evidence of cause-and-effect relationships between manual therapy and recovery of injured individuals. However, there is scientific support for much of the theory behind many forms of manual therapy, and the following sections include important components of the theoretical foundation for manual therapy. Before discussing individual therapies, the text will address one additional aspect of manual therapy that is neither anatomical nor clearly neurological: the power of touch and human interaction.

Certified athletic trainers often provide care to physically active people entering the medical system on an emergency basis, some for the first time. The high school athlete injured for the first time, the university freshman far from home, or the older individual whose work and family life have been disrupted present with more than an injured body part to be treated. These people come to the certified athletic trainer with anxiety, unanswered questions, and a sense of being lost in the health care system. Our increasingly bureaucratic and technology-driven health care system often leaves individuals wondering if anyone really cares about them. Manual therapy requires hands-on time with the individual. A caring touch and opportunity for conversation can ease anxiety and foster confidence that the individual is being cared for and will recover. A sense of being in good hands promotes compliance with a plan of care and a positive outlook, which in turn promote recovery. Some of the benefits of manual therapy are due to the psychological-affective responses to treatment rather than the anatomical-neurological responses. Some may call this a placebo response; however, improvement is improvement, and perhaps much of the failure of our medical system stems from the loss of the personal touch. Certainly, medical technology has advanced medical care, but at a price. The skilled manual therapist who provides a personal touch will help some physically active individuals whom others cannot.

## Massage

Massage, the rubbing or kneading of a part of the body, is one of the earliest recorded treatments of human suffering. Massage developed in many early cultures. The terminology and techniques of massage, as well as its acceptance as a therapy, have changed over time. Today, massage techniques are applied by several allied medical professionals as well as massage therapists.

Athletic trainers have used massage since the beginnings of the profession. Massage has been purported to relieve pain, increase blood flow, enhance lymphatic drainage, and stretch connective tissues. Experience and observation provide evidence of the effects of massage on pain and muscle spasm. Certainly relief of spasm may enhance lymphatic drainage, and mechanical energy can stretch connective tissues. However, blood flow to deep tissues is regulated by metabolic demand. The effect of massage on blood flow has not been extensively studied, but an understanding of circulatory regulation suggests that massage has little impact on blood flow to deeper tissues.

The primary benefits of massage in athletic training are pain relief, reduced muscle spasm, and increased tissue extensibility. But how does massage relieve pain and muscle spasm? Contact with the skin stimulates the cutaneous receptors and increases input along large-diameter afferent pathways. The gate control theory of spinal level pain modulation (figure 13.1) offers

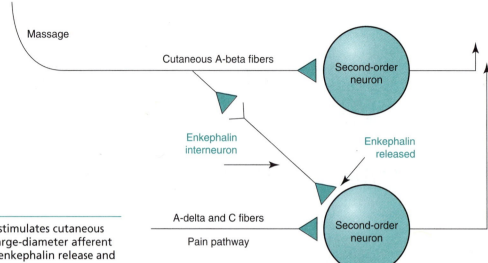

**Figure 13.1** Massage stimulates cutaneous receptors, increasing large-diameter afferent input and resulting in enkephalin release and inhibition of pain pathways.

a plausible explanation for the analgesic benefits of massage techniques employing gentle stroking motions **(effleurage)** and kneading **(petrissage)** of muscle. Because muscle guarding and spasm are the result of pain, massage alleviates the trigger for muscle spasm and mobilizes the muscle and surrounding connective tissues.

Deeper massage techniques over trigger points may result in a deep sensation of pain during massage yet provide extended relief. Painful stimulation activates the descending analgesic pathways described in chapter 4. Thus, the response to deep, kneading massage techniques also has a plausible explanation.

Relief of pain and muscle spasm and mobilization of connective tissues are important treatment goals. In theory, achieving these goals enhances lymphatic drainage. Certainly, pain relief and muscle relaxation promote free, active contraction of muscle, which is the primary means by which lymph is pumped through the body.

A massage is part of routine training and preparation for many endurance athletes. This is particularly true in professional cycling, and all of the European-based professional teams employ one or more *sorvoiners*, or massage therapists, to take care of their riders.

# Gamma Gain, Myofascial Release, and Strain–Counterstrain

Muscle is made up of two types of fibers. Extrafusal fibers are the contractile fibers that allow muscle to generate force. The extrafusal fibers are innervated by alpha motor neurons. Interspersed within the extrafusal fibers, which make up most of the substance of muscle, are intrafusal fibers. Intrafusal fibers house muscle spindles that are specialized mechanoreceptors; these send information regarding changes in muscle length, and therefore movement, to the central nervous system.

Intrafusal fibers receive neural stimulation from gamma efferent neurons. The efferent input allows for continual adjustment of the length of the spindle so that it is maintained at an optimum length to detect changes within the muscle.

In some circumstances, there may be excessive activity in the gamma efferent neurons to a particular muscle or portion of a muscle, which is referred to as **gamma gain.** The effect of gamma gain is to maintain the spindles in a hypersensitive state, resulting in normal movements causing reflexive contraction throughout a muscle via the reflex arc depicted in figure 13.2. The increased tension **(hypertonicity)** in a muscle will ultimately result in adaptive shortening in surrounding fascial tissues. The taut bands of tissues and hypersensitive trigger points associated with myofascial pain syndrome (MFPS) are thought to result from gamma gain.

*(continued)*

The question of what causes gamma gain has not been fully answered. The likely trigger is pain. Acute pain results in muscle spasm and guarding. Rapid movement of muscle in spasm results in a reflexive contraction of the affected muscle, suggesting that muscle spindles are in a hypersensitive state due to increased gamma efferent activity. The increase in gamma activity is the result of input from nociceptors. This explanation makes sense when applied to the response to acute injuries, but how does it relate to persistent pain problems such as MFPS?

The increased tone and resulting fascial adaptations found in MFPS are an insidious process. When fascia becomes shortened, it too becomes hypersensitive to stretch. Stretch of fascial tissue is painful; free nerve endings are being stimulated. Noxious input from the fascia triggers an increase in gamma efferent activity, perpetuating a cycle of spindle hypersensitivity, increased tone in muscle, fascial adaptations, and painful movement when the tight fascia is stretched. The cycle builds from mild discomfort into a pain pattern that can include referred pain and frequent headaches. Effective treatment of MFPS requires that the causes, which may include combinations of stress responses, muscle imbalance and poor posture, injury, and illness, must begin with breaking this cycle.

Breaking the cycle just described by arresting gamma gain is the focus of two manual therapy techniques, strain–counterstrain and indirect myofascial release. These techniques place muscles and fascia in shortened positions of comfort. Such positioning decreases gamma efferent activity and interrupts the cycle that is maintaining the body in a dysfunctional state.

## Myofascial Release

Myofascial release (MFR) is similar to massage in that the certified athletic trainer uses his or her hands to influence the connective tissues and neural input. There are multiple release techniques. The techniques and terminology of MFR overlap with those of other manual therapies. However, MFR, as a component of manual therapies, has a much more elaborate theoretical basis, which has resulted in a greater understanding of somatic dysfunction.

*Myo* refers to muscle and *fascia* to the system of supporting connective tissue that maintains the integrity of the human body. Injury, illness, stress, repetitive movements, poor posture, and fatigue can contribute to changes in the length–tension relationship of the fascia and muscles over time. For example, extensive swimming can strengthen and shorten the chest muscles while stretching and weakening the muscles of the upper back. The surrounding fascia adapts accordingly, setting the stage for a myofascial pain pattern.

Injuries such as whiplash can cause a pattern of guarding that in turn results in fascial adaptations. Psychological stress also results in tension and can contribute to the development of a myofascial pain pattern.

At the center of myofascial pain is gamma gain. When muscle is in spasm or protective guarding, it becomes hypersensitive to stretch due to increased input along gamma efferent nerves to the muscle spindles (figure 13.2). The cycles of pain, protective guarding, and fascial shortening gradually escalate until the athlete experiences myofascial pain.

The role of the certified athletic trainer is to break the cycle and address the physically active person's symptoms. Many modalities can be used to treat physically active individuals, and all treatment plans for myofascial pain should include active therapeutic exercises. However, these interventions do not directly address the problem of fascial restrictions and gamma gain.

Myofascial release techniques can be divided into direct and indirect techniques. In applying indirect techniques, the athletic trainer attempts to place muscle and fascia in positions that remove stress from the tissues, resulting in decreased noxious input from the fascia, which in turn diminishes activity in gamma efferent nerves. These techniques are gentle but require practice to master. Direct techniques attempt to stretch bound fascia to decrease the stress on and afferent input from the tissue. Both types of techniques can be used to treat a physically active individual's myofascial pain pattern. Practice and experience will improve your manual skills as well as your ability to integrate traditional modalities, manual therapy, and exercise into a comprehensive plan of care.

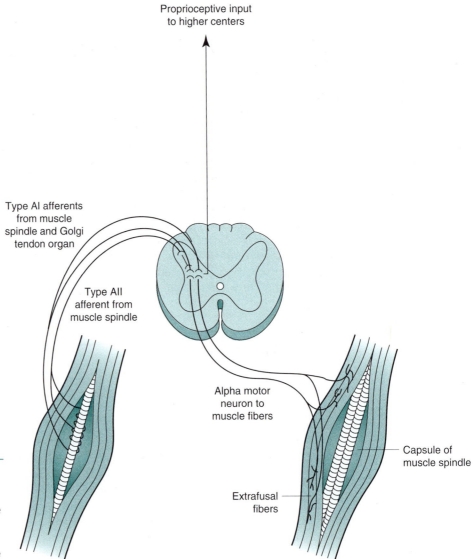

Proprioceptive input
to higher centers

Type AI afferents
from muscle
spindle and Golgi
tendon organ

Type AII
afferent from
muscle spindle

Alpha motor
neuron to
muscle fibers

Capsule of
muscle spindle

Extrafusal
fibers

**Figure 13.2** Sensory input from the muscle spindles and Golgi tendon organs affects motor function of same muscle via synapses at the spinal cord level.

Adapted by permission from Wilmore and Costill 1999.

Myofascial pain patterns are common in the neck, upper back, and shoulder. Poor posture, several hours spent driving or sitting in front of a computer, stress, and general fatigue slowly take a toll. Gentle release techniques often dramatically relieve pain, spasm, and accompanying headaches.

## Strain–Counterstrain

Strain–counterstrain, another type of manual therapy, was originated by Dr. Lawrence Jones (Jones et al. 1995). Like MFR, strain–counterstrain relieves pain and dysfunction by altering neural activity. Strain–counterstrain is a technique in which a body segment is passively moved into a position of greatest comfort, thereby relieving pain by reducing or arresting inappropriate proprioceptive activity that is responsible for the dysfunction.

Jones provided a holistic view of somatic dysfunction, recognizing that injury to one structure, such as a ligament, affects other tissues including muscle, fascia, blood vessels, lymphatic vessels, and neural elements. Strain–counterstrain techniques are directed toward treating not the primary lesion, such as the sprained ligament, but rather the resulting dysfunctions.

Strain–counterstrain techniques can increase pain-free range of motion following musculoskeletal injury. As with MFR, direct and indirect techniques of strain–counterstrain are described. Direct techniques involve applying force against a restrictive barrier to improve motion, whereas indirect techniques involve moving the body away from a motion-restricting barrier to a position of comfort and relaxation.

By placing a body segment in a position of comfort, the indirect techniques inhibit the cycle of pain and increased muscle guarding due to increased gamma efferent outflow (figure 13.3). One key element of indirect techniques is to slowly move the treated body segment back to a resting position after a period (90-120 sec) of passive positioning. The slow, painless movement prevents a surge of input from spindles and reestablishment of the movement dysfunction.

You need laboratory instruction and practice in order to become proficient at both MFR and strain–counterstrain techniques. Over the years athletic trainers have become increasingly interested in these manual therapies, probably because they address the notion of a pain–spasm cycle. Athletic trainers appreciate that modality applications do not repair injured tissue but are used to treat the signs and symptoms of injury, including loss of function. Strain–counterstrain techniques are most useful in short-duration pain patterns and during tissue repair and early maturation. Myofascial techniques, although similar, seem to be most effective in treating more long-standing pain patterns, especially those related to the spine.

Pain results in muscle guarding and spasm, which in turn causes pain. Sometimes this cycle persists despite adequate time for tissue repair. Strain–counterstrain can be used to place a body segment in a position of comfort and break the cycle. A slow return to anatomical or resting position prevents recurrence of pain, often leading to prolonged relief.

## Joint Mobilization

Muscle energy and joint mobilization are manual therapies primarily directed to restoring joint function. Joint mobilization is used to restore intrinsic joint motion or arthrokinetics. Joint mobilization also stimulates joint receptors and increases afferent input across large-diameter afferent fibers. Thus, joint mobilization may also ease pain and improve the individual's willingness to move a joint.

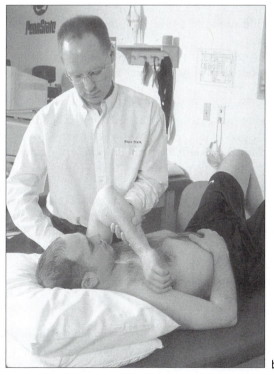 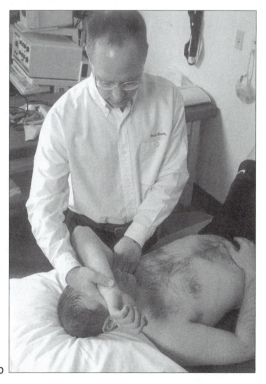

a                                    b

**Figure 13.3**  Strain–counterstrain for the short (a) and long (b) heads of biceps brachii dysfunction.

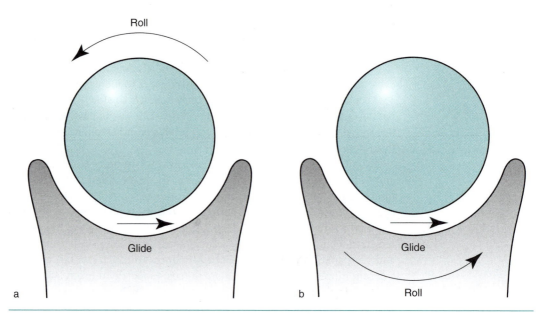

**Figure 13.4** When a convex surface moves on a concave surface, roll and glide are in opposite directions *(a)*. When a concave surface moves on a convex surface, roll and glide occur in the same direction *(b)*.

To appreciate the value of joint mobilization techniques, you must fully understand how joint movement occurs. Joints are formed by the articulating surfaces of bones. Muscles, through the attachments of tendons, cause bones to move upon one another at the joint. Outwardly, the articulating surface of one bone appears to pivot about a single, fixed axis, but few joint motions actually occur about a single axis. During most joint movements, the articulating surfaces slide and glide upon one another while the rolling or pivoting occurs about a moving axis.

The subtle slides and glides are referred to as **arthrokinematics,** whereas the observed motion created by movement of one bone upon another is referred to as **osteokinematics.** Joint mobilization involves the assessment and treatment of arthrokinematics. The "convex–concave rule," illustrated in figure 13.4, will help you assess and treat restricted arthrokinematic movements.

When arthrokinematic movement is limited, range of motion is limited and the joint is often painful. From the perspective of modality application and pain management, joint mobilization addresses the first two priorities in an injured person's plan of care: pain relief and restoration of range of motion. In fact, when pain and loss of motion are due to arthrokinematic dysfunction, joint mobilization is the treatment of choice.

A more thorough discussion of joint mobilization and treatment techniques is included in *Therapeutic Exercise for Musculoskeletal Injuries, Second Edition* (Houglum 2005). However, this technique is introduced in the context of therapeutic modalities because of its application in managing joint pain and loss of motion.

A loss of range of motion is common following musculoskeletal injury such as a sprain of the lateral ankle ligaments. A loss of dorsiflexion affects the ability to walk and run. Stretching of the gastrocnemius and soleus can help restore motion, but often the problem is related to a restriction of posterior glide of the talus in the mortise. In these cases, joint mobilization techniques in which the talus is manually moved posteriorly will be far more effective at restoring motion than stretching.

## Muscle Energy

Muscle energy techniques are manual procedures in which the injured person's muscles are actively contracted against a counterforce in a specific treatment position. Muscle energy techniques may be used to stretch tight muscles and fascia, strengthen weakened muscle, or mobilize restricted joints (Woerman 1989). These techniques may be used, for example, in the treatment of sacroiliac (figure 13.5) and lumbar facet dysfunction.

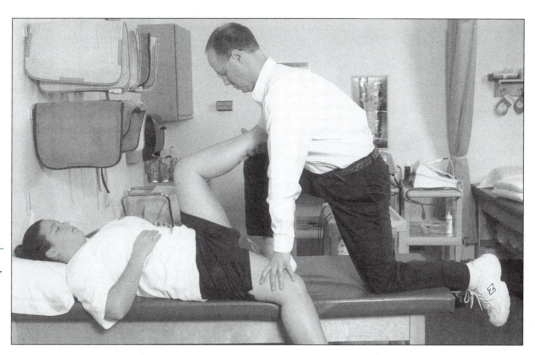

**Figure 13.5** Muscle energy technique for an anterior innominate rotation, a common source of sacroiliac dysfunction.

Like joint mobilization, a muscle energy technique can be considered a procedure rather than a modality application. However, when restricted joint movement causes pain and movement dysfunction, a therapeutic modality usually fails to improve the patient's situation. Muscle energy and joint mobilization techniques address the cause of the injured person's complaints and often speed the recovery of normal movement and function. You can use TENS and moist heat with most manual techniques, including MFR, muscle energy, and joint mobilization; TENS and heat relieve pain and reduce muscle spasm, so the injured person becomes more relaxed and comfortable, allowing for more effective manual therapy.

Like all modalities, manual therapy techniques are contraindicated in the treatment of some injured physically active individuals. These contraindications are summarized in table 13.1. Injuries to ligaments and bone are the most common contraindications for manual therapies. However, these contraindications are not absolute and require that the certified athletic trainer make sound clinical decisions. For example, if an athlete suffered a fracture and dislocation at the ankle, this injury would contraindicate all manual therapies. However, once the tissues have healed and the leg is removed from immobilization, massage, MFR, and joint mobilization could be used to restore range of motion in the foot-ankle complex. It is also possible that the prolonged use of crutches could result in sacroiliac dysfunction that may respond to muscle energy techniques.

The certified athletic trainer must also be able to recognize signs and symptoms of infections and diseases in the physically active individuals they treat. Treatment of infection and organic diseases is beyond the scope of athletic training practice. If the certified athletic trainer is unsure of the nature and etiology of musculoskeletal pain, an evaluation by a physician must be conducted before any manual therapy is attempted.

In addition to the specific precautions and contraindications discussed previously and in *Therapeutic Exercise for Musculoskeletal Injuries, Second Edition* (Houglum 2005), there are additional contraindications for joint mobilization and muscle energy procedures because of the greater force applied to the body during those procedures. Joint mobilization and muscle energy procedures should not be used in the presence of joint or bony instability or when degenerative changes result in a bony block to motion. Joint mobilization and muscle energy procedures also should not be used in the presence of malignancies or advanced osteoporosis; mobilization of the cervical spine should not be performed in the presence of advanced rheumatoid arthritis.

**Table 13.1  Indications and Contraindications for Manual Therapies, Traction, and Intermittent Compression**

| | Indications | Contraindications |
|---|---|---|
| Manual therapies | | General: Symptoms of organic disease or cancer must be followed up before a modality, including a manual procedure, is administered. |
| Massage | Pain<br>Muscle spasm<br>Edema | Infection<br>Skin breakdown or disease |
| Myofascial release | Persistent pain with fascial restrictions; taut bands or trigger points | Acute inflammation, recent fracture, or surgery<br>Caution with joint instability or joint prosthesis<br>Caution if pregnant |
| Strain–counterstrain | Persistent pain with well-localized tender points | Increased pain during treatment<br>Caution following fracture or if joint instability present |
| Muscle energy | Subluxation or malpositioning of a bony element | Recent fracture<br>Joint instability<br>Joint fusion<br>Bony instability<br>Severe osteoporosis |
| Joint mobilization | Loss of range of motion due to arthrokinematic restriction | Infection<br>Joint instability<br>Bone-on-bone end-feel<br>Recent fracture<br>Bony instability<br>Advanced osteoporosis<br>Mobilization of cervical spine in the presence of advanced rheumatoid arthritis |
| Traction | | |
| Cervical | Pain<br>Muscle spasm<br>Hypomobile facet<br>Disc herniation | Positive vertebral artery test<br>Positive alar ligament test<br>Acute neck injury (fractures, sprains with joint instability)<br>Advanced rheumatoid arthritis<br>Bone cancer<br>Increased pain or radicular symptoms with treatment<br>Advanced osteoporosis |
| Lumbar | Pain<br>Muscle spasm<br>Disc herniation<br>Hypomobile facet<br>Nerve root impingement | Pregnancy<br>Claustrophobia<br>Internal disc derangement<br>Fractures, sprains with joint instability<br>Bone cancer<br>Increased pain or radicular symptoms with treatment<br>Advanced osteoporosis<br>Hiatal hernia |
| Intermittent compression | Swelling and edema | Thrombophlebitis<br>Infection<br>Acute fracture<br>Pulmonary edema and congestive heart failure |

There is considerable debate as to whether dysfunction at the sacroiliac joint is a common cause of low back pain. Identification and treatment of asymmetry with muscle energy techniques does dramatically relieve pain and spasm for some individuals. Muscle energy techniques incorporated into a comprehensive plan of care can be the key to relief from weeks or months of pain and dysfunction.

# IS MANUAL THERAPY EFFECTIVE?

Unlike the modalities discussed in previous chapters, "manual therapy" is a collection of treatment techniques used for a broad spectrum of musculoskeletal problems. A search for evidence of effectiveness of manual techniques reveals that most studies have involved manipulative procedures (grade V mobilization) in the treatment of spine-related conditions. The results from a search of the Physiotherapy Evidence Database are found in table 13.2. The reader is reminded that manual therapy techniques require formal instruction and practice that are well beyond the scope of this text. There is relatively less information on the effects of grades I through IV mobilization; thus grade V or manipulative procedures were included in this review.

There is evidence that early posterior mobilization of the talus on the calcaneus (Green et al. 2002) speeds recovery from lateral ankle sprains and may prevent residual loss of normal arthrokinematic motion at the ankle (Denegar, Hertel, and Fonseca 2002). Restrictions of distal tibiofibular mobility have also been identified, but results from clinical trials of mobilization of this articulation have not been reported. Conroy and Hayes (1998) reported some benefit of joint mobilization in a small group of patients with glenohumeral impingement syndrome. While pain reduction was found at 24 h after treatment, a larger, longer-term study is needed to better assess the efficacy of this intervention.

Searches of PubMed and the Physiotherapy Evidence Database using search terms "myofascial release" and "strain–counterstrain" identified a single report from a clinical trial. Sucher (1993) reported on four patients with carpal tunnel syndrome that did not respond to conservative care. All improved and carpal tunnel dimensions changed following a regimen of "manipulative myofascial release" and self-stretching.

While much has been written about massage, clinical trials are sparse. Furlan et al. (2002) completed a systematic review of massage in the treatment of low back pain. These authors concluded that "massage might be beneficial for patients with sub-acute and chronic, nonspecific low-back pain, especially when combined with exercises and education." This conclusion is supported by the results reported by Preyde (2000), who found that patients with subacute low back pain treated by experienced massage therapists had less pain and greater functional improvement at the conclusion of treatment and 1-month follow-up. In a smaller study, Hernandez-Reif et al. (2001) reported that two 30-min massages per week were effective in decreasing pain and improving motion in women with at least 6-month histories of back pain. Low back pain is a complex syndrome, and no single treatment is completely effective. Massage offers a low-cost, low-risk adjunct to a comprehensive plan of care for many physically active individuals with back pain.

Clinical trials addressing the efficacy of massage on other musculoskeletal conditions are difficult to locate. Blackburn, Simons, and Crossley (1998) studied the effects of massage and stretching in a group of young athletes. Subjects received six sessions of massage over 5 weeks and performed a regimen of stretching. The authors reported an increase in work performed by the dorsiflexor muscles before symptoms of exertional compartment syndrome occurred. Measures of functional performance were not included in this study. Massage has been reported to decrease the frequency and duration, but not severity, of tension headaches, although control group comparison was not made (Quinn, Chandler, and Moraska 2002).

Clinical trials addressing the efficacy of manual therapy techniques in the treatment of specific musculoskeletal conditions are needed to maximize health care resources and improve treatment outcome. At present the clinician must rely heavily on personal experience and preferences in deciding if and when to include a manual technique in a plan of care and if so, which one.

**Table 13.2   Assessing the Efficacy of Manual Therapies: Main Conclusions From Recent Studies**

| Author | Type of report | Nature of problem | Main conclusion |
|---|---|---|---|
| **Cervical spine and headache** | | | |
| Coulter (1996) | Systematic review | Acute neck pain | Mobilization better than cervical collar and rest; exercise equally effective |
| | | Subacute and chronic neck pain | Manipulation effective in short term but benefit not sustained at 1 week; short-term pain relief with manipulation, increased motion |
| | | Tension headache | Data suggest short-term relief with manipulation or mobilization |
| | | Other conditions | Lack of evidence favoring or disfavoring intervention |
| Bronfort et al. (2001) | Systematic review | Chronic headache | Spinal manipulative therapy better than massage; lack of data to draw strong conclusions |
| Cassidy et al. (1992) | Clinical trial | Neck pain | Manipulation more beneficial than mobilization in immediate decrease in pain, no long-term follow-up |
| Mealy et al. (1986) | Clinical trial | Whiplash | Early efforts to restore motion more effective than collar and rest at 8 weeks posttrauma |
| **Thoracic spine** | | | |
| Schiller (2001) | Clinical trial | Mechanical thoracic spine pain | Greater decrease in pain and improved lateral flexion immediately and 1 month after six treatments (included control group comparison) |
| **Lumbar spine** | | | |
| Hsieh et al. (2002) | Clinical trial | Subacute low back pain | No difference in amount of improvement between manipulation, myofascial therapy, combined treatments, or completion of back school |
| Assendelft et al. (2003) | Meta-analysis | Acute/Chronic low back pain | Manipulation not found to be superior to other treatment approaches |
| Hurwitz et al. (2002) | Clinical trial | Low back pain | Chiropractic care and medical care resulted in similar 6-month outcome assessment; physical therapy provided somewhat greater benefit than medical care alone |
| Ferreira et al. (2002) | Systematic review | Chronic low back pain | Manipulation superior to sham treatment, response similar to that with NSAIDs |
| Aure et al. (2003) | Clinical trial | Chronic low back pain | 16 treatments of manual therapy superior to exercise therapy on several outcome measures at 0-, 1-, 6-, 12-month follow-up |
| Cherkin et al. (1998) | Clinical trial | Subacute low back pain | Chiropractic care and physical therapy more effective than education; observed differences small, and cost-effectiveness of these interventions questioned |

# TRACTION

Mechanical traction involves using a machine or apparatus to apply a traction force to the body (figure 13.6), whereas with manual traction the force is applied by the hands of the certified athletic trainer. Most traction treatments are administered to distract or separate segments of the cervical or lumbar spine. Research has demonstrated that vertebral separation occurs (Colachis and Strohan 1965, 1969). However, gravity reduces the separation as soon as the

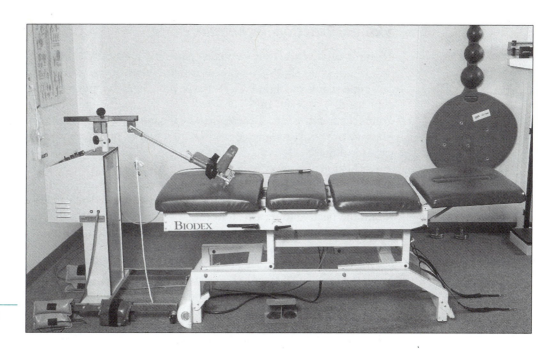

**Figure 13.6** A split traction table.

individual sits or stands. Thus, the efficacy of traction in the management of spinal dysfunction is questionable. The use of mechanical traction, in particular, has declined in all allied medical fields and has never been extensive in athletic training.

Although the use of mechanical traction by certified athletic trainers is limited, an understanding of the principles and applications of manual and mechanical traction is useful. Some cervical manual traction is necessary during joint mobilization. Traction, joint mobilization, and MFR techniques can be combined to treat cervical facet dysfunction and myofascial pain patterns. Some individuals with acute low back pain respond well to traction, especially when placed in a position of comfort.

## Cervical Traction

Distraction of the cervical spine can benefit individuals with cervical facet dysfunction or cervical disc pathology, degenerative changes that narrow the intervertebral foramen and cause myofascial pain. Manual traction should be performed before mechanical traction is considered. Manual traction allows you to carefully control force application and head position to maximize the relief of symptoms. Manual traction also allows you to combine manual techniques. If manual traction relieves pain or radicular symptoms, you can move to mechanical traction for longer treatments that require less of your time. Take care to reproduce the position and traction force that provided the greatest relief. You cannot precisely quantify the traction force that you apply through your hands. However, a force of 15 to 25 lb will result in a perceived elongation of the cervical spine. The best approach to adjusting the mechanical force is to gradually increase it until the individual reports relief similar to that experienced with manual traction.

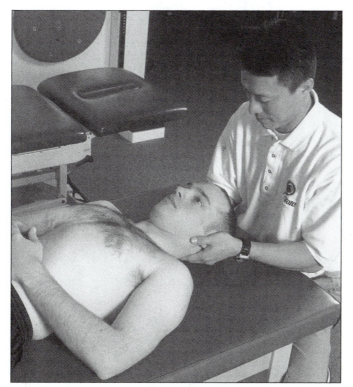

**Figure 13.7** Manual cervical traction.

## *Manual Traction Technique*

To apply cervical traction manually, place the physically active individual in a supine position. Place your hands in a position that allows distraction of the cervical spine without causing discomfort (figure 13.7). Relax your hands as much as possible, because tension in your hands will result in tension and guarding by the individual being treated. When this occurs the traction forces are resisted by the muscles, defeating the purpose of the treatment. Massage or release techniques can be used first to minimize tension in and guarding by the paraspinal muscles.

As traction is applied, the head can be positioned for greatest comfort. In neutral position, the greatest separation occurs in the upper cervical spine. As the neck is flexed to 30°, the traction forces are directed to the lower cervical spine. You can also carefully side-bend and rotate the head and neck to find the position of greatest relief. Side-bending is especially useful in relieving pressure on spinal nerves in individuals with degenerative changes that result in radicular symptoms.

Traction treatment does not structurally change the spine. However, the treatment can break the cycle of pain, muscle spasm, and guarded movement. Postural training and upper body reconditioning can result in long-term management of symptoms in some individuals.

## *Mechanical Traction Technique*

In people who respond well to manual traction, mechanical traction is an option that requires less of your time. The physically active individual should be positioned supine, with the neck flexed and side-bent to a position of greatest comfort. A halter or Saunder's traction device (figure 13.8) can be used to transmit the traction forces. A Saunder's device is easier to set up than the halter, especially for those who rarely apply cervical traction. To apply the device, position the individual's head so that the pads align with the base of the occiput; then adjust the pads securely at the base of the occiput. If the pads are too tight, the person will complain of pain. If they are too loose, the pads will slide and pinch the ears, and little traction force will be transferred to the spine.

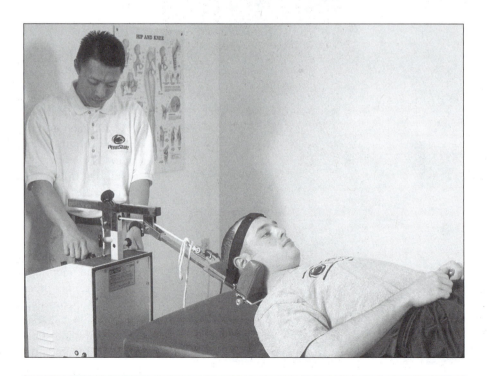

**Figure 13.8**    Cervical traction with Saunder's device.

You can select continuous or intermittent traction. Intermittent traction, in which the maximum traction force is applied for a set time period (typically 30 sec) and then a reduced force is applied, is more comfortable and better tolerated in most cases. The period of reduced force, or rest period, is usually about the same duration as the length of time the maximum force is applied. The traction force during rest is usually 50% of the maximum traction force.

The amount of traction force should be gradually increased to provide a tolerable distraction. Begin with 15 lb on smaller individuals and those with more pain and 25 lb on larger individuals with more long-standing pain. Treatment time can be adjusted up to 20 to 30 min depending on the individual's response. Traction can be combined with moist heat to control pain and promote muscle relaxation.

Irritation of a nerve root due to herniation of an intervertebral disc or stenosis causes pain that radiates along the course of the nerve. This pain, referred to as radicular pain, can be excruciating. Manual and mechanical traction can relieve radicular symptoms. Often relief is temporary at first; however, short-term relief offers hope. A combination of appropriate positioning, exercise, and the frequent use of cold or superficial heat at home can reduce stress on damaged and irritated tissues and result in long-term resolution.

## Precautions and Contraindications

Mechanical cervical traction is not appropriate for everyone and could result in catastrophic injury when applied inappropriately. In general, mechanical or manual traction is contraindicated following acute injury to the neck, the term *acute* implying that trauma caused the symptoms. Trauma to the head and neck may damage bone, ligament, and musculotendinous structures, resulting in laxity or instability. Fracture and injury to the stabilizing soft tissues must be ruled out or allowed to heal before you use traction. If traction is applied too early, the result may be greater permanent laxity and instability or, in the worst case, subluxation and injury to the spinal cord. As a rule, use manual traction rather than mechanical traction for individuals with a history of traumatic injury to the cervical spine.

One additional consideration of extreme consequence is fracture of the dens or odontoid process of the second cervical vertebra (axis) (figure 13.9). Trauma, especially with a whiplash mechanism, can fracture the dens. Unfortunately, this fracture is not always recognized and may not be particularly painful. If traction is applied in the presence of a dens fracture, dislocation of the first or second cervical vertebra could result, an often fatal injury. The alar ligament test allows you to evaluate the integrity of the dens. The alar ligament attaches to the occiput and the dens (figure 13.10). When the head is rotated or side-bent, the pull through the alar ligament causes a palpable rotation of C2. If the dens is fractured, the leverage to rotate C2 is lost. Thus, to assess the integrity of the dens, you can palpate the spinous process

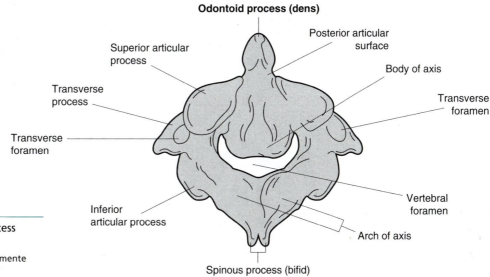

**Figure 13.9**  Odontoid process (dens).

Reprinted by permission from Clemente 1981.

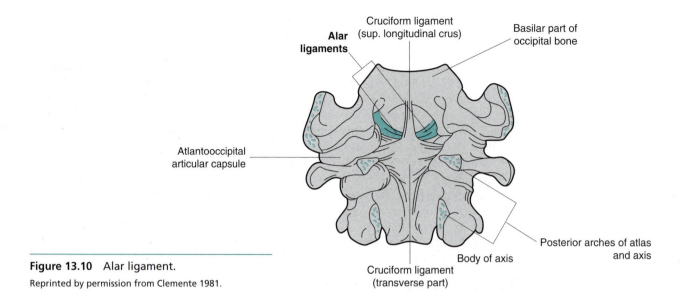

**Figure 13.10**   Alar ligament.

Reprinted by permission from Clemente 1981.

of C2 and passively side-bend or rotate the individual's head. If the spinous process does not move, the individual should be evaluated for fracture of the dens by the team or referring physician. You should perform the alar ligament test before using cervical traction when treating an individual with a history of traumatic injury to the neck, especially if a whiplash mechanism was involved.

Another concern related to cervical traction involves the potential to place the head in a position that compromises the vertebral arteries. The vertebral arteries pass through the foramen in the transverse processes of the fifth to second cervical vertebrae. These vessels ascend to the circle of Willis, which distributes blood supply to a large area of the brain (figure 13.11). Rotation and extension of the head will diminish blood flow through the vertebral artery on the side to which the head is rotated. Normally this does not pose a problem, because the vertebral arteries are paired and sufficient blood supply is provided through the contralateral side. However, some individuals present with a compromised vertebral artery on one side. Prolonged positioning of the head can lead to an insufficient blood supply to the brain and pose the risk of stroke. To test the integrity of the vertebral arteries, extend and rotate the head (figure 13.12). If the individual notes dizziness or blurred vision, or you note

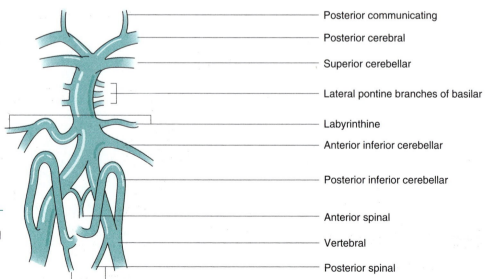

**Figure 13.11**   The vertebral arteries and their intracranial branches.

Reprinted by permission from Hollinshead and Rosse 1985.

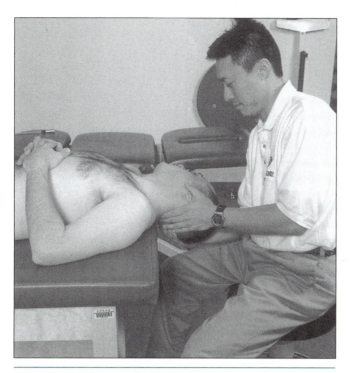

**Figure 13.12** The vertebral artery test.

nystagmus or slurred speech, the vertebral artery on the opposite side may be compromised. The situation can be quickly reversed by repositioning the head in neutral and restoring flow through the vertebral artery system. A positive vertebral test is not common, yet you should perform a vertebral test on any individual before you administer mechanical cervical traction. A positive vertebral artery test contraindicates mechanical traction where long-term positioning of the head poses a risk.

Traction is also contraindicated in some individuals with osteoporosis and rheumatoid arthritis, conditions that may render the bone or connective soft tissues of the cervical spine unable to withstand traction forces. If you have any concerns when treating people with these conditions, consult with the referring physician. It is much better to err on the side of caution than risk injury to the cervical region. The contraindications to cervical traction are summarized in table 13.1 on page 226.

## Lumbar Traction

Distraction of the lumbar spine can also be accomplished with mechanical traction. The traction forces can separate or distract the facet joints and relieve pressure on spinal nerves caused by disc injury. Most facet dysfunction, or mechanical low back pain, responds better to manual techniques such as mobilization and muscle energy.

Most physically active individuals with disc pathology need help to find a resting position that alleviates symptoms. Most disc injuries involve the posterior lateral aspect of the disc. Lumbar extension is believed to encourage the nucleus to migrate anteriorly, away from the spinal nerves. Thus, lying prone with a tolerable extension of the lumbar spine often alleviates the radicular symptoms associated with disc injury. The advantage of finding positional relief is that the individual can control symptoms at home.

Because of the nature of managed care and success in treating low back problems without mechanical lumbar traction, it is not used often. However, it may be very useful in the management of acute conditions when manual techniques and positioning fail to bring relief.

### Setup

Setting a physically active person up for lumbar traction is somewhat involved. Two wide harnesses must be applied, one above the iliac crests and one over the lower ribs. The belts must be snug or the traction force will cause the belts to slide, diminishing the traction forces at the lumbar spine. The belts can be applied with the individual supine but might be much easier to apply with the person standing (figure 13.13). Once the belts are in place, you can position the individual on the traction table. Those whose symptoms are worse in sitting or improved with lying or lumbar extension should be positioned prone (figure 13.14*a*). If sitting is more comfortable or lying and lumbar extension more painful, position the individual supine with the hips and knees flexed (figure 13.14*b*).

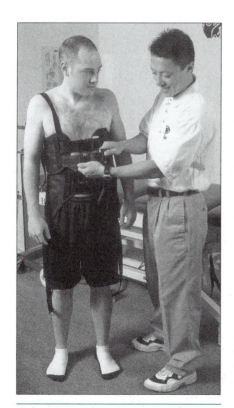

**Figure 13.13** Placing lumbar traction harnesses.

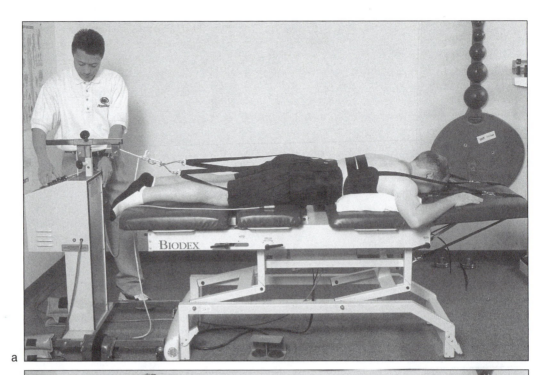

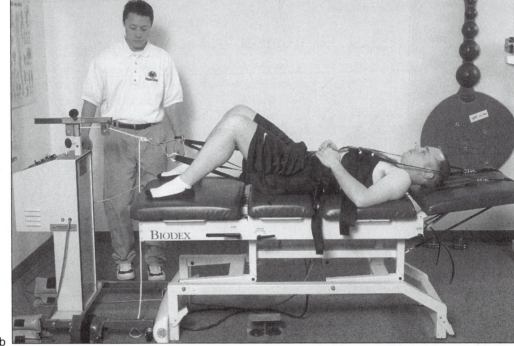

**Figure 13.14**
Mechanical lumbar traction: an individual in the prone position with a pillow under the abdomen to help control lumbar spine extension *(a)*, and an individual in the supine position with hip flexed to approximately 90° *(b)*.

Once the person is positioned, traction forces are administered in either a continuous or an intermittent mode. Intermittent traction (30-45 sec on, 15-30 sec rest) is better tolerated. Shorter "on" times (15 sec) have been suggested for treating facet dysfunction and longer "on" times (60 sec) for disc injury. Unfortunately, little research supports the efficacy of mechanical lumbar traction or provides well-substantiated treatment parameters.

An initial traction force of 25% of body weight is a reasonable starting force. If the initial force is tolerated, increase the traction force up to 50% of body weight. Treatment times usually range from 10 to 20 min, depending upon the nature of the problem and the response to treatment.

### *Precautions and Contraindications*

There are fewer contraindications for lumbar traction (summarized in table 13.1 on p. 226) than for cervical traction. Pregnancy, hiatal hernia, and advanced osteoporosis are absolute contraindications. Fractures and medical conditions, such as cancer, that affect the integrity of the connective tissues also contraindicate mechanical traction. Occasionally individuals experience a significant increase in pain during traction, in which case traction must be terminated. This is particularly common in persons suffering from internal disc derangement.

In daily practice, practical considerations such as belt adjustment and an inability to tolerate treatment affect decisions about the application of mechanical lumbar traction more often than do absolute contraindications. The harness used to apply lumbar traction is adjustable; however, it is often difficult to fasten the belts snugly on very thin individuals, and often the belts cannot be fitted on obese individuals. Furthermore, some people experience claustrophobia when the belts are tightened to prevent sliding.

# INTERMITTENT COMPRESSION

Intermittent compression involves the use of a pneumatic device that intermittently inflates a sleeve around an injured joint or limb. Intermittent compression devices are used to reduce edema and posttraumatic swelling. In athletic training, the primary cause of fluid accumulation in the tissues is trauma. Chapter 3 reviewed the mechanism for posttraumatic swelling and covered the role of the lymphatic system in resolving swelling. Elevation of an injured extremity and contraction of the skeletal muscles can reduce swelling. Intermittent compression may speed the resolution of posttraumatic swelling in some situations. The limited evidence, as discussed further on, does not support the use of intermittent compression in the management of some common musculoskeletal injuries.

Therapeutic modalities that relieve pain and muscle spasm—followed by active exercise—reduce swelling more effectively than does intermittent compression. The exercise activity must be well tolerated and must not cause further tissue damage. However, simple active range of motion exercises within the limits of pain are sufficient to increase lymphatic drainage over that in a resting state. Thus, intermittent compression is better reserved for treating complicated problems such as persistent swelling and wounds caused by venous insufficiency.

## Setup

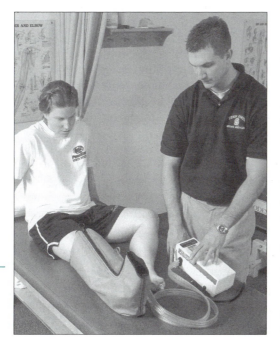

**Figure 13.15** Intermittent compression pump with sequential air filling.

Intermittent compression is easy to administer. A compression stocking is applied to the limb to be treated (figure 13.15). Once the stocking is in place, the intermittent compression unit is adjusted for duty cycle and maximum pressure. No duty cycle has been established as the most effective. Inflation times of 30 to 40 sec are well tolerated when interspersed with 20- to 30-sec off or deflation periods.

There is some disagreement regarding the optimal inflation pressure. Manufacturers have developed guidelines for various conditions (Fond and Hecox 1994). The maximum pressure recommended in treating posttraumatic edema is 50 to 90 mmHg (Fond and Hecox 1994; Hooker 1998). A setting just below diastolic blood pressure is well tolerated by physically active individuals and appears to reduce edema. Once the duty cycle and pressure have been set, the injured individual remains with the affected limb elevated throughout a 20- to 30-min treatment.

## Contraindications

There are few contraindications for intermittent compression (table 13.1). Certainly all situations in which tissue movement is restricted, such as healing fractures and gross joint instability, would contraindicate intermittent compression. Infection, thrombophlebitis, pulmonary edema, and congestive heart failure also contraindicate intermittent compression.

Intermittent compression is a relatively safe, passive approach to reducing posttraumatic edema. However, setup is somewhat time-consuming, and the individual is not actively engaged in the rehabilitation process. Thus, the injured person will likely improve faster by performing pain-free active exercises to encourage lymphatic drainage during treatment in the clinic or athletic training room, and three to four times daily at home, as long as the swelling persists.

## TRACTION AND INTERMITTENT COMPRESSION: EFFECTIVE THERAPIES?

Clinical trials of traction have involved patients with pain in the lumbar and cervical regions. Beurskens et al. (1995, 1997) and Pal (1986) concluded that traction was ineffective in the treatment of patients with low back pain. These investigators had follow-up as long as 6 months posttreatment. Not all the evidence is unsupportive of the use of traction. Van der Heijden et al. (1995) reported that high-dose traction (44% of body weight) was more effective in reducing back pain and improving function than low-dose (19% of body weight) continuous lumbar traction at 5 and 9 weeks posttreatment. The sample size for the study was small (12 and 13 subjects per group), and the differences reported did not reach statistical significance. Furthermore, the treatments were not compared to rest or active interventions. Similarly, Mesarzos et al. (2000) reported that 5 min of static lumbar traction applied in supine at 30% and 60% body weight increased the pain-free range of a straight leg raise immediately after treatment in patients with back pain. However, the duration of this change in motion was not established.

Cervical traction may be effective in the management of patients with radicular symptoms associated with cervical dysfunction. Moeti and Marchetti's (2001) case series on patients with radicular symptoms reported complete resolution of pain in 7 of 11 patients with symptom duration of less than 12 weeks but in only 1 of 4 with longer-duration symptoms. Constantoyannis et al. (2002) came to similar conclusions in a series of four patients. Swezey, Swezey, and Warner (1999) reported that home over-the-door traction devices were effective in helping a large percentage of patients classified on the Quebec Task Force of Whiplash Associated Disorders Cohort Study scale. None of these studies involved comparison to control groups. Two reports comparing cervical traction to no-treatment controls provide conflicting results. Zylbergold and Piper (1985) reported that treatment with intermittent traction over 6 weeks was more effective than no traction in reducing pain and improving motion in patients with cervical spine disorders. Klaber-Moffett, Hughes, and Griffiths (1990) found that similar patients treated with traction "improved slightly more" than no-traction controls. While the design of this study was of high-quality, traction forces were limited to 6 to 15 lb. The use of greater traction forces might have yielded different results.

The use of intermittent compression has been studied in a variety of patients, including those with lymphedema following mastectomy and venous insufficiency. However, few studies could be located that addressed the efficacy of intermittent compression in the management of musculoskeletal conditions. Stockle et al. (1997) reported that intermittent compression reduced postoperative swelling more effectively than a cold compression unit or periodic ice bag application in patients suffering foot and ankle trauma. Airaksinen et al. (1991) reported that intermittent compression decreased lower limb edema following 6 to 12 weeks of cast immobilization in patients with leg fractures. However, this intervention was not compared with active exercise. Griffin et al. (1990) reported decreases in hand edema immediately following intermittent compression in patients suffering from trauma to the hand. Measurements were obtained only immediately following 30 min of treatment.

The timing of measurements is important. Tsang et al. (2001) reported that intermittent compression decreased effusion at the ankle following ankle sprains. The reduction in effusion, however, was very brief. Within 5 min of weight bearing, limb volumes had returned to pretreatment levels. Rucinski et al. (1991) found that intermittent compression increased effusion following ankle sprain.

At this time there is a lack of evidence to recommend the routine use of either lumbar traction or intermittent compression in the treatment of musculoskeletal conditions. When contraindications and precautions are observed, these interventions might be beneficial adjuncts to a comprehensive plan of care in selected circumstances. The certified athletic trainer should, however, consider the time required and the cost of treatment before applying these and other interventions for which much of the evidence suggests that treatment outcomes are not improved. The evidence for management of radicular symptoms of cervical origins is somewhat more favorable. Certainly when treatments can be safely rendered through low-cost home devices, the use of cervical traction may be an important component of a comprehensive treatment strategy.

## SUMMARY

1. Discuss the potential benefits of using manual therapy techniques in rehabilitation.

   Because manual therapies require hands-on treatments, they offer time for conversation and an opportunity develop open communication and mutual understanding. Manual therapies offer additional approaches to relieving pain and muscle spasm and restoring range of motion.

2. Describe massage, myofascial release, strain–counterstrain, muscle energy, and joint mobilization.

   Massage is a collection of techniques that involve rubbing or kneading part of the body. Myofascial release (MFR) is similar to massage in that the certified athletic trainer uses the hands to influence the connective tissues and neural input. However, MFR is directed at specific trigger points and areas of fascial tension and restriction. Strain–counterstrain involves placing the body into a position of greatest comfort, thus relieving pain by reducing or arresting inappropriate proprioceptive activity. Joint mobilization is used to restore intrinsic joint motion or arthrokinetics. Using the convex–concave rule, you can apply joint mobilization techniques to identify and treat motion restriction resulting from the loss of normal gliding between bones during rotation at a joint. Muscle energy techniques are manual procedures that involve active contraction of the individual's muscles against a counterforce in a specific treatment position. Muscle energy techniques can be used to stretch tight muscles and fascia, strengthen weakened muscle, or mobilize restricted joints.

3. Describe the afferent and efferent innervation of intrafusal and extrafusal muscle fibers and the relationship between the gamma and alpha motor neurons.

   Muscle is made up of contractile, extrafusal fibers and sensory, intrafusal fibers called muscle spindles. The contractile fibers are innervated by alpha motor neurons. When an impulse is transmitted down an alpha motor neuron, all of the extrafusal muscle fibers it innervates contract. When many alpha motor neurons are stimulated, many extrafusal fibers contract and the muscle generates force. The length and tension of a muscle are perceived by the muscle spindles. Gamma afferent fibers send information from the spindle to the central nervous system. The length of a muscle spindle must be constantly adjusted in order for it to optimally sense changes in muscle length and tension. The gamma efferent motor nerves innervate the spindle to adjust the resting length.

4. Apply the "convex–concave rule" in performing joint mobilization.

   Joint mobilization is used to restore normal joint arthrokinematics. In normal joint function, when a convex surface, such as the head of the humerus, moves on a concave surface, such as the glenoid, the convex surface glides in the direction opposite to the direction of roll. For example, during abduction of the arm, the head of the humerus rolls upward but glides downward. If a concave surface such as the tibial plateau moves on a convex surface, such as the femoral condyles, roll and glide occur in the same direction. For example, during knee flexion, the tibia rolls and glides posteriorly.

5. Describe the manual and mechanical traction techniques used to treat cervical spine dysfunction.

The cervical spine can be distracted manually or using a traction device. Manual traction offers the advantage of finding the position and traction force that provide the greatest relief. Mechanical traction, with the recipient lying supine, can be accomplished with a traction harness or a Saunder's traction device.

6. Identify contraindications for manual therapies and mechanical traction.

Symptoms of organic diseases such as cancer must be followed up before treatment with any modality, including manual therapies. Massage is contraindicated if infection or skin breakdown or disease is present. Release techniques should not be used during acute inflammation or shortly after a fracture or surgery. Caution is advised if the recipient is pregnant or has a joint replacement or joint instability. Strain–counterstrain should be discontinued if pain increases and should be used with caution following a fracture or if a joint is unstable. Muscle energy is contraindicated in those with a recent fracture or when there is joint instability or a joint fusion. Infection, joint instability, recent fracture, and a "bone-on-bone" end-feel contraindicate joint mobilization; also mobilization of the cervical spine is contraindicated in the presence of advanced rheumatoid arthritis. Both muscle energy and joint mobilization are contraindicated in the presence of bony instability and advanced osteoporosis. There are several contraindications for cervical traction, including a positive vertebral artery or alar ligament test, acute neck injury including fracture and joint instability, advanced rheumatoid arthritis, bone cancer, and advanced osteoporosis. Cervical traction should be discontinued if pain increases or radicular symptoms are exacerbated by treatment. Lumbar traction is contraindicated by pregnancy, claustrophobia, internal disc derangement, fractures and sprains with joint instability, bone cancer, advanced osteoporosis, and hiatal hernia. Lumbar traction should also be discontinued if pain is increased or radicular symptoms are exacerbated by treatment.

7. Describe the mechanical traction techniques used to treat lumbar spine dysfunction.

Traction to the lumbar spine can be administered with the individual in prone or supine position. If symptoms are reduced when the individual is sitting, as is often the case with foraminal or spinal stenosis, having the individual lie supine with the hip flexed is preferred. If symptoms decrease when the spine is extended, as is the case when the individual lies prone, the person should be treated in prone position. A traction force of one-fourth to one-half of body weight with intervals of traction (e.g., 40 sec) and rest (e.g., 20 sec) is generally recommended.

8. Describe the application of, and contraindications for, intermittent compression therapy.

Intermittent compression involves the use of a pneumatic device that intermittently inflates a sleeve around an injured joint or limb. Intermittent compression facilitates lymphatic drainage, which will reduce swelling. Intermittent compression should not be applied in the presence of thrombophlebitis, infection, or acute fractures or in cases in which the individual has pulmonary edema or congestive heart failure.

# CITED SOURCES

Airaksinen O, Partanen K, Kolari PJ, Soimakallio S: Intermittent pneumatic compression therapy in posttraumatic lower limb edema: Computed tomography and clinical measurements. *Arch Phys Med Rehabil* 72:667-670, 1991.

Assendelft WJ, Morton SC, Yu EI, Suttorp MJ, Shekelle PG: Spinal manipulative therapy for low back pain. A meta-analysis of effectiveness relative to other therapies. *Ann Intern Med* 138:871-881, 2003.

Aure OF, Hoel Nilsen J, Vasseljen O: Manual therapy and exercise therapy in patients with chronic low back pain. A randomized, controlled trial with 1-year follow-up. *Spine* 28:525-531, 2003.

Beurskens AJ, de Vet HC, Koke AJ, Lindeman E, Regtop W, van der Heijden GJ, Knipschild PG: Efficacy of traction for non-specific low-back pain: A randomized clinical trial. *Lancet* 346:1596-1600, 1995.

Beurskens AJ, de Vet HC, Koke AJ, Regtop W, van der Heijden GJ, Linderman E, Knipschild PG: Efficacy of traction for non-specific low back pain. 12 week and 6 month results of a randomized clinical trial. *Spine* 22:2756-2762, 1997.

Blackburn PG, Simons LR, Crossley KM: Treatment of chronic exertional anterior compartment syndrome with massage: A pilot study. *Clin J Sport Med* 8:14-17, 1998.

Bronfort G, Assendelft WJ, Evans R, Haas M, Bouter L: Efficacy of spinal manipulation for chronic headache: A systematic review. *J Manip Physiol Ther* 24:457-466, 2001.

Cassidy JD, Lopes AA, Yong-Hing K: The immediate effect of manipulation versus mobilization on pain and range of motion in the cervical spine: A randomized controlled trial. *J Manip Physiol Ther* 15:570-575, 1992.

Cherkin DC, Deyo RA, Battie M, Street J, Barlow W: A comparison of physical therapy, chiropractic manipulation, and provision of an educational booklet for the treatment of patients with low back pain. *N Engl J Med* 339:1021-1029, 1998.

Clemente CD. Anatomy- A regional atlas of the human body. Baltimore. Urban & Swartzenberg 1981. Fig. 465, 467.

Colachis SC, Strohan BR: Cervical traction relationship of time to varied tractive force with constant angle of pull. *Arch Phys Med Rehabil* 46:815-819, 1965.

Colachis SC, Strohan BR: Effects of intermittent traction on separation of lumbar vertebrae. *Arch Phys Med Rehabil* 50:251-258, 1969.

Conroy DE, Hayes KW: The effect of joint mobilization as a component of comprehensive treatment for primary shoulder impingement syndrome. *J Orthop Phys Ther* 28:3-14, 1998.

Constantoyannis C, Konstantinou D, Kourtopoulos H, Papadakis N: Intermittent cervical traction for cervical radiculopathy caused by large-volume herniated disks. *J Manip Physiol Ther* 25:188-192, 2002.

Costill JH, Wilmore JH. Physiology of sport and exercise. Champaign, IL. Human Kinetics. 1999. pg. 60-61.

Coulter I: Manipulation and mobilization of the cervical spine: The results of a literature survey and consensus panel. *J Musculoskeletal Pain* 4:113-123, 1996.

Denegar CR, Hertel J, Fonseca J: The effect of lateral ankle sprain on dorsiflexion range of motion, posterior talar glide, and joint laxity. *J Orthop Sports Phys Ther* 32:166-173, 2002.

Ferreira M, Ferreira P, Latimer J, Herbert R, Maher CG: Does spinal manipulative therapy help people with chronic low back pain? *Australian J Physiother* 48:277-284, 2002.

Fond D, Hecox B: Intermittent pneumatic compression. In Hecox B, Mehreteab TA, Weisberg J (Eds), *Physical Agents*. Norwalk, CT, Appleton & Lange, 1994, 419-428.

Furlan AD, Brosseau L, Imamura M, Irvin E: Massage for low back pain (Cochrane review). *The Cochrane Library* 2, 2002.

Furlan AD, Brosseau L, Imamura M, Irvin E: Massage for low back pain. Abstract www.cochrane.org/cochrane/revabstr/AB001929.htm.

Green T, Refshauge K, Crosbie J, Adams R: A randomized controlled trial of passive accessory joint mobilization on acute ankle inversion sprains. *Phys Ther* 81:984-994, 2002.

Griffin JW, Newsome LS, Stralka SW, Wright PE: Reduction of chronic posttraumatic hand edema: A comparison of high voltage pulsed current, intermittent pneumatic compression, and placebo treatments. *Phys Ther* 70:279-286, 1990.

Hernandez-Reif M, Field T, Krasnegor J, Theakston H: Lower back pain is reduced and range of motion increased after massage therapy. *Int J Neurosci* 106:131-145, 2001.

Holingshead Wh, Rosse C. Textbook of Anatomy. Philadelphia. Harper & Row, 1985. pg. 928.

Hooker D: Intermittent compression devices. In Prentice WE (Ed), *Therapeutic Modalities for Allied Health Professionals*. New York, McGraw-Hill, 1998, 392-403.

Houglum PA: *Therapeutic Exercise for Musculoskeletal Injuries*, 2nd ed. Champaign, IL, Human Kinetics, 2005.

Hseih CY, Adams AH, Tobis J, Hong CZ, Danielson C, Platt K, Hoehler F, Reinsch S, Rubel A: Effectiveness of four conservative treatments for subacute low back pain. A randomized clinical trial. *Spine* 27:1142-1148, 2002.

Hurwitz EL, Morgenstern H, Harber P, Kominski GF, Belin TR, Yu F, Adams AH: A randomized trial of medical care with and without physical therapy and chiropractic care with and without physical modalities for patients with low back pain: 6 month follow-up outcomes from the UCLA low back pain study. *Spine* 27:2193-2204, 2002.

Jones LH, Kusunose R, Goering E: *Jones Strain-Counterstrain*. Boise, ID, Jones Strain-Counterstrain, Inc., 1995.

Klaber-Moffett JA, Hughes GI, Griffiths P: An investigation of the effects of cervical traction. Part 1: Clinical effectiveness. *Clin Rehabil* 4:205-211, 1990.

Mealy K, Brennan H, Fenelon GC: Early mobilization of acute whiplash injuries. *BMJ* 292:656-657, 1986.

Meszaros TF, Olson R, Kulig K, Creighton D, Czarnecki E: Effect of 10%, 30% and 60% body weight traction on straight leg raise test of symptomatic patients with low back pain. *J Orthop Sports Phys Ther* 30:595-601, 2000.

Moeti P, Marchetti G: Clinical outcome from mechanical intermittant cervical traction for the treatment of cervical radiculopathy: A case series. *J Orthop Sports Phys Ther* 31:527-538, 2001.

Pal B, Mangion P, Hossain MA, Diffey BL: A controlled trial of continuous lumbar traction in treatment of back pain and sciatica. *Br J Rheumatol* 25:181-183, 1986.

Preyde M: Effectiveness of massage therapy for subacute low-back pain: A randomized controlled trial. *CMAJ* 162:1815-1820, 2000.

Quinn C, Chandler C, Moraska A: Massage therapy and frequency of chronic tension headaches. *Am J Public Health* 92:1657-1661, 2002.

Rucinski TJ, Hooker DN, Prentice WE Jr., Shields EX Jr., Cote-Murray DJ: The effects of intermittent compression on edema in postacute ankle sprains. *J Orthop Sports Phys Ther* 14:65-69, 1991.

Schiller L: Effectiveness of spinal manipulative therapy in the treatment of mechanical thoracic spine pain. A pilot randomized clinical trial. *J Manip Physiol Ther* 24:394-401, 2001.

Stockle U, Hoffmann R, Schultz M, von Fournier C, Sudkamp NP, Haas N: Fastest reduction of posttraumatic edema: Continuous cryotherapy or intermittent impulse compression? *Foot Ankle Int* 18:432-438, 1997.

Sucher BM: Myofascial manipulative release of carpal tunnel syndrome: Documentation with magnetic resonance imaging. *J Am Osteopath Assoc* 93:1273-1278, 1993.

Swezey RL, Swezey AM, Warner K: Efficacy of home traction therapy. *Am J Phys Med Rehabil* 78: 30-32, 1999.

Tsang KKW, Hertel JH, Denegar CR, Buckley WE: The effects of elevation and intermittent compression on the volume of injured ankles (Abstract). *J Athl Train* 36:S-50, 2001.

Van der Heijden GJM, Beurskens AJH, Dirx MJM, Bouter LM, Lindeman E: Efficacy of lumbar traction. A randomized clinical trial. *Physiotherapy* 81:29-35, 1995.

Woerman AL: Evaluation and treatment of dysfunction in the lumbar-pelvic-hip complex. In Donatelli R, Wooden MJ (Eds), *Orthopaedic Physical Therapy*. New York, Churchill Livingstone, 1989, 403-483.

Zlybergold RS, Piper MC: Cervical spine disorders. A comparison of three types of traction. *Spine* 10: 867-871, 1985.

## ADDITIONAL READINGS

Dutton M: *Manual Therapy of the Spine*. New York, McGraw-Hill, 2002.

Dvorak J, Dvorak V: *Manual Medicine: Therapy*. New York, Thieme Medical, 1988.

Dvorak J, Dvorak V: *Manual Medicine: Diagnostics*, 2nd ed. New York, Thieme Medical, 1990.

King R: *Performance Massage*. Champaign, IL, Human Kinetics, 1993.

Kuprian W: *Physical Therapy for Sports*, 2nd ed. Philadelphia, Saunders, 1995.

# Treatment Plans for Acute Musculoskeletal Injuries

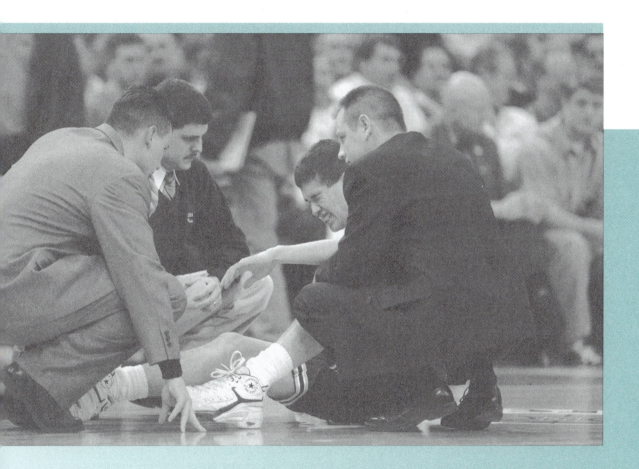

## *Objectives*

After reading this chapter, the student will be able to

1. develop rehabilitation plans of care to control the signs and symptoms of acute inflammatory response;

2. provide a rationale for the application of therapeutic modalities to treat the signs and symptoms of acute inflammation;

3. provide guidelines for progression of a rehabilitation plan of care through the repair and maturation phases of tissue healing; and

4. discuss the role of therapeutic modalities during the repair and maturation phases of tissue healing.

It is a busy Monday in the athletic training room. A baseball pitcher sustained an acromioclavicular sprain of his throwing shoulder while horseback riding over the weekend. A soccer player also sustained a shoulder injury. A wide receiver sustained a sprain of the tibial collateral ligament of his right knee, and a field hockey player sprained her left ankle. All are acute injuries, but each will require a unique rehabilitation plan of care.

To safely return these athletes to competition, you must do more than apply therapeutic modalities or instruct the athlete in therapeutic exercises. First you have to consider the injury, the healing process, and the demands placed on the body by each athlete's sport. The initial goal of treatment for each athlete will be to control pain and swelling and protect the damaged tissues, and the next goal will be to restore range of motion and neuromuscular control. Therapeutic modalities can help achieve early treatment goals. Each athlete, however, will return to sport at a different time. The soccer player will return sooner than the pitcher because of the stresses that throwing places on the shoulder. The field hockey player is found to have a mild ankle sprain and may return to play in only a week because the injured ligaments can be protected with taping and bracing. The football player has sustained a complete tear of the ligament and will miss more time. This chapter integrates the information presented on inflammation and healing, pain, and the therapeutic modalities discussed in the previous six chapters and establishes the framework for applying specific therapeutic exercises and procedures.

The practicing clinician must make decisions about the patients he or she serves. The recipient of care should be provided the rationale for a recommended treatment and information regarding alternatives. The certified athletic trainer should also be able to justify his or her decisions to referring physicians and those that reimburse health care providers. The decision to apply or not apply therapeutic modalities is part of a comprehensive evaluation and treatment process.

In this chapter, our focus is on acute musculoskeletal injuries. The schematic (figure 14.1) provides an overview of the decision sequence and plausible rationale for interventions following acute musculoskeletal injury. The certified athletic trainer may encounter patients at various stages in the recovery process. These contacts may include immediate on-the-field care as well as referrals into an outpatient setting days, or in some cases, weeks after the injury. Thus, certified athletic trainers must be able to identify where in the decision sequence they first encounter each patient seeking care. To accomplish this task and properly manage acute musculoskeletal injuries, you must understand the inflammatory process. Although the physiological events that occur from the time of injury to the maturation of regenerated or scar tissues occur sequentially, the timing of the events varies with the extent of injury and the general health of the injured person. Neither are there absolute boundaries between the stages of the inflammatory process (figure 14.2). However, the principal purpose of the inflammatory, repair, and maturation phases, and the symptoms experienced during each, provide a framework for a plan of care.

The acute inflammatory response initially limits the loss of red blood cells from the vascular system through clotting and vasoconstriction. The initial response, mediated through epinephrine and thromboxane, begins at the moment of tissue damage. Unless larger vascular structures are damaged or the skin is lacerated, your actions probably have little impact on this initial response. Thus, it is unlikely that you can apply a modality quickly enough to influence these early events in the inflammatory response.

Once further loss of red blood cells is prevented, the acute inflammatory response proceeds to remove damaged tissues and set the stage for repair. During this time the cardinal signs of inflammation appear. It has long been suggested that modalities, particularly cold, can be applied to limit inflammation. At this point you must ask whether the goal of treatment is to inhibit inflammation or to relieve pain, minimize loss of function, and limit the secondary cell death associated with acute inflammation.

Acute musculoskeletal injury

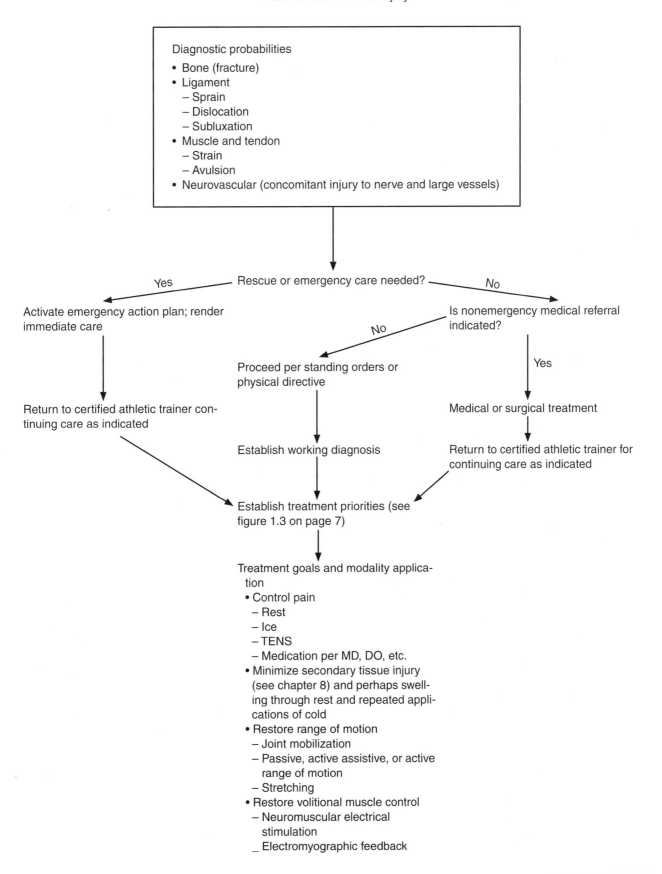

**Figure 14.1**  Schematic of decision sequence.

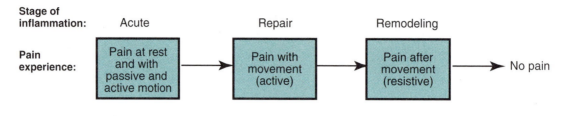

**Figure 14.2**    The pain experience through the phases of inflammation.

The cases presented at the opening of this chapter further illustrate the challenges of clinical decision making. Efforts to relieve pain, limit swelling, and preserve neuromuscular control are warranted in each case. However, in each case the damaged ligaments will heal because of the physiological process of inflammation. Return to competition often depends upon the ability of the sports medicine team to protect healing tissues. The soccer player with the injured shoulder may return to play sooner than the baseball player because a pitcher cannot throw without stressing the acromioclavicular joint. The soccer player may return sooner than the football player because taping and bracing will adequately protect the ankle but not the knee. An individualized, goal-oriented plan of care must be developed for each injured person. Therapeutic modalities should be applied when they can help the individual achieve specific treatment goals.

# Acute Injury and Acute Onset of Pain—Are They the Same?

The following case studies further illustrate some of the considerations in the management of acute problems. In the first, the onset of pain is associated with tissue damage. Is this necessarily true in the second case?

## Case Study 1

A soccer player is assisted into the athletic training room. Examination by you and later by the team physician reveals that she has suffered a Grade II sprain of the tibial collateral ligament. The physician believes that the player will be able to return to soccer in about 6 weeks. What are the short-term treatment goals for this athlete? Which modalities should be applied?

## Case Study 2

A 43-year-old club hockey player is referred to your care because of acute recurrence of low back pain. The player states that he twisted his back when he collided with two opponents in a game early this morning. He experienced immediate pain and chose not to continue playing, because there were only a few minutes left to play. He was evaluated by his personal physician because he began experiencing increased pain and muscle spasm while at work. He was provided with analgesic medications and referred for treatment of mechanical low back pain.

On presentation he is in obvious discomfort but states the pain is well localized to the mid-lumbar spine. He denies radicular symptoms or significant medical problems except for one previous episode of back pain experienced while he was cutting wood last year. He reports that he received treatment on three occasions consisting of superficial heat, manual therapies, and therapeutic exercise, and that his back pain resolved within 2 weeks. What are the short-term treatment goals for this athlete? Which modalities should be applied?

# MANAGEMENT IN THE ACUTE STAGE: REST, ICE, COMPRESSION, ELEVATION

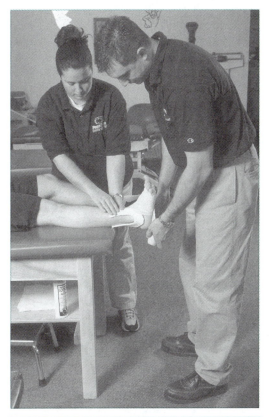

**Figure 14.3** A felt horseshoe-shaped pad provides an excellent compress when held in place by an elastic wrap.

If the inflammatory process is not completed, tissue is not repaired. Thus, the initial treatment goals following tissue damage should be to protect the damaged tissues, limit secondary cell death, and control swelling, pain, and loss of function. Although a greater understanding of secondary cell death is needed, it is reasonable to believe that these goals can be accomplished with *a combination of* rest, elevation, compression, and cryotherapy. The RICE recipe (rest, ice, compression, elevation) is well known by athletic trainers, and it makes sense. However, elevation and rest are often overlooked, perhaps because it is assumed that ice—because of an anti-inflammatory effect—is the only really important treatment intervention. There is evidence from an animal model that cold alone may also limit swelling (Dolan et al. 1997), although the efficacy of cryotherapy in controlling swelling following musculoskeletal injury in humans has not been substantiated. Elevation may have a greater effect on swelling than does ice. External compression promotes rest of the injured tissue and can potentially limit swelling. However, most compressive dressings applied following athletic injuries do not provide sufficient counterforce to effectively limit swelling. Felt pads, donuts, and horseshoes (figure 14.3) can increase the effectiveness of external compression.

To summarize, cold application should be viewed as a component of the RICE recipe that controls pain, limits the loss of function associated with acute inflammation, and minimizes secondary cell death. The injured individual should be *instructed in each component* of the RICE recipe to maximize the effect of early injury management (figure 14.4).

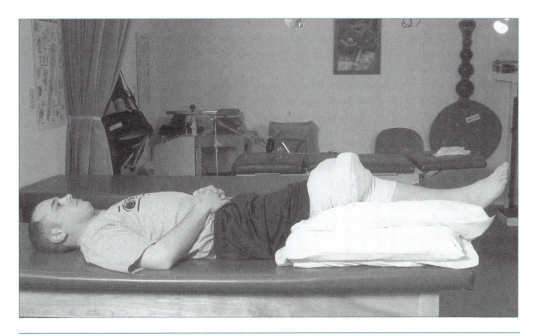

**Figure 14.4** Protect damaged tissues and control swelling, pain, and loss of function with rest, ice, compression, and elevation.

Furthermore, while the analgesic effect of cold is rapid and readily apparent, secondary cell death is not. *Repeated applications* of ice and rest are needed for a period of time after the injury. Research is needed to better determine the optimal frequency and duration for cold applications. As noted in chapter 8, a 20-min application of cold is sufficient to decrease tissue temperatures for more than 2 h when the person is at rest (Knight 1995; Knight et al. 1980). Thus, a 20-min application every 2 h while at rest may reduce secondary cell death and provide pain relief. For how long should cold applications be repeated? This question remains unanswered. The activity of neutrophils is greatest in the 6 to 8 h after injury. Neutrophils are potent sources of tissue-damaging free radicals. Thus, at minimum it seems prudent to repeat ice applications for 6 to 8 h after acute musculoskeletal injuries when possible.

## MODALITIES USED IN ADDITION TO RICE

You are not limited to RICE in managing the symptoms of the acute inflammatory response. Microcurrent has been proposed as a treatment that limits the retraction of endothelial cells and minimizes increases in capillary membrane permeability. Studies involving animal models support the effects of these modalities (Bettany, Fish, and Mendel 1990). However, the effects of this intervention on the injury response over several days following tissue damage in humans have not been fully investigated.

One must remember that the increased capillary membrane permeability promotes movement of leukocytes from the circulation to phagocytize necrotic tissue. It is likely that modality intervention with cold or microcurrent might slow this response. However, the presence of necrotic tissue stimulates continuation of the acute inflammatory phase. Thus, the question remains: Will minimizing increases in capillary membrane permeability limit the development of swelling, delay tissue repair, neither, or both? Further study should be completed before these modalities are used to manage acute inflammation.

Transcutaneous electrical nerve stimulation (TENS) can be applied as an adjunct to RICE. Although it seems illogical to use a modality that relieves pain by increasing sensory input in conjunction with cryotherapy, which decreases sensory input, the combination of these modalities may be more effective in decreasing pain and muscle spasm than either used alone. This observation has not been fully explained; however, it may be that cold has a greater effect on the thinly myelinated and unmyelinated afferent fibers that transmit pain information than on the heavily myelinated A-alpha and A-beta afferent fibers. Research has indicated that cryotherapy has little impact on proprioception and pressure sensation, supporting the notion that large-diameter afferent fiber impulse transmission is not slowed by cold application (Ingersoll, Knight, and Merrick 1992; West 1998). Thus, TENS with conventional parameters may block pain through ascending pathways while the cold slows transmission along pain-carrying fibers, decreases the sensitivity of muscle spindles, and relieves muscle spasm.

Therefore, RICE is usually the treatment of choice following acute musculoskeletal injury; TENS appears to be a useful adjunct to relieve pain and reduce muscle spasm. During the acute inflammatory response, movement of the injury area is restricted. As pain subsides, the individual's rehabilitation program should be modified to address losses in range of motion and neuromuscular control. There is no single physiological landmark that signals the end of acute inflammation and the beginning of repair, so how do you know when you can initiate treatments to restore range of motion and neuromuscular control? In general, you must be certain that therapeutic activities do not compromise tissue repair, and you should let pain guide the advancement of exercise. In some situations, such as a mild to moderate lateral ankle sprain, the individual can progress toward functional exercise rapidly because the healing tissues are not stressed during weight bearing. In other cases, such as mechanical low back pain, the pain–spasm response is more disabling than the tissue damage. However, in situations such as a tibial collateral ligament sprain or a fracture, tissue repair must occur before many exercises can be initiated because valgus stress to the knee could disrupt the repair process.

# REPAIR PHASE

As the physiological events of an acute inflammatory response proceed, necrotic tissue is phagocytized and a new vascular network to support repair is established. The injured area is less hot and swollen. Pain is experienced with movement but not while the injured part is at rest.

During the repair phase, new treatment goals are established. Restoring range of motion and neuromuscular control become the focus of treatment. As range of motion and neuromuscular control improve, muscular strength and endurance emerge as the new short-term treatment priorities.

The transition from treatment directed at controlling pain and the other symptoms of acute inflammation to treatment that addresses losses of motion, neuromuscular control, endurance, and strength is no more clear-cut than the physiological events that distinguish acute inflammation from early tissue repair. However, a few simple guidelines are available.

When the injured person no longer experiences pain at rest and demonstrates a willingness to move the injured part, you can initiate efforts to restore motion and neuromuscular control provided that the therapeutic activities do not jeopardize the repair process. You may find that modality application before or during manual therapies and therapeutic exercises can help you reach treatment goals. The goals of modality application have changed subtly at this point. Controlling pain *during motion* and recovering motion and function become the central focus. Since the events leading to secondary cell death have ended, the clinician now has a wider range of therapeutic modalities to choose from.

For example, after spraining the lateral ankle ligaments, an individual often experiences a loss of ankle range of motion, especially dorsiflexion. Once active motion can be initiated, you can use cold water immersion (figure 14.5), contrast therapy, or superficial heat in the form of whirlpool at the beginning of treatment. These modalities reduce pain and stiffness and allow for more aggressive therapeutic exercises, in terms of active range of motion and weight bearing, as well as less muscle guarding during manual procedures such as joint mobilization.

If healing tissues can be protected, the rehabilitation program can be progressed as rapidly as tolerated. For example, if the sprain is isolated to the lateral ligaments, activities such as balance, walking, and jogging will not significantly stress the damaged ligaments. Thus, the individual can be progressed from partial weight bearing to walking and jogging as rapidly as tolerated. In general, therapeutic exercises should not be painful; pain indicates that the acute inflammatory response has not resolved or that the stress of the exercise exceeds the capacity of the damaged tissues. Painful exercise will inhibit neuromuscular control and slow the return to sport.

One dilemma you will face is defining the limits of pain. All injuries hurt, and individuals differ in their sensitivity to and tolerance of pain. In addition, most competitive athletes train intensely with the attitude of "no pain, no gain." Therefore, follow these guidelines for therapeutic exercise: The exercise is inappropriate if the pain experienced alters proper movement mechanics and if the injured individual is unable to do tomorrow what was done today.

If we continue to use a lateral ankle sprain as an example, an individual may rapidly progress to full weight bearing and be able to walk without a limp. It may be, however, that as the athlete begins to jog, a limp becomes apparent. You must now choose from the following four options: (1) Continue the exercise if instructional or visual feedback (a mirror is good for this) corrects the faulty mechanics; (2) apply a modality such as

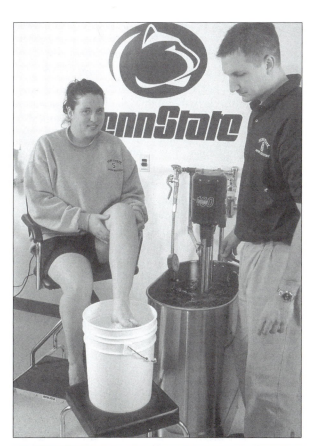

**Figure 14.5**  Cold water immersion and active range motion can be used to reduce pain and stiffness and allow for more aggressive therapeutic exercises.

cold to allow for pain-free activity; (3) limit the individual to exercises that are pain free; or (4) terminate the exercise session. There isn't a single right answer, and clinical experience will help you make the best decision. If the mechanical flaws are minor and the athlete feels able to continue exercise, it may be possible to correct faulty mechanics. If mild pain appears to be altering the movement mechanics, the analgesic (not anesthetic) response to cryotherapy may allow progression to jogging. If pain and altered gait pattern are more substantial, the individual may need more time to master less demanding tasks or may have reached his or her limit for activity that day.

The skilled clinician will usually err on the side of caution. Overstressing the tissues will stimulate an acute inflammatory response and can slow recovery by days. The master athletic trainer advances a program of rehabilitation at just the right rate, using pain and quality of movement as guides.

The issue of faulty movement mechanics noted in the previous paragraph warrants another mention. The restoration of normal neuromuscular control may be a treatment goal in the management of acute musculoskeletal injuries as well as patients suffering from persistent pain. Not all injured athletes will demonstrate impaired neuromuscular control and specific therapeutic exercises are often sufficient to overcome these deficits when they are identified. Some individuals will, however, benefit from additional treatment strategies that promote restoration of neuromuscular control.

One such strategy is biofeedback. Electromyographic (EMG) biofeedback requires specific equipment, but since no energy is delivered to the body, EMG differs from all of the modalities previously discussed. Since neuromuscular control deficits affect a broad range of injured athletes and patients, we elected to introduce EMG biofeedback and further discuss restoring neuromuscular function in the next chapter.

# MATURATION

The point of transition from repair to maturation is no better defined than that from the acute response to the repair phase. However, several distinctions delineate repair from maturation. Clinically, the individual will experience pain after, but not during, movement. Physiologically, the quality of the collagen formed during maturation is better than that formed during the repair phase, and the alignment of the protein fibers permits greater tensile strength. The vascular network needed to support repair retracts.

In general the tissue maturation phase is a long, gradual process during which the rate of new tissue growth is gradually matched by the rate of tissue resorption. The intensity, duration, and complexity of therapeutic exercise can be increased, and the body responds to the demands imposed upon it. Appropriate levels of activity will facilitate the maturation process, but excessive activity will result in pain and perhaps other symptoms of acute inflammation.

The goals of treatment during tissue maturation differ from those established earlier. During the maturation phase, pain control is no longer required. The individual should be well along in terms of regaining full range of motion and neuromuscular control. At this stage, functional progression back to practice and competition becomes foremost in the plan of treatment. Thus, there should be little need for therapeutic modalities during this period of recovery.

## Tissue Restrictions and Rest–Reinjury

Modality application during tissue maturation may be necessary, however, in selected circumstances. Occasionally an athlete may have difficulty regaining full motion and tissue pliability due to scarring and the formation of adhesions. In these cases, modalities such as ultrasound, diathermy, massage, joint mobilization, and fascial stretching can be used.

Perhaps the most common example is the use of joint mobilization with postoperative scarring. For instance, after anterior cruciate ligament reconstruction there is a tendency for loss of patellar mobility and the formation of a tight, dense scar. If patellar mobilization is not addressed early in the postoperative care, loss of mobility can restrict knee range of motion and cause knee pain with functional activity.

The surgical incision cuts across tissue boundaries, and the scarring process can result in adhesion between dermal and fascial layers. These adhesions can become hypersensitive and restrict normal tissue movement. Optimal treatment involves early tissue mobilization. However, if tissue maturation is under way when the scar and capsular tissue restrictions are identified, successful treatment is still possible. Heating the tissue with ultrasound or, in some cases, superficial heating modalities can increase tissue elasticity and enhance the response to manual therapies.

Modality application also may be indicated when overuse of the injured area results in postexercise pain, swelling, and stiffness. These minor exacerbations can be controlled with cold and occasionally TENS. Repeated bouts of therapeutic exercise and athletic activity that aggravate the condition should be avoided through the establishment of appropriate guidelines for return to unrestricted participation. Failure to follow such guidelines will ultimately slow the athlete's return to competition (see "Rest–Reinjury Cycle" in chapter 5).

# Delayed and Failed Tissue Healing

The human body possesses a truly amazing ability to recover from injury and repair itself. Knowledge of the processes by which the body heals is fundamental to effective athletic training. However, despite the body's innate ability to heal and an ever-increasing understanding of the physiology of tissue repair, sometimes the process fails. Over the last 25 years there has been an increase in the treatment of delayed and slowed healing responses with modalities. The failure to heal indicates a breakdown in the acute inflammatory, tissue repair, and tissue maturation processes.

## *Nonhealing or Slow-to-Heal Skin Wounds*

The most common and costly nonhealing wounds are skin wounds. You are unlikely to encounter a nonhealing or slow-to-heal skin wound in the athletic training room; however, certified athletic trainers working in nontraditional settings may observe these wounds.

Slow-to-heal and nonhealing skin lesions are caused by pressure (decubitus ulcers) and vascular compromise (arterial or venous insufficiency). Medical complications, limited mobility, and poor nutrition contribute to the development and compromised healing of these wounds. At one time many of these wounds were treated with regular cleansing in a whirlpool. Unfortunately, many of the additives used to prevent infection, as well as the action of the water, actually damaged fragile granulation tissues and delayed healing. Wound management has been extensively investigated. New wound dressings and treatment regimens have been developed.

The application of electrical, acoustic (ultrasound), and light (laser) energy has been shown to speed wound healing through increased collagen production by fibroblasts (figure 14.6). The wound healing literature indicates that optimal responses occur within a fairly narrow range of energy delivery. Dyson's (1990) summary of the findings of several studies from the 1970s and 1980s revealed that wounds respond to pulsed ultrasound delivered at an amplitude of 1.0 W/cm² or less. Kloth and Feeder's (1990) summary of clinical trials with electrical energy yielded similar conclusions. Slow-to-heal wounds respond favorably to low-amplitude (<800 μA) direct current as well as pulsed monophasic currents with low average current. There is some indication that wound healing responses to laser treatment are similar, in that low average energy stimulates the greatest response.

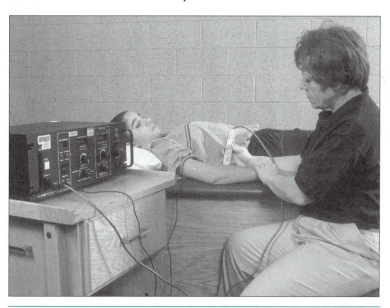

**Figure 14.6** Treating a wound with a laser to speed collagen production.

## Delayed Healing and Nonunion Fractures

Unlike nonhealing skin ulcers, nonunion fractures can affect otherwise healthy physically active people. Delayed or nonunion fractures of the scaphoid, fifth metatarsal, and tibia are not uncommon in physically active people. Nonunion of scaphoid fractures is related to the vasculature surrounding the bone and the potential for disruption of blood supply to a portion of the bone following fracture. Early recognition and proper management greatly minimize the risk of nonunion following scaphoid fracture. The causes of nonunion in other areas are less well defined; infection, poor nutrition, or other medical conditions may contribute. In some cases, the cause of delayed healing or nonunion is never identified.

As noted in chapter 11, small electrical currents and pulsed ultrasound have been reported to promote healing in delayed and nonunion fractures. This section briefly reviews modalities in wound and fracture healing as well as potential implications for treatment of physically active individuals.

Researchers studying the healing of nonunion fractures following treatment regimens with pulsed ultrasound (Heckman et al. 1994; Kristiansen et al. 1997) and pulsed electromagnetic fields (Heckman et al. 1994; Holmes 1994; Marcer, Musati, and Bassett 1984) report that the optimal response requires low levels of energy. These devices are used upon physician prescription. In states where law permits, athletic trainers can apply these modalities if there is access to the devices. Exogen Inc. (Piscataway, NJ) manufactures a pulsed ultrasound unit to stimulate fracture healing (figure 14.7). The device delivers a low average power of 117 mW, and clinical treatment consists of one 20-min application daily. If more research is conducted and the use of these modalities increases, athletic trainers may more frequently administer them.

The study of modality application and healing is not limited to skin lesions and fractures. Researchers are also investigating the impact of electrical current introduced through indwelling electrodes on ligament and tendon repair. The vascularity of some areas of tendon is limited, which compromises healing through a normal inflammatory response. It is possible that devices similar to those used to stimulate fracture healing will be developed for use on ligaments and tendons.

The discussion in the previous three paragraphs gives rise to one important question: If modalities can speed healing of slow-to-heal skin wounds and nonunion fractures, can it speed healing of tissues damaged by athletic injury and promote an earlier return to sport? At present there is no evidence that any of the modalities discussed in this text can speed tissue repair in a healthy individual who is free from conditions known to compromise the repair process. However, work is in progress to answer this question more definitively.

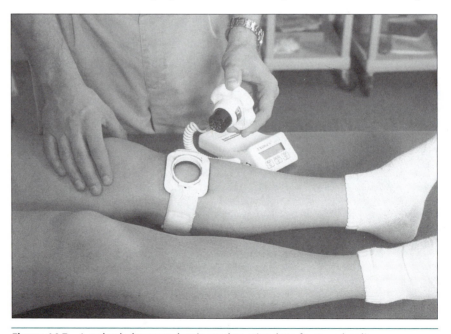

**Figure 14.7**  A pulsed ultrasound unit used to stimulate fracture healing.

## SUMMARY

1. Develop rehabilitation plans of care to control the signs and symptoms of acute inflammatory response.

   Acute inflammation is associated with pain, swelling, and loss of function. Rest, ice, compression, and elevation, used in combination, will alleviate pain and minimize swelling. Early pain-free range of motion can be initiated to enhance lymphatic drainage if motion does not disrupt tissue repair.

2. Provide a rationale for the application of therapeutic modalities to treat the signs and symptoms of acute inflammation.

   Cold pack application and TENS can be used following injury to relieve pain. Cold slows nerve conduction velocity, whereas TENS increases large-diameter afferent nerve input into the central nervous system. The decrease in pain message transmission may be accompanied by enkephalin release at the dorsal horn; each has an analgesic effect. Elevation decreases capillary hydrostatic pressure, and compression may raise interstitial pressure. Cold causes vasoconstriction. Used in combination, ice, compression, and elevation will limit swelling. Cold also reduces metabolic activity and may protect against secondary tissue injury.

3. Provide guidelines for progression of a rehabilitation plan of care through the repair and maturation phases of tissue healing.

   It is impossible to know exactly how much stress healing tissues can tolerate without being reinjured. Pain, however, offers the best guide for progression of a rehabilitation program. If pain is defined as a discomfort that alters normal movement mechanics, then two guidelines for progression can be established: Active therapeutic exercise should be pain free, and the injured individual should be able to do tomorrow what was done today. Pain during or following exercise is a sign that excessive stress is being applied to the healing structure and that the frequency, duration, or intensity of the activity (or more than one of these) should be reduced.

4. Discuss the role of therapeutic modalities during the repair and maturation phases of tissue healing.

   During tissue repair, cold or superficial heat may be applied to reduce pain and facilitate completion of therapeutic exercises. There is no clear choice, although as time passes and pain and spasm give way to soreness and stiffness, superficial heat may be preferred. During this time, whirlpools and fluidotherapy provide an environment where cold and heat can be combined with active range of motion exercises. As repair gives way to maturation, pain, swelling, and limited motion no longer affect therapeutic exercises and attention turns toward functional, sport-specific exercise. During this time, modality application is no longer indicated.

## CITED SOURCES

Bettany JA, Fish DR, Mendel FC: Influence of high volt pulsed direct current on edema formation following impact injury. *Phys Ther* 70:13-18, 1990.

Dolan MG, Thornton RM, Fish DR, Mendel FC: Effects of cold water immersion on edema formation after blunt injury to the hind limbs of rats. *J Athl Train* 32:233-237, 1997.

Dyson M: Role of ultrasound in wound healing. In Kloth LC, McCullough JM, Feeder JA (Eds), *Alternatives in Wound Healing*. Philadelphia, Davis, 1990, 259-286.

Heckman J, Ryaby JP, McCabe J, Frey JJ, Kilcoyne RF: Acceleration of tibial fracture-healing by noninvasive, low-intensity pulsed ultrasound. *J Bone Joint Surg* (American Volume) 76:26-34, 1994.

Holmes Jr. GB: Treatment of delayed unions and nonunions of the proximal fifth metatarsal with pulsed electromagnetic fields. *Foot Ankle Int* 15:552-556, 1994.

Ingersoll C, Knight KL, Merrick MA: Sensory perception of the foot and ankle following therapeutic applications of heat and cold. *J Athl Train* 27:231-234, 1992.

Kloth LC, Feeder JA: Electrical stimulation in tissue repair. In Kloth LC, McCullough JM, Feeder JA (Eds), *Alternatives in Wound Healing*. Philadelphia, Davis, 1990, 221-257.

Knight KL: *Cryotherapy in Sport Injury Management*. Champaign IL, Human Kinetics, 1995.

Knight KL, Aquino J, Johannes SM, Urban CD: A re-examination of Lewis' cold-induced vasodilation in the finger and ankle. *Athl Train* 15:238-250, 1980.

Kristiansen T, Ryaby JP, McCabe J, Frey JJ, Roe LR: Accelerated healing of distal radius fractures with specific, low-intensity ultrasound. *J Bone Joint Surg* (American Volume) 79:961-973, 1997.

Marcer M, Musati G, Bassett CA: Results of pulsed electromagnetic fields (PEMFs) in ununited fractures after external skeletal fixation. *Clin Orthop Related Res* 11(190):206-265, 1984.

West TF: The role of diminished cutaneous sensory information and cryotherapy on haptic determination of rod length. Doctoral dissertation. The Pennsylvania State University, 1988.

## ADDITIONAL READING

Kloth LC, McCulloch JM, Feeder JA: *Wound Healing: Alternatives in Management*. Philadelphia, Davis, 1990.

# CHAPTER 15

# Neuromuscular Control and Biofeedback

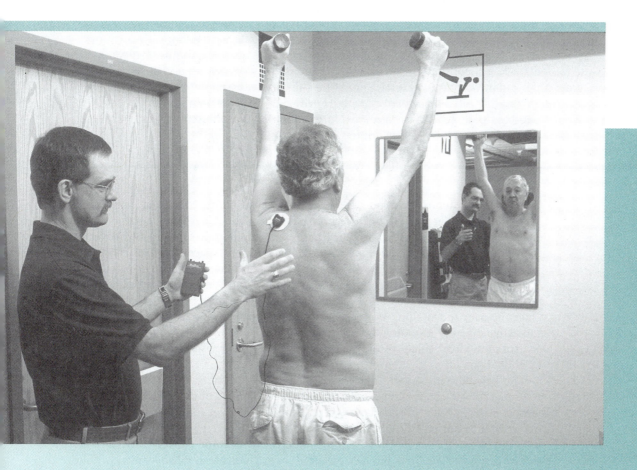

## *Objectives*

After reading this chapter, the student will be able to

1. define biofeedback;

2. describe the application of electromyographic biofeedback in treating impaired neuromuscular control;

3. describe the instrumentation and signal processing related to electromyographic biofeedback; and

4. describe the use of biofeedback in relaxation training.

**A**high school cross country runner complains of anterior knee pain. She states that her family physician diagnosed her as having patellofemoral pain syndrome. She was advised to wear arch supports because of excessive pronation and to work with her coach to strengthen her quadriceps muscles. Despite the use of arch supports and strengthening exercises, her knee pain has persisted.

Evaluation by the team orthopedic surgeon confirms the diagnosis of patellofemoral pain syndrome, and the runner is referred to the athletic training room for evaluation and treatment. Examination reveals a hypermobile patella, bilateral hyperpronation, and obvious inhibition of the vastus medialis muscle with active quadriceps setting. You decide to use biofeedback to improve recruitment of the vastus medialis. First biofeedback is used during quadriceps setting and straight leg raises. As neuromuscular control improves, the therapeutic exercise program is progressed to include mini-squats, step-ups, resisted balance exercises, leg extensions, and leg presses. Initially, biofeedback is used during each exercise. After a few treatments, the athlete demonstrates control over the vastus medialis in all exercises, and biofeedback is discontinued. She also reports much less pain during and after running. After a few weeks of regular therapeutic exercise her knee pain resolves completely.

What was missing from the initial treatment program? Why did the knee pain improve following treatments that included biofeedback? This chapter explores impaired neuromuscular control and the use of biofeedback in treating musculoskeletal injuries.

Neuromuscular control incorporates the efferent neural output to skeletal muscles with the afferent neural input received by the central nervous system. Coordinated, purposeful movement requires precise feedback from the periphery to allow for refined control over muscle contractions and ultimately movement of the body through space.

The basic concepts of neuromuscular control, as well as the impact of pain and injury on neuromuscular control, were discussed in chapter 6. As described in chapters 1 and 14, neuromuscular control is an important component in a comprehensive rehabilitation plan. Once the pain and swelling associated with acute inflammation or persistent pain subside and active range of motion is sufficiently restored, it is necessary to assess neuromuscular control and address deficits before the patient advances into resistance training and functional rehabilitation.

The paradigm presented in chapter 6 included three levels of neuromuscular control: volitional muscle contractions, reflex responses, and control of more complex, coordinated movement. The focus of this chapter is on volitional control and the instrumentation that can assist in restoring volitional control. Included are the general concepts of biofeedback followed by a more detailed description of **electromyographic (EMG)** biofeedback. Electromyographic biofeedback can help physically active individuals regain control of volitional muscle contractions and transition to functional activities. Several examples of clinical strategies to promote control of volitional contractions and more complex movements are provided to illustrate functional progression.

If no impairment of volitional control is identified or an impairment has been successfully addressed, attention turns to reflex control. Reflex responses are rapidly generated muscle contractions in response to changes sensed by the receptors found in tendon, muscle, ligaments, and joint capsules. The simplest is the spinal reflex elicited with tapping on a tendon. These responses occur very rapidly, and biofeedback is not useful in retraining them.

Reflex responses may be impaired due to damage to the peripheral receptors, pain, or swelling. A program of progressively greater challenges to reflex responses can improve performance and reduce the rate of reinjury. For example, balance training on disks and wobble boards has been reported to decrease the sense of instability in athletes with chronic ankle instability (Tropp et al. 1984), decrease postural sway (suggesting greater control of balance) (Gauffin, Tropp, and Odendrick 1988; Mattacola and Lloyd 1997; Bernier and Perrin 1998), and decrease the incidence of recurrent ankle sprain (Wester et al. 1996; Holme et al. 1999). Mattacola and Dwyer (2002) identified intermediate and advanced rehabilitative exercises for the treatment of ankle injuries. Similar exercise progressions have been suggested in the rehabilitation of the injured knee (Houglum 2005).

Myers and Lephart (2000) described the impairment of proprioception and neuromuscular control following capsuloligamentous injury at the shoulder. Several open and closed chain exercises directed at enhancing neuromuscular control over the scapulothoracic are depicted by Paine and Voight (1993). Exercises to improve function of the scapulothoracic and glenohumeral joints are pictured in Houglum's (2005) *Therapeutic Exercise for Musculoskeletal Injuries, Second Edition*. The importance of identifying and treating deficits in reflex control in the shoulder complex following injury through a progressive exercise regimen cannot be overemphasized. Ultimately the exercise program advances to exercises integrating controlled motion throughout the kinetic chain, especially in work with "throwing athletes" including racket sport players and golfers. McMullen and Uhl (2000) provided a thorough review of the theoretical basis for and progression of kinetic chain exercises for shoulder rehabilitation, as well as several illustrations of specific exercises.

Progression from reflex retraining to sport-specific functional activities is the final transition in the neuromuscular control progression. At this point the rehabilitative activities become more sport specific and individualized. Clearly the demands of sports such as gymnastics and soccer differ markedly. Take, for example, the rehabilitation of a gymnast and a soccer player following a lateral ankle sprain. The gymnast might be required to perform on a beam, complete a floor routine, or "stick" landing after vaulting or completing a bar routine—all very demanding tasks. The soccer player, however, might have to play on wet, slippery surfaces and must redevelop touch with the ball. Knowledge of the demands of the athlete's sport is essential in completing the rehabilitation progression.

# VOLITIONAL CONTROL AND BIOFEEDBACK

Biofeedback is the use of instrumentation to bring physiological events to conscious awareness. Electromyographic biofeedback permits awareness of neural recruitment of muscles by transducing the electrical activity during muscular contractions into audio or visual signals. Biofeedback devices can also measure heart rate and galvanic skin response (sweating) during relaxation training. Visual feedback during therapeutic exercise can be enhanced with mirrors. Sometimes a combination of feedback devices is used in neuromuscular reeducation following musculoskeletal injury.

Although EMG biofeedback is used more commonly to increase tension and force production by a muscle or groups of muscles, it can also be used with other types of biofeedback to help individuals learn to control tension and stress responses. An introduction to this aspect of enhancing neuromuscular control is provided at the end of this chapter.

## Why Is Biofeedback Effective?

Biofeedback is really a teaching aid. Effective learning requires precise and timely information about the quality of performance. This is true in the cognitive, psychomotor, and affective domains. Feedback must be timely, so the individual can assess performance and identify areas for improvement. As a student, you know that tests returned months after you take them lose their value as a learning tool because your focus has shifted to other coursework and new information.

The feedback provided must also be as precise as possible, as illustrated by the process of learning golf. Everyone in sports medicine should attempt to learn golf, because proficiency in this game requires considerable coordination, and the learning process is a study in neuromuscular education. Step up to the tee, swing the club, and see what happens. Unless you are truly gifted, your first swing will result in the ball's rolling forward or slicing wickedly, or perhaps in no contact at all. You're not sure what went wrong, only that the outcome was flawed. Slowly you improve through trial and error. To speed the acquisition of the basic skills, find a good golf coach and watch the improvement. Effective coaching provides far more precise information as to the reasons for poor shots. Swing speed, swing plane, head and hand position, and other factors can be quickly assessed and improved. Thus, precision of feedback is as important as timeliness.

Chapter 6 addressed the reasons for impaired neuromuscular control. At this point we hope you appreciate the certified athletic trainer's role in restoring volitional control during simple and more complex motor tasks. In addition, biofeedback in relaxation training must be introduced. Before we proceed further with neuromuscular control and the use of biofeedback in relaxation training, a review of instrumentation, especially for EMG biofeedback, is needed.

## Instrumentation

If EMG biofeedback is to provide useful information, the electrical activity of the muscle must be recorded and transformed into visual and auditory signals. This process begins with the detection of electrical activity by electrodes. In clinical practice, surface electrodes are used. In some research applications, the electrodes consist of fine wires inserted into the muscle. The indwelling electrodes provide very specific information from a portion of a muscle but are not appropriate for clinical use. Surface electrodes provide less specific information, but the convenience of these electrodes and their ability to quantify activity of muscles and muscle groups make them ideal for sport rehabilitation.

There are several configurations of surface electrodes. All consist of two active leads and a ground. The self-adhesive electrode with a single three-pole attachment is illustrated in figure 15.1. These electrodes are easy to apply, stay in place, and are inexpensive.

Once the raw electrical signal is detected at the electrode, it is conducted to the electrical circuitry within the EMG biofeedback unit. Within the unit, the raw EMG signal received through the electrodes is filtered, amplified, rectified, integrated (figure 15.2), and transduced into visual and audio output that is proportional to the amount of electrical activity in the muscle. Advances in technology allow for signal processing with much smaller components, permitting greater portability of the unit and expanding the applications of EMG biofeedback in rehabilitation.

Filtering removes "noise" from high- and low-frequency sources. Electrical activity of muscles falls into the 80- to 250-Hz range. It is important that electrical activity below and above this range is filtered before the signal is processed. For example, the electrical current that runs the lights and equipment in athletic training rooms and clinics is 60 Hz, so without effective filtering, turning on an ultrasound or a TENS unit could cause signal fluctuation.

Effective signal processing requires that the raw EMG signal be amplified. Actual electrical activity in muscle falls in the microvolt range, so a signal amplifier is used to amplify the signal into the millivolt range.

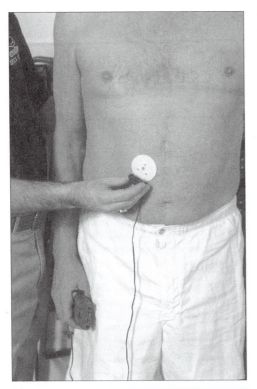

**Figure 15.1**   An electromyography electrode.

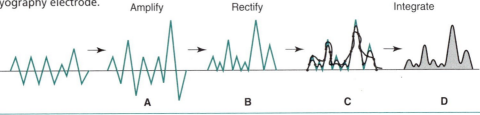

Amplify          Rectify          Integrate

A          B          C          D

**Figure 15.2**   Electromyographic signal processing. Electrical signal detected at an electrode is amplified (**A**) and rectified (**B**). The signal is then integrated (**C**) by taking samples at specific time intervals (i.e., every 0.1 sec for sampling rate of 100 Hz). The sampling points are connected, and the electrical activity is quantified by calculating the area under the curve (*d*).

When a signal is rectified, all deflections from the isoelectric line are made positive or negative. Signal integration involves sampling the rectified signal and fitting a curve through the sampled points. This process essentially "smoothes" the signal, allowing for the area under the curve to be quantified (integrated). The integrated electrical signal is then used to power lights, sound, or a signal meter to provide immediate and highly specific feedback about the amount of electrical activity within the target muscle.

Other forms of biofeedback operate in a similar manner. Heart rate monitors detect the electrical activity of heart muscle contractions. Changes in the conductivity of the skin (galvanic skin response) can provide feedback regarding the body's response to stress. Feedback is provided through measurement of changes in conductivity of a small, imperceptible electrical current and conversion of the electrical signal into visual and auditory feedback.

Skin temperature can also provide valuable feedback. Surface temperature monitoring does not require electrical signal processing but does require thermometers that can be attached to the skin and very sensitive temperature gauges.

# CLINICAL APPLICATIONS: RESTORING CONTROL OF VOLITIONAL CONTRACTION

Restoring control over isolated, volitional muscle contraction is often an early goal of rehabilitation, especially following knee injuries and surgeries. If you examine an injured physically active person the day before arthroscopic knee surgery, you will probably find that all of the quadriceps muscles contract strongly during active quadriceps sitting and straight leg exercises. Reexamine the knee the day after surgery, and a decrease in active control of the vastus medialis is often evident with these activities. The effect is more dramatic following arthrotomy.

The affected muscles have not atrophied. Rather, the individual has lost the ability to contract the muscles fully because of neural inhibition. As in learning to play golf, precise and immediate feedback speeds neuromuscular reeducation. Electromyography provides positive feedback when the appropriate neural pathways are activated, eliminating much trial and error in this early stage of rehabilitation (figure 15.3).

Neuromuscular inhibition is not limited to postoperative applications. Many physically active people with patellofemoral pain syndrome also demonstrate inhibition of the vastus medialis. Furthermore, many individuals with shoulder pain due to glenohumeral impingement, instability, and rotator cuff lesions fail to properly stabilize their scapula or activate their rotator cuff during shoulder flexion and abduction. Shoulder pain appears to inhibit neuromuscular control in these muscles, leading to altered movement patterns, losses in motion, and greater losses of shoulder function. Electromyographic biofeedback, mirrors (figure 15.4), and, occasionally, shoulder taping can be used to restore neuromuscular control throughout the shoulder range of motion.

Rarely, individuals are unable to generate a muscle contraction despite the use of biofeedback and their best effort. In these situations, resort to neuromuscular stimulation (NMS) to induce a muscle contraction. Using an electrical current to contract a target muscle (usually the quadriceps following knee injury or surgery; figure 15.5) generates afferent input. The object of NMS in these situations is to restart the motor efferent-proprioceptive feedback loop by inducing muscle contraction. Be aware, however, that strong electrically stimulated contractions are poorly tolerated.

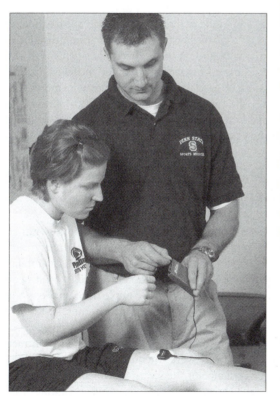

**Figure 15.3** An individual performing a quadriceps set with biofeedback.

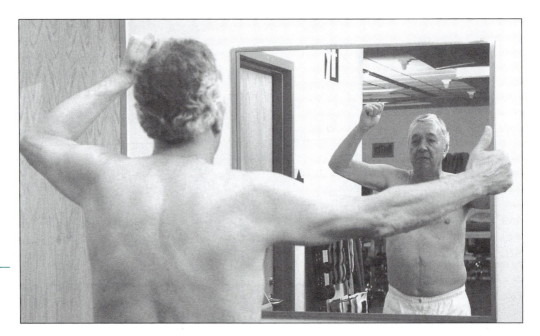

**Figure 15.4** Shoulder hiking with abduction of the arm.

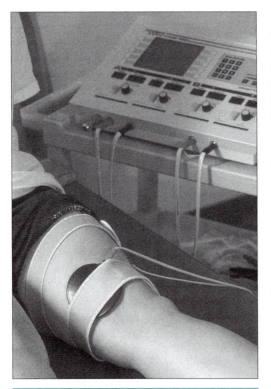

**Figure 15.5** Neuromuscular stimulation of quadriceps.

Using a stimulus with the phase duration and frequency described in chapter 10, apply a 10- to 15-sec "on" time with a 4- to 5-sec ramp and a 10- to 15-sec "off" time. Longer recovery between contractions is not necessary because of the submaximal nature of the muscle contractions; in addition, longer "off" time promotes boredom. In 10 min the injured physically active person will experience 20 to 30 muscle contractions. The individual should be encouraged to contract the affected muscle volitionally during the stimulation. Some people are very timid at first and must be encouraged to adjust the amplitude of the stimulus during the treatment. Allowing the individual to control the strength of the stimulus reduces apprehension and makes the treatment more effective.

Once the injured person can contract the affected muscle volitionally, EMG biofeedback can be used to enhance neuromuscular control. You can use NMS and EMG biofeedback in a single treatment session depending on how quickly the individual responds to NMS and how much exercise he or she can tolerate.

## CLINICAL APPLICATIONS: FUNCTIONAL PROGRESSION

Sport, work, and daily tasks require coordinated, complex motions rather than isolated control of a single muscle or muscle group. Performing quadriceps sitting and straight leg raises has little carryover to walking, climbing stairs, running, cutting, and jumping. The rapid, coordinated recruitment of all the muscles needed to complete relatively complex motor tasks is not generated through conscious control of each individual muscle. Rather, complex motor tasks are executed from a motor pattern.

Again using the golf swing as an example, it is evident that many muscles must contract at precisely the right moment to hit the ball well. If one were to concentrate on controlling only one muscle, let alone several muscles, performance of the swing would suffer badly. Yet the accomplished golfer can consistently hit good shots. Why? The accomplished golfer can execute a complex movement generated from higher centers and continuously adjusted through afferent feedback. Injury, pain, swelling, and instability inhibit execution of the coordinated, complex movement. Thus, rehabilitation cannot end with restoration of volitional control over muscles or proprioceptive training. Once the early goals of rehabilitation are met, a functional progression of increasingly complex tasks must be introduced. Functional or sport-specific rehabilitation and work hardening are advanced stages of rehabilitation, in which coordinated, complex movements are refined and the stamina and strength needed to return to sport and work are built.

As the movement patterns executed during therapeutic exercise become more rapid and complex, the value of EMG biofeedback declines. Concentration on biofeedback inhibits the automated nature of complex movements. However, biofeedback is useful in the early transition from retraining of volitional muscle control to rehearsal of more simple movements requiring contraction of multiple muscles and movement of multiple joints.

The treatment of patellofemoral pain syndrome (PFPS) provides an example of the use of EMG biofeedback in an exercise progression. The initial assessment of an injured person with PFPS often reveals inhibited recruitment of the vastus medialis, which is more affected by knee pain and swelling than the other quadriceps muscles. Selective inhibition of the vastus medialis worsens PFPS in some individuals because the imbalance between the forces generated by the vastus medialis and lateralis results in lateral glide of the patella. This, in turn, is believed to irritate the patellofemoral joint, resulting in more pain, swelling, and neuromuscular inhibition and perpetuating the condition.

Early treatment of PFPS should focus on relieving pain and swelling. As these treatment goals are accomplished, EMG biofeedback during open chain exercises such as quadriceps sitting and straight leg raises will restore volitional control over the vastus medialis. Although volitional control in open chain activities is an important goal, the lower extremity rarely functions in an open chain. Thus, the therapeutic exercise program must be progressed to closed chain and to work- and sport-specific activities: namely, pattern-generated movements.

## Open Versus Closed Chain Exercises

open chain exercises—Exercises in which the distal segment is free to move. For example, leg extension exercises are considered open chain because the foot is free to move rather than remaining firmly in contact with the ground.

closed chain exercises—Exercises in which the distal segment is fixed in place. For example, leg press exercises are considered closed chain because the foot is firmly in contact with the exercise device.

Early restoration of neuromuscular control is most effective when activity is isolated to a particular muscle or muscle group such as the quadriceps. Open chain exercises allow individuals to isolate their effort on a single muscle group and then proceed to closed chain exercises in a progressive exercise program. Failure to establish volitional control in the open chain before beginning closed chain exercises often reinforces substitute motor patterns. Some individuals are able to perform a leg press after anterior cruciate ligament reconstruction yet struggle to move an 8-lb plate in open chain 90° to 60° quadriceps contraction, because they substitute gluteal and hamstring force generation for the quadriceps function they lack. Thus, it is important to assess and retrain volitional control in an open chain before progressing to more functional, closed chain movements.

After more complex movements are initiated, EMG biofeedback provides valuable information regarding muscle recruitment. If we continue to use PFPS as an example, once the individual has gained control over the vastus medialis in the open chain, EMG biofeedback can be used during activities such as step-ups, lunges, 1/4 squats, and balance exercises (figure 15.6). Electromyographic biofeedback is also useful when you are instructing individuals to use machines for resistance exercises including leg extensions and leg presses (figure 15.7) and for gait training. The EMG biofeedback permits you and the injured person to monitor the quality of motor recruitment in these more advanced and functional exercises. Once

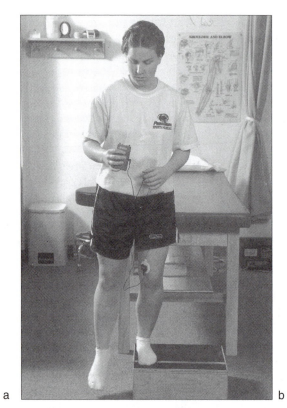
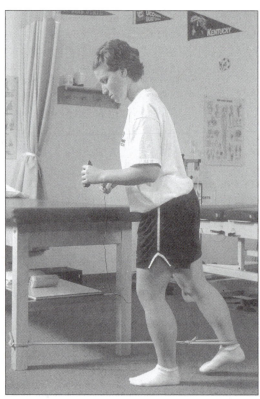

**Figure 15.6** Biofeedback during step-ups *(a)* and tubing-resisted kickers *(b)* .

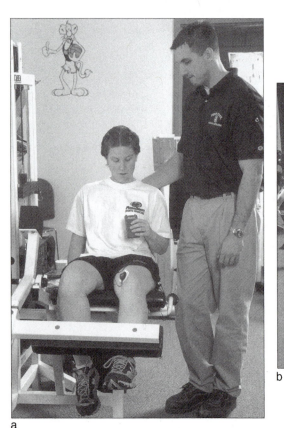
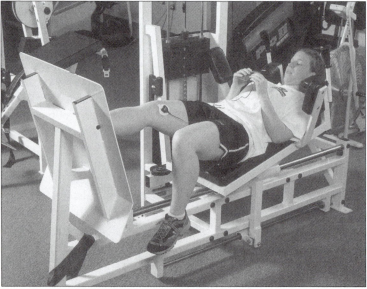

**Figure 15.7** Biofeedback during short arc leg *(a)* extension and leg press *(b)*.

the appropriate motor pattern has been established, EMG biofeedback is no longer needed. This process is very important for individuals who will complete a home-based or independent exercise program during their rehabilitation. Practicing faulty or substitute motor patterns will ingrain the pattern and slow recovery or even exacerbate the injury.

The use of EMG biofeedback is not limited to rehabilitation of the lower extremity. Biofeedback is useful for individuals with back pain who struggle to gain control over the abdominal musculature during pelvic tilts, abdominal curls, and standing pelvic tilts (figure 15.8).

Electromyographic biofeedback is useful in treating many types of shoulder dysfunction. Impingement syndrome, rotator cuff tendinitis, and glenohumeral ligament laxity are similar in that tissues in the subacromial space become inflamed. The resulting pain appears to cause neuromuscular inhibition of the rotator cuff muscles, especially supraspinatus and to a lesser degree infraspinatus.

The use of EMG biofeedback during exercises that isolate these rotator cuff muscles, such as scaption, empty can, and active external rotation (figure 15.9), speeds neuromuscular rehabilitation. Using a mirror (figure 15.10) to provide visual feedback is helpful when the injured person demonstrates a "shoulder-hiking" pattern with glenohumeral abduction. This substitution pattern, which develops to avoid a painful arc during glenohumeral abduction and flexion, can be difficult to suppress without visual, and sometimes EMG, biofeedback.

The role of the scapula in shoulder dysfunction has received much attention in the past 15 years (Kibler 1991). Many physically active individuals with impingement syndrome demonstrate weakness in the scapular stabilizers, especially middle and lower trapezius and serratus anterior. People with myofascial pain patterns involving the neck and upper back frequently present with similar dysfunction. Most of these individuals also have poor postural awareness. Thus, improved scapular stabilization is a common treatment goal. Once again, EMG biofeedback (figure 15.11) can speed neuromuscular reeducation and recovery. Visual feedback through the use of mirrors on videotaping can also facilitate recovery of postural and neuromuscular control.

As with the treatment of knee injuries, EMG biofeedback for the shoulder can be used as the therapeutic exercise program becomes more work and sport specific. This is especially true when scapular stabilization is being developed. Electromyographic biofeedback helps the individual relearn how to "set" the scapula before and during throwing and lifting.

# LEARNING RELAXATION

This chapter has been devoted to the topic of restoring neuromuscular control and an introduction to EMG biofeedback. However, increasing neuromuscular activity is only one of many possible treatment goals and is not the sole application of biofeedback. Many people who suffer from myofascial pain find that their symptoms are exacerbated when they are fatigued or under stress. Unfortunately, many people seem unable

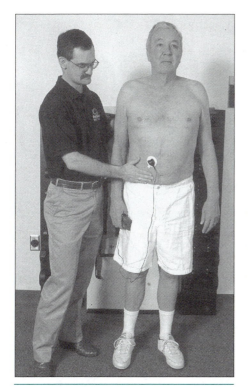

**Figure 15.8** Biofeedback at the abdominal site during standing pelvic tilt.

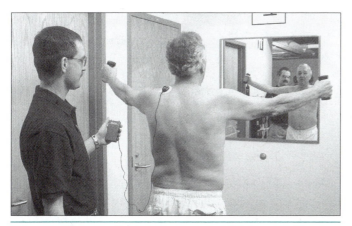

**Figure 15.9** Biofeedback during active abduction.

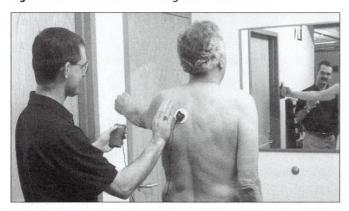

**Figure 15.10** Biofeedback at middle trapezius and mirrors for scapular stabilization.

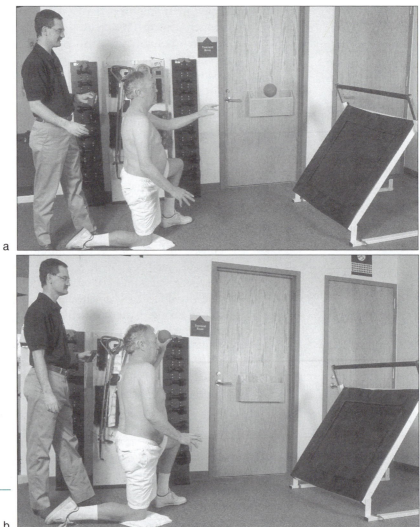

**Figure 15.11** Biofeedback at middle trapezius in throwing *(a)* and catching *(b)*.

to relax. Biofeedback from EMG, galvanic skin response, heart rate, and skin temperature can be used in relaxation training.

Multiple forms of feedback are often used because individuals vary in their responses to stress. Some people experience an increase in neuromuscular activity in response to stress. Others may experience a galvanic skin response or a drop in temperature. By identifying thoughts or events that increase stress, and strategies to decrease it, physically active individuals can improve their ability to relax and break the cycle of stress, pain, and spasm.

These strategies can also be used to help individuals return to competition following injury. Psychological preparation to return to sport following injury has been receiving increased attention, and it is recognized that physical rehabilitation following serious injury is not enough to enable a person to return to the environment where the injury occurred. Biofeedback can help the individual, and the sports medicine team, assess the stress response to returning to competition. Videotape of competition, biofeedback, and thought stopping can be very effective in managing this stress response.

Physicians, physical therapists, and certified athletic trainers typically have not devoted much attention to the psychological aspects of rehabilitation. Clinical psychologists and sport psychologists can be invaluable in the successful management of persistent pain and the individual's psychological response, respectively. The certified athletic trainer with experience in stress management and biofeedback can assist members of the health care team with this aspect of rehabilitation.

# Biofeedback and Relaxation

## Biofeedback Techniques

Muscle tension

Galvanic skin response

Temperature

Heart rate

Often, several forms of biofeedback are used simultaneously to identify how individuals respond to stress and to train them in relaxation.

## Relaxation Techniques

Thought stopping

Visual imagery

Breathing exercises

Isolated muscle contraction and relaxation

Specialized preparation in relaxation training is needed to effectively use these techniques. Do not attempt intervention with these techniques without appropriate training or with individuals whose psychological or psychiatric dysfunction is beyond your scope of practice.

## SUMMARY

1. Define biofeedback.

   Biofeedback is the use of instrumentation to bring physiological events to conscious awareness. Electromyographic (EMG) biofeedback permits awareness of neural recruitment of muscles by transducing the electrical activity during muscular contractions into audio or visual signals.

2. Describe the application of EMG biofeedback in the treatment of impaired neuromuscular control.

   An EMG biofeedback device monitors electrical activity of muscle through electrodes applied to the skin. The individual is asked to contract the targeted muscle, such as the vastus medialis. The biofeedback unit is adjusted to indicate successful recruitment of the target muscle through audio or visual feedback. As neuromuscular control improves, greater recruitment of the target muscle is required to induce positive feedback, and more complex activities are added to the therapeutic exercise regimen.

3. Describe the instrumentation and signal processing related to EMG biofeedback.

   When a raw electrical signal is detected at the electrode, it is conducted to the electrical circuitry within the EMG biofeedback unit. Within the unit, the raw EMG signal received through the electrodes is filtered, amplified, rectified, integrated, and transduced into visual and audio output that is proportional to the amount of electrical activity in the muscle. Filtering removes "noise" from high- and low-frequency sources. Electrical activity of muscles ranges from 80 to 250 Hz. Electrical activity below and above this range is filtered before the signal is processed. Effective signal processing requires that the raw EMG signal be amplified. Actual electrical activity in muscle falls in the microvolt range. The signal is amplified into the millivolt range by a signal amplifier. When a signal is rectified, all deflections from the isoelectric line are made positive or negative. Signal integration involves sampling the rectified signal and fitting a curve through the sampled points. This process essentially "smoothes" the signal, allowing the area under the curve to be quantified (integrated). The integrated electrical signal is then used to power lights, sound, or a signal meter to provide immediate and highly specific feedback about the amount of electrical activity within the target muscle.

4. Describe the use of biofeedback in relaxation training.

Biofeedback can be used to teach relaxation and management of tension and stress. Biofeedback can be used to make an individual aware of muscle tension (EMG biofeedback), heart rate, sweating, galvanic skin response, and temperature—areas that reflect the stress response in most individuals. By identifying thoughts or events that increase the physiological response to psychological stress, and strategies to decrease this response, individuals can improve their ability to relax and break the cycle of stress, pain, and spasm.

## CITED SOURCES

Bernier JN, Perrin DH: Effect of coordination training on proprioception of the functionally unstable ankle. *J Orthop Sports Phys Ther* 27:264-275, 1998.

Gauffin H, Tropp H, Odendrick P: Effect of ankle disc training on postural control in patients with functional instability of the ankle joint. *Int J Sports Med* 9:141-144, 1988.

Holme E, Magnusson SP, Becher K, Bieler T, Aagaard P, Kjaer M: The effect of supervised rehabilitation on strength, postural sway, position sense, and re-injury after lateral ligament sprain. *Scand J Med Sci Sports* 9:104-109, 1999.

Houglum PA: *Therapeutic Exercise for Musculoskeletal Injuries*, 2nd ed. Champaign, IL, Human Kinetics, 2005.

Kibler BW: Role of the scapula in the overhead throwing motion. *Contemp Orthop* 22:525-532, 1991.

Mattacola CG, Dwyer MK: Rehabilitation of the ankle after acute sprain or chronic instability. *J Athl Train* 37:413-429, 2002.

Mattacola CG, Lloyd JW: Effects of a 6-week strength and proprioception training program on measures of dynamic balance: A single-case study design. *J Athl Train* 32:127-135, 1997.

McMullen J, Uhl TL: A kinetic chain approach for shoulder rehabilitation. *J Athl Train* 35:329-337, 2000.

Myers JB, Lephart SM: The role of the sensorimotor system in the athletic shoulder. *J Athl Train* 35: 351-363, 2000.

Paine RM, Voight M: The role of the scapula. *J Orthop Sports Phys Ther* 20:386-391, 1993.

Tropp H, Ekstrand J, Gillquist J: Factors affecting stabilometry recordings of single limb stance. *Am J Sports Med* 12:185-188, 1984.

Wester JU, Jespersen SM, Nielsen KD, Neumann L: Wobble board training after partial sprains of the lateral ligaments of the ankle: A prospective randomized study. *J Orthop Sports Phys Ther* 23: 332-336, 1996.

## ADDITIONAL READINGS

Basmajian J: *Biofeedback: Principles and Practice for Clinicians.* Baltimore, Williams & Wilkins, 1989.

# CHAPTER 16

# Clinical Management of Persistent Pain

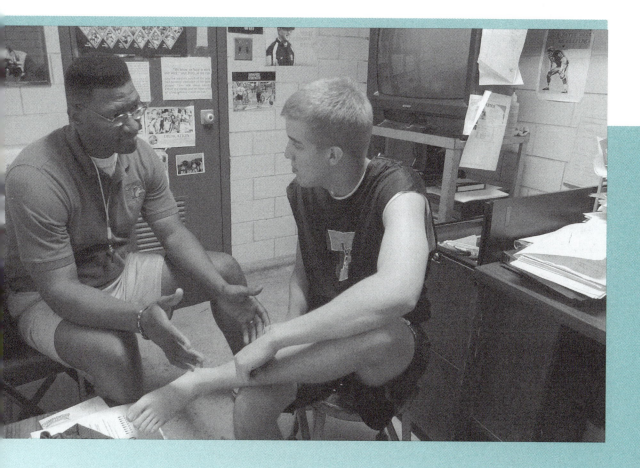

## *Objectives*

After reading this chapter, the student will be able to

1. identify sources of persistent pain through a medical history and physical examination; and

2. develop appropriate rehabilitation plans of care or referral to appropriate health care professionals for individuals with persistent pain due

to (a) diagnostic errors, (b) faulty plans of rehabilitation, (c) faulty biomechanics, (d) rest–reinjury cycle, (e) complex regional pain syndrome, (f) myofascial pain, and (g) depression and somatization.

The certified athletic trainer must be prepared to evaluate a broad spectrum of physically active people. Often an individual presents with a history of long-standing, or persistent, pain with no single identifiable cause. Consider the following cases and related questions.

A recreationally active financial aid officer presents to a sports medicine clinic with a history of many months of neck and shoulder pain with frequent headaches. She has no history of trauma, and a previous medical evaluation had revealed no structural problem. She was diagnosed with myofascial pain syndrome. What other questions should be included in the medical history? What factors are contributing to the problem? What would you expect to find on physical examination? What are the short- and long-term treatment goals? Will the use of therapeutic modalities help her achieve treatment goals?

A freshman college track athlete with a history of "shinsplints" throughout high school is evaluated in the athletic training room. She has very tight fascia in her legs and multiple tender trigger points. She states that recent x-rays and a bone scan revealed normal results. Why has her problem persisted for so long? Is there an underlying cause? How should this athlete be treated?

A freshman high school baseball pitcher presents to a sports medicine clinic complaining of 4 months of shoulder pain that has limited his ability to pitch. He states that he took 3 weeks off from pitching but the shoulder did not heal. He was concerned that he had a torn rotator cuff despite assurances to the contrary by an orthopedic surgeon. Why had this injury failed to heal?

The complaints of these physically active people are not uncommon. The questions raised in each case must be answered to develop an effective rehabilitation plan. In some cases therapeutic modalities may help resolve the problem but in other cases may be of little benefit. As stated in the beginning of this text, application of a therapeutic modality does not constitute a treatment but is part of a comprehensive plan of care. Developing a plan of care requires that you identify the underlying causes of symptoms. Thus, this final chapter was written to help you evaluate and treat physically active individuals with persistent pain and identify situations in which therapeutic modalities may help the individual achieve treatment goals.

Perhaps we can best introduce the challenges of treating persistent and chronic pain by recalling our discussion of the management of acute musculoskeletal injuries in chapter 14. The signs and symptoms associated with these injuries, selection of modalities, and decisions regarding progression of the plan of care were closely linked to the inflammatory response to tissue injury. When symptoms persist, occur in the absence of a history of trauma, or are unrelated to our current understanding of inflammation (e.g., tendinosis), decisions related to modality application must be made on criteria other than the stage of inflammation. Figure 16.1 provides an overview of the diagnostic possibilities and the decisions that the clinician must make in the management of patients presenting with complaints of lasting pain and pain of insidious onset.

Through experience and application of the available research, the clinician's evaluation and treatment of individuals with persistent pain evolve. In a high school or college athletic training room, the majority of individuals treated seek care for acute, sport-related, musculoskeletal injuries. The certified athletic trainer will certainly be called on to evaluate some athletes with overuse injuries and persistent symptoms caused by poor mechanics. On occasion, those seeking care will have other causes for their symptoms, and some may be suffering from truly chronic pain. An outpatient sports medicine center is very different. Many patients referred to a sports medicine center for treatment of a musculoskeletal problem, whether they are physically active or not, have experienced pain for weeks, months, and occasionally years. Unfortunately, the exposure of many athletic training students to this clinical population is limited. Furthermore, many students receive little classroom instruction from certified athletic trainers who have worked in this clinical setting.

This is a very important issue in athletic training. The role of the athletic trainer has changed over the past 20 to 30 years The changing role of the certified athletic trainer is part

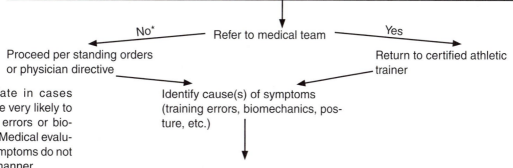

Patient presenting with pain

1. of insidious onset,
2. that is persistent or chronic, or
3. that is recurrent

Diagnostic probabilities

- Bone (stress fracture); potential contributors are training error and biomechanics
- Muscle and tendon (tendinopathy); potential contributors are training error and biomechanics
- Joint; potential contributors are training error and biomechanics
  - Osteoarthritis
  - Systemic disease (e.g., rheumatoid arthritis)
  - Infection
  - Somatic/biomechanic dysfunction
- Medical conditions
  - Cancer
  - Rheumatic diseases
  - Multiple other sources (e.g., Lyme disease)
- Neurological; potential contributors are history of trauma, recent surgery
  - Neural symptoms related to disc pathology, stenosis, etc.
  - Complex regional pain syndrome
- Vascular
  - Ischemic conditions (e.g., thoracic outlet syndrome)
  - Thrombus
- Myofascial pain syndrome; potential contributors are history of trauma, stress, posture
- Psychological conditions
  - Depression
  - Somatization
  - Fear avoidance

No*  Refer to medical team  Yes

Proceed per standing orders or physician directive

Return to certified athletic trainer

*May be appropriate in cases where symptoms are very likely to result from training errors or biomechanical factors. Medical evaluation is needed if symptoms do not resolve in a timely manner.

Identify cause(s) of symptoms (training errors, biomechanics, posture, etc.)

Treatment priorities will depend on diagnosis and causative factors

For transient pain relief and treatment of myofascial pain: cold, superficial heat, TENS

For calcific tendinopathy: ultrasound

For carpal tunnel syndrome: laser

- Modalities (modality application may be warranted in some cases but certainly not all)
- Appropriate rest
- Therapeutic exercise
- Biomechanical correction (e.g., orthotics)
- Counseling

Remember: Treatment must be goal directed and based on diagnosis, likely causative factors, and treatment goals.

**Figure 16.1**  Evaluating patients with nonacute pain and selecting those appropriate for treatment with a therapeutic modality.

of the evolution of the profession. Sports medicine clinics, practically unheard of in 1970, provide athletic training services to vast numbers of high school and amateur athletes. Today's certified athletic trainers must be prepared to work in the changing health care environment and to care for physically active people from all walks of life.

This preparation does not require lots of new skills but rather new applications for existing skills. Persistent pain is a large part of most clinical athletic trainers' practice, and most of their professional development involves refining the basic skills learned as an athletic training student in order to treat those with persistent pain.

Because persistent and chronic pain can be related to multiple factors, successful management demands a complete health history. During the physical examination the clinician must not forget that the sources of dysfunction may be distant to the area of pain. Decisions related to the plan of care, including if and which modalities are indicated, cannot be made without a working hypothesis related to causes, rather than a diagnostic label, for the persistent symptoms. This chapter is devoted to the clinical management of persistent pain and the appropriate use of therapeutic modalities in treating lasting pain.

# TREATING PERSISTENT PAIN

The rehabilitation plan of care is developed from the medical history and physical examination. Within the plan of care, treatment goals are arranged on a hierarchy from entry into the health care system to full recovery. Therapeutic modalities may facilitate achievement of one or more treatment goals in the plan of care.

These statements are true whether you are treating an acute injury or persistent pain; however, in the case of persistent pain the medical history and physical examination are more detailed, and the data gathered are analyzed more extensively. All of this information is then combined to develop a progressive plan of care. Unfortunately, when these steps are not fully completed, multiple modalities are often administered in the hope that "something works." On rare occasions the problem resolves despite the lack of a sound plan of care; usually, however, such treatment fails.

## Medical History

Perhaps the single biggest problem in the clinical management of persistent pain is the failure to obtain, evaluate, and act upon a thorough medical history. Taking a medical history, which is reviewed thoroughly in *Examination of Musculoskeletal Injuries, Second Edition* (Shultz, Houglum, and Perrin 2005), appears to be simple. However, a great deal of practice and attention to detail are needed to maximize the information gleaned from a medical history taken from individuals with persistent pain. In college and high school environments, certified athletic trainers know the athletes from day-to-day contact and gain important information from the preparticipation examination. Furthermore, most of the athletes seeking treatment are suffering from acute musculoskeletal injuries, for which the time and often the mechanism of injury are easily identified. Individuals with persistent pain may relate an insidious onset of symptoms without an identifiable cause.

Contrast, for example, the medical histories required from two individuals. One is a 17-year-old basketball player for a team you have covered all season who sprained her ankle when she stepped on another player's foot during a practice that you attended. The other is a 38-year-old tennis player, computer programmer, and mother of two small children who has a 6-month history of right shoulder and neck pain of insidious onset. In the first case you know the athlete, her recent injury history, and the nature of her off-court activities, and you probably have established a rapport with her. In the second case you are establishing a plan of care for a person you have never met who may be entering a new health care environment. During the 15 min or so allotted for the initial examination, you must collect a lot of information. You need to know when and how the problem started, what seems to make it better and worse, and the impact of work and child care on her symptoms. You must learn what other medical evaluation has been made and what treatment has been administered (and if it helped). You must learn about the tennis player's general health and medical history. In addition, you must learn what her goals are in terms of outcome priorities. In short, you need to quickly establish communication with this individual so that you can obtain all of the information you need. Furthermore, you must respond to the patient's concerns and questions. As this example illustrates, obtaining a medical history from someone with persistent pain, compared to an athlete you know who has an acute injury, is much more involved, but far more critical to developing an effective plan of care.

At the completion of the medical history, you should have one or more working diagnoses. Developing a working diagnosis requires you to analyze information provided during the history as the interview proceeds. Thus, you must organize the interview, develop the questions, and analyze the responses while listening carefully to what is being said. Completing a thorough, informative medical history requires good clinical skills and lots of practice. A sample format for evaluating musculoskeletal injuries is included here (figure 16.2). Individual items may not be appropriate for all cases (e.g., documentation of gait following a shoulder injury).

# Evaluation Document

Name: _____    Age/date of birth: _____    Sport/position: _____

Date: _____    Physician ID or medical record #: _____

Diagnosis: _____

Diagnostic tests/medications/surgical procedure: _____

Pertinent medical history: _____

## Subjective Report

Ask about onset, recent improvement, or worsening of symptoms; pattern of symptoms; rating of pain and dysfunction; description of pain; report of radicular or distant pain sites; and previous experience with treatments for musculoskeletal injuries (what seemed to work or not work).

## Objective Findings

Observation: General appearance; obvious guarding of movement or alteration from normal movement pattern (e.g., limping); presence of swelling; discoloration; and appearance of incisions, wounds, and scars.

Range of motion: Active and passive range of motion.

Circulation, motor function, and sensory function in affected limb or area.

Strength: Results of manual muscle and instrumented resistance tests.

Girth: Swelling at joint or loss of muscle mass.

Gait: Limping, appropriate use of crutches or cane, and evidence of excessive or limited pronation.

Posture: Posture, postural awareness, and postural control.

Results of special tests:

Problem list: Develop a hierarchy of problems that must be overcome to progress the rehabilitation program and return the individual to athletics.

Short-term goals and treatment plan: Develop a short list of goals to be achieved in the next few days to 2 weeks and the treatments to be used to achieve these goals.

Long-term goals with criteria for progression.

Figure 16.2    A sample format for evaluating musculoskeletal injuries.

## Physical Examination

The physical examination should yield information that confirms or refutes the working diagnoses established from the medical history. Conducting a physical exam without a working diagnosis is a time-consuming and usually fruitless endeavor.

The structure of the physical examination will vary based on the medical history and plausible diagnoses. Observation, range of motion assessment, strength assessment, and neurovascular assessment are fairly universal components. However, the order in which tests are performed and the specific tests conducted will differ depending on the nature of the problem. In a well-conducted physical examination you will complete necessary testing in an organized manner while avoiding the tendency to "test for everything" and unnecessarily increase suffering.

Some clinicians complete a physical examination in a cookbook fashion. Rather than focusing on confirming or refuting the preliminary diagnosis, they collect a quantity of data. Unfortunately, the data are not very useful because they were not collected in the context of testing the working diagnosis.

A second common flaw in a physical examination for persistent pain is the failure to examine joint, nerve, vascular, and muscle function throughout the painful region. The screening exams described in *Examination of Musculoskeletal Injuries, Second Edition* (Shultz, Houglum, and Perrin 2005), often yield key findings that confirm the cause and therefore identify the solution to the persistent pain. You must consider and assess for the presence of radicular and referred pain patterns as well as biomechanical causes of persistent pain.

Once you have made a diagnosis and identified the causes of the persistent pain, a plan of treatment can be established. In some cases, therapeutic modalities can be used to achieve goals identified in the plan of care. In other cases, the application of therapeutic modalities may be detrimental because they promote a passive, rather than active, role of the individual in the plan of care.

In chapter 5 the causes of persistent pain were categorized (figure 16.3). The remainder of this chapter reviews treatment strategies, including effective use of therapeutic modalities, in the clinical management of these persistent pain problems.

# DIAGNOSIS AND PLAN OF CARE PROBLEMS

When pain persists, the first step in reevaluation is to confirm the medical diagnosis and review the plan of care. A sports medicine team approach to reevaluation is necessary to review the original diagnosis, the response to medications and surgery, and the response to and compliance with the rehabilitation program.

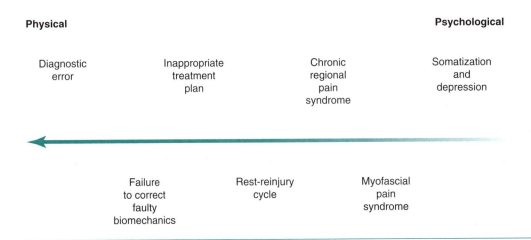

**Figure 16.3** Sources of persistent pain.

In the context of therapeutic modalities, a failure to improve can provide useful information. Transient (hours or days) relief of pain and swelling following treatment may indicate an underlying structural lesion or a rest–reinjury cycle. For example, persistent knee pain with recurrent swelling may be due to a torn meniscus or a loose body within the joint. Persistent back pain may have many causes, including cancer (see "Case Report and Signs of Cancer" below). Thus, the issue of a failure to respond to treatments as expected over a few days or weeks is a serious matter. In these cases, consultation with the patient's physician is warranted so that appropriate care can be rendered.

# Case Report and Signs of Cancer

An older golfer presented to a sports medicine clinic complaining of back pain. He was treated with transcutaneous electrical nerve stimulation (TENS) and received some short-term relief. His back pain, however, progressively worsened over the next 10 days. The underlying cause of the back pain, identified during this period of treatment, was cancer of the liver. Two lessons were learned: (1) Pain that appears to be orthopedic in nature can be due to organic pathologies, and (2) you must know the signs and symptoms of cancer and explore this possibility in individuals with chronic pain.

## Signs and Symptoms of Cancer

You should be aware of signs and symptoms of cancer so you can arrange appropriate medical follow-up. The presence of one or more signs or symptoms associated with cancer does not confirm a diagnosis. The signs and symptoms listed here should not raise alarm but rather should prompt consultation with a physician to identify the cause (Goodman and Snyder 1995).

- Change in bowel or bladder function
- Unusual bleeding or discharge
- A lump or mass in breast or elsewhere
- Obvious changes in a wart or mole or a sore that fails to heal
- Persistent cough or hoarseness
- Night pain or night sweats
- Weight loss
- Difficulty swallowing or loss of appetite
- Jaundice
- Unexplained muscular weakness or loss of coordination
- Fever
- Headaches, memory loss, poor concentration
- Fatigue, increased sleeping
- Onset of seizures

# Interrupting a Rest–Reinjury Cycle

A rest–reinjury cycle develops due to excessive stress to damaged tissues during the repair and, most commonly, remodeling phases. Some individuals misinterpret the absence of pain as indicating that damaged tissues are fully healed. When the level of exercise, work, and athletic activity exceeds the capacity of the remodeling tissue, microtrauma occurs and inflammation and pain result.

A rest–reinjury cycle has some similarities with inappropriate plans of care. For example, consider a middle-aged man seeking treatment following an arthroscopic meniscectomy. He and his surgeon were concerned about a pattern of recurrent pain and swelling in the knee that was always worse following therapeutic exercises. A review of his therapy indicated that he was riding on a stationary bicycle with a very low seat and doing full-range leg extensions with a heavy weight three times per week. The exercise program was aggravating long-standing, mild patellofemoral pain. The treatment consisted of discontinuing the offending activities and starting a simple home exercise program. The pain and swelling were completely resolved at a 2-week follow-up appointment. Problems related to rest–reinjury cycles need to be addressed through a careful review of the individual's activities and education. As with issues related to diagnosis and plans of care, the continued application of the same or different therapeutic modalities is unlikely to facilitate recovery and may delay essential treatments.

Pain is a warning that the tissues are not ready to withstand the stresses being placed on them. The key to breaking the rest–reinjury cycle is education. The individual must accept the responsibility of avoiding activities that reinjure the healing tissues. However, the certified athletic trainer and other members of the sports medicine team need to provide a reasonable rationale for following a plan of care that will safely return physically active individuals to their desired level of performance.

Therapeutic modalities have a limited role in clinical management of a rest–reinjury cycle. Therapeutic modalities can alleviate pain following reinjury, but the pain relief must not be misinterpreted as indicating a full recovery.

## Biomechanics

The mechanics of activities are also closely linked to issues of plan of care and rest–reinjury. In the context of this discussion, biomechanics is presented as a subsection to emphasize that improper execution of sport-specific tasks may be the underlying cause of persisting symptoms. Take the case of the freshman baseball pitcher with shoulder pain. A careful history obtained from the baseball pitcher revealed that his pain began shortly after he "learned" to throw a curveball the previous summer. He did not experience pain at rest and was asymptomatic the day he came to the clinic. Physical exam revealed tightness in the posterior rotator cuff, weak scapular stabilizers, and a few mildly tender trigger points. His throwing mechanics, which were evaluated in the parking lot, were poor, especially when he attempted to throw a curveball. Fortunately he was to attend a baseball camp at a nearby university in 10 days, and arrangements were made with the coaches to evaluate and correct his mechanical flaws. Two treatments with manual therapy, exercises to condition the scapular stabilizers and rotator cuff, and improved throwing mechanics resolved his shoulder pain. Each component of the plan of care contributed to recovery; however, the correction of the faulty throwing mechanics was essential to the long-term success of treatment. As with other categories of persistent pain, finding the cause sets the stage for successful management.

## Evaluation and Treatment of Myofascial Pain Syndrome

The recognition and treatment of myofascial pain syndrome (MFPS) were presented in chapter 5. The concepts from these earlier chapters can now be applied to developing a plan of care for the individual with MFPS. Myofascial pain syndrome is complex, and the cause is usually multifactorial. Thus, the first step in developing a plan of care is to complete a thorough medical history and physical examination. Once the diagnosis of MFPS is made and causes are identified, a plan of care can be established (figure 16.4).

Because there is no single cause of MFPS and the condition is not completely understood, there is no single treatment approach. Each injured individual is an experiment of one. The plan of treatment needs to address the primary complaint of pain, provide a progressive plan of therapeutic exercises to improve posture and correct faulty movement mechanics, and help the individual recognize when stress and fatigue are contributing to pain. The injured individual should become an active member of the sports medicine team as the factors contributing to MFPS are identified and a plan of care evolves.

There are several approaches to pain control in treating MFPS. Myofascial release techniques can be used to alter neural input from painful areas and alleviate fascial restrictions.

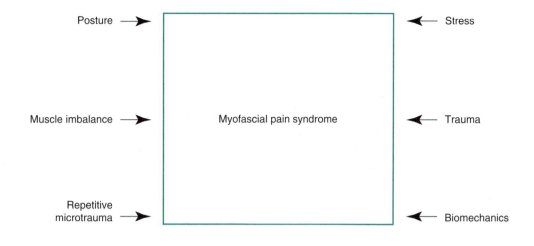

**Figure 16.4**   Contributors to myofascial pain syndrome.

Conventional modalities including heat, cold, ultrasound, and TENS are effective adjuncts to manual therapies.

Direct stimulation of trigger points often relieves pain. Trigger point massage (acupressure) and TENS over trigger points can result in dramatic, initially transient relief of pain. Deep circular massage of a trigger point can be done with the eraser end of a pencil or an index finger. The massage will elicit a deep burning sensation that is difficult to describe. However, with experience you will be able to help injured individuals recognize the difference between pressure and the exquisite sensitivity of trigger points. Generally trigger points are massaged bilaterally for 30 to 40 sec each. The number of trigger points that are sensitive varies depending on the painful region and the individual. However, trigger point stimulation can usually be completed in less than 10 min.

TENS is an alternative to massage and may be somewhat more effective. The stimulus should be intense but tolerable. A low frequency (2 to 4 pulses per second) with a long phase duration (>250 µs) or burst mode should be used. A probe-style electrode (approximately the size of a pencil eraser) such as a Neuroprobe (Physiotechnologies, Topeka, KS) is ideal. The intensity should be adjusted to produce a burning, needling sensation within individual tolerance. Each trigger point is treated for 30 to 40 sec.

Pain relief with TENS is usually rapid. Some individuals experience a dull, numbing sensation after treatment. The initial relief usually lasts for 1 to 2 h, although it can last longer. With subsequent treatments, the duration of relief increases, and complete relief can be obtained in as few as four treatments. In those whose pain continues to return, TENS with conventional parameters may also provide relief. A home TENS unit provides the individual a measure of control over pain.

Myofascial release, conventional heat and cold modalities, and trigger point therapy do not cure MFPS. However, these techniques, used individually or in combination, can break the pain cycle. If pain can be controlled, the individual generally will accept therapeutic exercise regimens and will be open to suggestions regarding stress management. Programs of pain-free exercise, improved postural awareness, correction of faulty movement mechanics, and stress management need to be combined with pain control techniques to resolve MFPS.

Although MFPS has multiple causes, there are a few basic components to an effective plan of care. The first is to correct for repetitive physical stresses that aggravate the problem. This may include modifying a workstation, providing an orthotic device, or altering how someone performs a task.

The case studies presented at the opening of this chapter illustrate the challenges of treating MFPS. The initial interview with the financial aid officer revealed that she spent much of her workday talking on a telephone while looking up account information on a computer. The risk management office of her employer evaluated her work requirements, provided a headset telephone and a new chair, and rearranged her workstation to decrease the number of repetitive movements during her workday. Without this intervention, her plan of care consisting of pain management, manual therapy, postural retraining, and conditioning of the upper back and paraspinal musculature would not have been effective.

Despite the persistence of the track athlete's "shinsplints," the ultimate biomechanical source of her problem had never been identified and addressed. Examination of her foot structure and running gait revealed hyperpronation due to a hypermobile first ray and rearfoot varus. Treatments with cryotherapy and TENS decreased her pain but did not resolve the condition. Orthotic control of her hyperpronation and a very gradual (5 months) progression to unrestricted training and competition formed the foundation for an effective plan of care. Although carefully controlling her training and doing extensive cross-training was frustrating, she was able to resume her track career, setting a school record in the 100-m hurdles as a freshman.

Each case was resolved primarily because the source of the persistent pain was identified and addressed. In addition, however, each plan of care contained a program of progressive, pain-free exercise. Therapeutic and conditioning exercises are nearly universal in a plan of care for MFPS. The key to success is pain-free exercise. The neuromuscular adaptations to painful movement were addressed in earlier chapters. To break the cycle of motion, pain, and myofascial adaptation, therapeutic exercises must be pain free; that is, pain must not alter proper movement mechanics, and activities done today can be repeated tomorrow. The role of therapeutic modalities and manual therapies in the management of MFPS is to alleviate pain, desensitize trigger points, and eliminate fascial restrictions; these changes in turn promote pain-free motion.

The benefits of therapeutic modalities and manual therapy in the clinical management of MFPS were demonstrated in the previous case studies. In the case of the financial aid officer, moist heat and TENS (figure 16.5) decreased tenderness of the trigger points and decreased muscle guarding. Myofascial release (figure 16.6), including suboccipital release and indirect techniques, further decreased the sensitivity and guarding. In theory, the pain–gamma gain cycle was broken (see chapter 13). The relief of pain, fascial restrictions, and muscle guarding

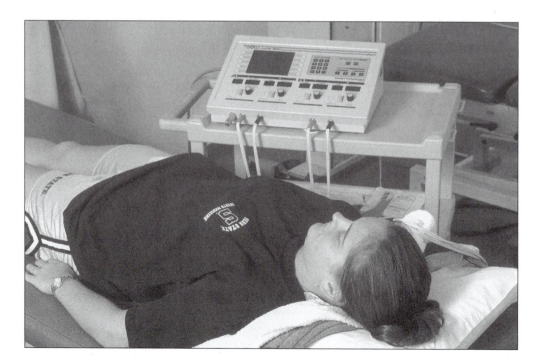

**Figure 16.5** Moist heat and transcutaneous electrical nerve stimulation in the treatment of myofascial pain syndrome in the upper trapezius and cervical spine.

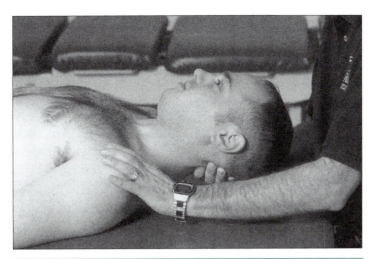

**Figure 16.6** Myofascial release in the treatment of myofascial pain syndrome in the upper trapezius and cervical spine.

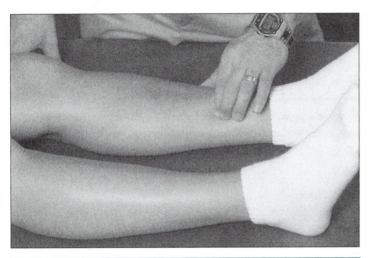

**Figure 16.7** Trigger point treatments for myofascial pain syndrome in the lower extremity.

fostered compliance with a program of postural exercises. In conjunction with her modified workstation, the plan of care resolved this physically active person's persistent pain within 4 weeks. Although 4 weeks may seem like a long time, the pain pattern had existed for several months and was gradually worsening. The certified athletic trainer and the physically active individual suffering from MFPS must have patience. Myofascial pain patterns are resolved by breaking the pain–gamma gain cycle, decreasing stresses on affected tissues, building elasticity in tight tissues, and improving endurance and strength in weak muscles. These changes occur over time and require continued compliance with a plan of care following discharge from formal rehabilitation.

Trigger point therapy (figure 16.7) and soft tissue massage broke the pain pattern in the track athlete described earlier. With repeated treatments, the trigger points became less sensitive and her pain decreased. As her pain decreased she was gradually able to tolerate more intense track workouts. Cryotherapy controlled her symptoms when she trained beyond her tolerance. This athlete's coaches supported the efforts of the sports medicine team and were very helpful in developing and monitoring a carefully controlled, progressive reconditioning program. Thus, the routine use of cryotherapy to control postexercise pain was avoided, and the athlete's recovery proceeded at a steady rate with only a few minor setbacks.

In the case of the freshman baseball pitcher, poor throwing mechanics was the central source of his shoulder pain. Myofascial adaptations, however, were present. He responded well to strain–counterstrain for the posterior rotator cuff and stretching of the external rotators (figure 16.8). He did not experience muscle spasms or pain at rest. In this case, throwing mechanics and posterior shoulder weakness were the primary problems, and treatment goals were established to address these issues. Because other therapeutic modalities would not have helped achieve treatment goals, none were applied. This case reinforces the value of developing manual therapy skills, and it is a reminder that therapeutic modalities should be applied to facilitate specific treatment goals rather than as a habit.

## Treating Complex Regional Pain Syndrome

Successful management of complex regional pain syndrome (CRPS) requires the cooperative efforts of a team of health care professionals. As stated in chapter 5, the most important role of the certified athletic trainer in treating CRPS is recognition. Those with unrecognized CRPS can languish in programs of rehabilitation, delaying comprehensive medical management. Sympathetic blocks and medications are usually needed to prevent the progression of CRPS, alleviate pain, and resolve the condition.

A progressive program of pain-free therapeutic exercise is also needed to allow full recovery from CRPS. Thus, the certified athletic trainer and physical therapist play an important role in

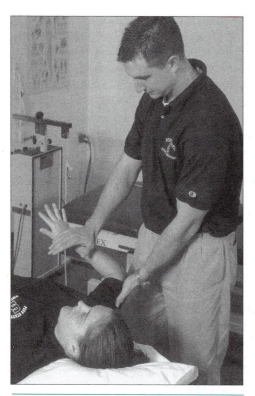

**Figure 16.8** Contract–relax stretch of external rotators.

treating physically active individuals with CRPS. Therapeutic modalities can exacerbate or alleviate the symptoms of CRPS. In general, modalities that are uncomfortable must be avoided. Cryotherapy should not be used. Sometimes superficial heat or the weight of a hydrocollator pack causes extreme pain; thus, these treatments should be used with caution. TENS, gentle massage techniques, and pulsed ultrasound sometimes can relieve the pain of CRPS. TENS offers the advantage of an adjustable level of sensory stimulus that can be controlled by the individual. Light touch and gentle massage decrease the hypersensitivity of the tissues. In some cases, TENS and massage deliver too much sensory stimulus and increase pain. Pulsed ultrasound offers another alternative; because the cold of the sound head can increase pain, the sound head should be warmed prior to treatment. Pulsed ultrasound delivers less total energy and is better tolerated than continuous ultrasound. TENS and manual techniques are preferable in treating CRPS; however, no treatment approach has proven universally effective. In treating an individual with CRPS, communicate with the individual's physician, be certain that treatments do not exacerbate the condition, and use the resources that afford the greatest relief of pain.

## Depression and Somatization

When physical symptoms are the result of psychological or psychiatric dysfunction, one would expect therapeutic modalities to have little effect. However, bear in mind the difficulty of identifying the link between depression or somatization and complaints of musculoskeletal symptoms. When an individual fails to respond to a plan of treatment that was developed to treat a somatic lesion or dysfunction, you must reassess the problem. Once the more physical causes of persistent pain discussed earlier are ruled out, the sports medicine team must consider nonphysical causes. Thus, the failure to respond as expected may provide important information during reevaluation.

Physically active individuals suffering from depression and somatization may react negatively to changes in a plan of care that decrease or discontinue treatment by a certified athletic trainer or physical therapist. These patients commonly manipulate caregivers and demand special attention from health care professionals. Be attentive to such behavior patterns, because they provide additional information in the evaluation and treatment of individuals with depression and somatization.

# TREATING CHRONIC PAIN

Despite the best diagnostic and treatment efforts, some patients continue to experience pain on a daily basis. As noted in chapter 4, changes in nervous system function may be responsible for pain that is not alleviated by therapies or medications other than narcotics. While there is a definition of chronic pain, medical science is searching for effective treatments. When a patient with true chronic pain is encountered, it is important that the clinician

1. appreciate that chronic pain is the result of altered neural function,
2. appreciate that continued palliative treatment is unlikely to be beneficial, and
3. refer the patient to those best trained in pain management.

Certainly the diagnosis of chronic pain is disheartening; however, the patient must ultimately accept that the lasting pain is due to complex and not fully understood changes in how pain signals are processed and that, at present, no treatment is fully effective. Medicine is devoting greater attention to pain experiences and the challenge of chronic pain; and new, more effective, treatments are likely to emerge.

## SUMMARY

1. Identify sources of persistent pain through a medical history and physical examination.

   Careful questioning of an injured physically active person often reveals the sources of persistent pain and provides direction for the rehabilitation plan. The certified athletic trainer should obtain a history of previous injuries and surgeries as well as information regarding the onset, location, characteristics, and timing of symptoms. The results of medical testing and responses to medications and other interventions should be reviewed. Thorough questioning may lead to consideration of diagnostic error, treatment error, rest–reinjury cycle, biomechanics flaws, myofascial pain, CRPS, or somatization as the cause of persistent pain.

2. Develop appropriate rehabilitation plans of care or referral to appropriate health care professionals for individuals suffering persistent pain due to (a) diagnostic errors, (b) faulty plans of rehabilitation, (c) rest–reinjury cycle, (d) faulty biomechanics, (e) complex regional pain syndrome, (f) myofascial pain, and (g) depression and somatization.

   Diagnostic error must be considered when a physically active individual fails to respond to rehabilitation. The sports medicine team must consider the possibility of diagnostic error and should thoroughly reevaluate exam findings and request additional testing as indicated. Faulty plans of care simply require restructuring the individual's treatment regimen, which may include adding or deleting therapeutic modality application. Rest–reinjury cycles require recognition and education to reverse. The injured physically active person must understand why symptoms are recurring and follow through with a complete plan of care before returning to unrestricted training and competition. Identifying and correcting faulty biomechanics often requires the assistance of experienced coaches and conditioning specialists. Consultation with coaches, as well as the analysis of videotaped performances, may identify and help correct the underlying source of persistent symptoms. Pain out of proportion to that expected following an injury or surgery is usually the first and most telling symptom of CRPS. Swelling, changes in skin color and temperature, and loss of motion also indicate referral to a physician. Early recognition is the key to successful treatment of CRPS. Treating myofascial pain requires identification of contributing factors, desensitization of trigger points, and release of fascial restrictions. Depression and somatization are complex problems, often requiring referral to health care professionals trained to treat psychological and psychiatric dysfunction. The certified athletic trainer should treat existing musculoskeletal dysfunction; however, comprehensive care of the individual is beyond the scope of athletic training practice.

## CITED SOURCES

Denegar CR, Peppard A: Evaluation and treatment of persistent pain and myofascial pain syndrome. *Ath Ther Today*, July 1997:40-45.

Goodman CC, Snyder TEK: Overview of oncologic signs and symptoms. In Goodman CC, Snyder TEK (Eds), *Differential Diagnosis in Physical Therapy*. Philadelphia, Saunders, 1995, 387-441.

Shultz SA, Houglum PA, Perrin DH: *Examination of Musculoskeletal Injuries*, 2nd ed. Champaign, IL, Human Kinetics, 2005.

## ADDITIONAL READINGS

Goodman CC, Snyder TEK: *Differential Diagnosis in Physical Therapy*. Philadelphia, Saunders, 1995.

McCance KL, Huether SE: *Pathophysiology: The Biologic Basis for Disease in Adults and Children*, 3rd ed. St. Louis, Mosby, 1998.

Wall PD, Melzack R: *Textbook of Pain*. New York, Churchill Livingstone, 1985.

# Glossary

**accommodation**—A decrease in the response of a nerve to an electrical impulse.

**afferent**—Conducting from the periphery toward the center (as in conduction of nerve impulses to the central nervous system).

**alpha motor neuron**—Efferent nerve innervating the myofibril.

**alternating current (AC)**—Continuous current with positive and negative phases.

**ampere**—A measure of electrical current (abbreviated A).

**amplification**—To increase in magnitude.

**analgesia**—Without pain.\QQ AU: Ideally this definition should be a noun construction—e.g., "a condition…"XQQ\

**anaphylactic reaction**—A severe, potentially fatal systemic response to a substance that an individual is highly sensitive to.

**anesthesia**—The loss of physical sensation.

**arthrogenic muscle inhibition**—A loss of muscle function caused by an injury or condition affecting a joint.

**arthrokinematics**—Sliding, rolling, and gliding of joint surfaces during motion (e.g., during abduction at the glenohumeral joint, the head of the humerus rolls superiorly and glides inferiorly); also called accessory motion.

**atrophy**—A wasting away or loss of muscle cell mass.

**avascular**—Without or having lost blood supply.

**average current**—The amount of current supplied over a period of time, which takes into consideration both the peak amplitude and the phase duration.

**beam nonuniformity ratio (BNR)**—A measure of the quality of the ultrasound head.

**beta endorphin**—A 31-peptide chain endogenous opioid that is important in the body's pain control system.

**bifurcated**—Divided.

**biomodulation**—The normal physiological function of a cell is stimulated by the administration of energy (either light, electrical, sound or thermal).

**biphasic current**—A pulsatile current with positive and negative phases.

**capacitance**—Ability to store an electrical charge.

**carrier frequency**—The frequency of pulsed energy for the period of time that the laser is emitted.

**cavitation**—The formation of cavities within the body; used in the context of ultrasound, the formation of gas bubbles within cell walls.

**chemotactic**—To chemically attract.

**chemotaxis**—A chemical attraction.

**chondroblasts**—Cartilage-forming cells.

**chronaxie**—The phase duration required to depolarize a nerve fiber when the amplitude is $2 \times$ rheobase.

**clinical trial**—A prospective study of treatment efficacy or effectiveness conducted with patients.

**coherence**—A property of laser light where all discharged photons are in sync with each other and travel in parallel.

**cold urticaria**—An allergic reaction to cold exposure.

**collagen**—Principal protein found in ligament, tendon, and scar tissues.

**collimation**—A property of laser light where the light travels in one direction without diverging. Once a medium change is encountered, there is a possibility for reflection, refraction and absorption of the light.

**complex regional pain syndrome (CRPS)**—Symptom complex characterized by pain that is disproportional to the injury.

**conduction**—Transfer of heat through the direct contact between a hotter and a cooler area.

**convection**—Transfer of heat by the movement of air or liquid between regions of unequal temperature.

**conversion**—Term implying that energy is changed from one form to another, for example, acoustic energy to thermal energy through the administration of ultrasound.

**coulomb**—Measure of electrical charge or a quantity of electrons (abbreviated C).

**cryokinetics**—Use of cryotherapy to facilitate therapeutic exercise.

**cryotherapy**—Therapeutic use of cold.

**depolarization**—To change from a polarized state.

**depression**—State of deep sadness, dejection, and gloom; distinguished from grief, which is an appropriate response to personal loss.

**diathermy**—Heating of tissue with electromagnetic energy.

**dipole**—A molecule with areas of opposite electrical charges.

**direct current (DC)**—Continuous current without alternating positive and negative phases.

**disability**—All limitations on performance of normal daily tasks, including those related to schoolwork, employment, family responsibilities, and sport participation, due to disease or injury.

**dorsal horn**—Area of synapse between first- and second-order afferent nerves.

**duty cycle**—Ratio of "on" and "off" time.

**effective radiating area (ERA)**—Area of the ultrasound head emitting acoustic energy.

**effectiveness**—A response to treatment applied during routine clinical practice.

**efferent**—Conducting from the center toward the periphery (as in conduction of nerve impulses from the central nervous system).

**efficacy**—A response to treatment administered in a controlled setting or under ideal conditions.

**effleurage**—A massage technique using long stroking motions.

**electromotive force**—A potential difference in electrical charges that results in a flow of electrical current.

**electromyography (EMG)**—A measure of the electrical activity in muscle.

**enkephalin**—A family of five-peptide chain transmitter substances that inhibit synaptic transmission in nociceptive pathways.

**etiological factors**—Factors that cause a condition.

**evidence-based health care**—The integration of the best research evidence with clinical expertise and patient values.

**fibrin**—A protein converted from fibrinogen to form the meshlike foundation of a clot.

**fibroblasts**—Cells that produce collagen and elastin.

**free radical**—A molecule containing an odd number of electrons, which can injure healthy tissues.

**frequency**—Number of cycles or sinusoidal waves per second.

**functional limitations**—Inability to perform physical tasks; in physically active individuals, specific examples could include sport-specific activities such as running and jumping.

**galvanic**—Direct current.

**gamma gain**—An increase in gamma motor neuron discharge.

**ground state**—The atom is in its most stable form and no electrons are in an elevated valence level.

**hemoconcentration**—Concentration of red blood cells.

**hyperemia**—An increase in blood flow to a part of the body.

**hypertonicity**—An increase in the resting tension of muscle.

**hypomobility**—Less than normal mobility.

**hypovolemic**—Referring to low blood volume.

**hypoxia**—Lack of oxygen.

**impairment**—Anatomical, physiological, psychological, and emotional aftereffects of disease and injury.

**inflammation**—Series of physiological events that occur in vascularized tissue.

**intensity**—Dose of sound energy delivered to the tissue; measured in watts per square centimeter (W/cm$^2$) of area of sound head transmitting energy.

**interstitium**—Space between the cells.

**iontophoresis**—Use of an electrical current to drive medications into the tissues.

**labile**—Changeable, fluctuating.

**lasing chamber**—An enclosed area where stimulated emissions may take place. This usually has mirrors on either side to reflect the photon energy.

**leukocytes**—White blood cells, of which there are five types: neutrophils, macrophages, basophils, esinophils, and lymphocytes.

**maladaptive behavior**—Faulty, self-defeating, or injurious intrapersonal adaptation to stress or change.

**mast cell**—Type of cell found in connective tissue that releases several chemical mediators of inflammation.

**mechanoreceptors**—Superficial receptors that respond to stroking, touch, and pressure.

**monochromatic**—Being only of one color.

**monophasic current**—Pulsatile current with only positive or negative pulses.

**muscle spindle**—Sensory receptor of length–tension changes in muscle.

**myofascial pain syndrome (MFPS)**—Persistent pain of soft tissue, origins characterized by taut fibrous bands and focal areas of hypersensitivity called trigger points.

**necrotic**—Dead.

**negligence**—Entails (1) doing something that a similarly qualified person under like circumstances would not have done (a negligent act or act of commission) or (2) failing to do something that a similarly qualified person would have done under similar circumstances (act of omission).

**neuromuscular control**—Use of sensory neural input and motor output to exert volitional control of skeletal muscle.

**neuromuscular stimulation**—Use of TENS to cause a muscle contraction.

**nociceptive**—Pain sensing.

**nociceptors**—Superficial receptors that are stimulated by potentially damaging mechanical, chemical, and thermal stress.

**noxious**—Pain producing.

**ohm**—A measure of resistance to the flow of electrons (abbreviated $\Omega$).

**opiates**—A substance derived from opium.

**opioid**—A naturally occurring or synthetic substance having an opiate-like effect.

**osteoblasts**—Bone-forming cells.

**osteokinematic**—Referring to movement of one bony segment on another; for example, glenohumeral abduction results in movement of the humerus on the glenoid.

**palliative care**—Treatments that relieve symptoms, often temporarily, without curing.

**peak current**—The maximum amplitude of the current at any point during the pulse without regard to its duration.

**permanent**—Unchangeable, as in permanent tissues that last through life but cannot be repaired.

**petrissage**—A massage technique in which the skin is lifted, squeezed, or kneaded.

**phagocyte**—A cell that engulfs and digests microorganisms and cellular debris.

**phonophoresis**—Method of driving medications into tissues with sound waves.

**photon**—A measurement of electromagnetic energy that lacks mass, lacks an electrical charge, and has an indefinite lifetime. Photons contain a specific amount of energy depending on its wavelength.

**physical agents**—Treatments that cause some change to the body.

**physiochemical effect**—To alter bodily functions by changing chemical balance (e.g. softening of scar under negative direct current).

**physiological effect**—To alter bodily functions by changing specific tissue activity (e.g. trigger the release of endogenous opiods through nerve stimulation).

**placebo effect**—Improvement in a condition not related to the effect of a treatment or medication.

**population inversion**—Atoms are excited so that the majority of the atoms in a particular environment are in this high-energy state. This allows the creation of a laser.

**practice act**—State law regulating the practice of a profession.

**pulsatile current**—Noncontinuous current; the flow of current is broken by intervals between pulses.

**pulse train**—Method of delivering laser energy so that the energy is pulsed for short periods of time. The end result is packets of pulsed energy to be emitted.

**radiation**—The emission of energy; radiant energy may be emitted from a source such as a heat lamp and absorbed by the body.

**rest–reinjury cycle**—Pattern of injury in which physically active individuals return to activity only to aggravate a condition from which they have not fully recovered.

**rheobase**—The minimum amplitude required to depolarize a nerve fiber.

**root mean square (RMS)**—A means of determining phase charge or the effective area contained in the waveform that results in the physiochemical effects.

**signs**—Indicators of illness or injury that the clinician measures, for example fever.

**somatization**—A somatic (bodily) manifestation of psychological dysfunction.

**somatosensory information**—Neural input that allows for sensation such as temperature, pressure, and pain as well as allowing for awareness of how the body is oriented in relation to time and space.

**spontaneous emissions**—Random discharge of a light wave that occurs naturally. An atom absorbs energy to raise its valence level and the same amount of energy is emitted spontaneously when the atom releases a photon.

**stable**—Slowly changing or resistant to change; opposite of labile.

**stimulated emissions**—A discharge of a light wave is stimulated by another light wave. When the photon strikes another excited atom, two identical photons are released.

**substance P**—A facilitatory transmitter substance in the nociceptive pathways.

**symptoms**—Indicators of injury or illness that the patient discloses, for example, "My shoulder hurts."

**synapse**—Junction between nerves.

**tetanic muscle contraction**—A sustained contraction of a muscle.

**therapeutic modality**—Literally, a device or apparatus having curative powers.

**thermoreceptors**—Superficial receptors that respond to temperature and temperature change.

**transcutaneous electrical nerve stimulation (TENS)**—The use of a therapeutic device that stimulates peripheral nerves by passing an electrical current through the skin.

**transmitter substance**—Chemical that influences transmission of neural impulses across a synapse; the substance may facilitate or inhibit transmission.

**trigger point**—A hypersensitive fibrous band of tissue.

**tort**—Private, civil legal action brought by an injured party, or the party's representative, to redress an injury caused by another person.

**ultrasound**—High-frequency acoustic energy.

**vascularized**—Having a blood supply; perfused.

**vasodilation**—An opening of the capillary beds.

**viscera**—The organs of thoracic, abdominal and pelvic organs.

**voltage**—Measure of electromotive force (abbreviated V).

**Wedenski's inhibition**—An action potential failure in a nerve caused by a medium frequency electrical current.

# Index

chronic 70-71, 79
defined 44
low-level laser therapy for 212
multidimensional nature of 46-49, 66
neuromuscular control and 87-88
persistent 70-79
physical exam and 45-46t, 270
referred 46t
transmission of 49-59
pain charts 47f
pain control theories
  gate control theory 59, 60, 61f-63, 219-220f
  pattern theory 59
  peripheral pain modulation 60
  specificity theory 59
  supraspinal and descending pain modulation 63-66
Pain Disability Index 47, 48f
pain scale 47
Paine, R.M. 255
Pal, B. 236
paleospinothalamic tract pain 49, 50-51f
paraffin baths 120, 121f
patellofemoral pain (PFP)
  biofeedback for 259-260f
  case study 254
  neuromuscular control and 88
patient pain and activity inventory 10f
patient self-report instruments 96
Patton, N.J. 190
peak current 134f
Peppard, A.P. 116
periaqueductal gray (PAG) 50, 51f, 57, 58f, 63, 64, 65f
peripheral pain modulation 60
peripheral sensory receptors
  deep tissue receptors 52t, 53f-54
  defined 52t
  superficial receptors 52t-53
persistent pain. *See also* chronic pain
  biomechanics and 72-73, 272
  case study 72
  chronic versus 70-71, 79
  complex regional pain syndrome (CRPS) 74, 275-276
  defined 70-71
  depression and somatization 70, 72f, 77-79, 276
  myofascial pain syndrome (MFPS) 72f, 74-77f, 272-275f
  rest-reinjury cycle and 72f, 73-74, 271-272
  sources of 71-79, 270f
  summary on 80
persistent pain management
  cancer symptoms 271
  common complaints 266
  cryotherapy and 116-117
  diagnosis and plan of care 72, 270f-276

evaluation of patients 266, 267f
  medical history 268-269
  physical examination 45-46t, 270
  summary on 277
petrissage 220
phagocytes 31f
phase duration 135f-138
phonophoresis 178, 186-187
phospholipid breakdown 32-33
photons 199, 200, 201f
physical agents 2
physical examination
  common referred pain patterns 46t
  for persistent pain 270
  P-Q-R-S-T format 45
Piper, M.C. 236
pituitary gland 50, 51, 57, 63, 64f
placebo 24, 66, 96
plantar fasciitis 46, 72
point application 209-210
Pownall, R. 118
P-Q-R-S-T format 45
premodulated interferential stimulation 158-159
Preyde, M. 227
proprioceptors 52t, 88
prostaglandins 30, 31t, 32, 33f, 60
psychological aspects of rehabilitation
  barriers to rehabilitation 20-22
  biopsychosocial models 15
  case study 22
  cognitive appraisal models 15-16
  death-and-dying model 15
  depression 16, 22, 276
  focus on today 19
  goal setting 17-18f
  minimizing suffering 19-20
  personality and environmental influences 16-17
  placebo 24
  secondary gain 20-21
  sharing responsibility 18-19
  social and environmental barriers 21-22
  substance abuse 21
  suffering 19-20
  summary of 24-25
pulsatile currents 132, 133f
pulsed electromagnetic fields (PEMF)
  defined 189
  fracture healing and 191
  musculoskeletal conditions and 190-191

**Q**
quadripolar electrode configuration 145, 146f
**R**
radiant energy 106-107
randomized controlled clinical trials (RCTs) 96, 100t, 101

# About the Authors

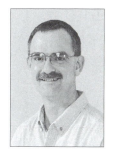

**Craig R. Denegar, PhD, ATC, PT,** is associate professor of orthopedics and rehabilitation and kinesiology at Pennsylvania State University. He has more than 25 years of experience as an athletic trainer and extensive clinical practice experience related to persistent orthopedic pain.

Dr. Denegar is a member of the National Athletic Trainers' Association (NATA) and is the former vice chair for free communications on the NATA Research and Education Foundation Research Committee. He is also a member of the American Physical Therapy Association and the recipient of the William G. Clancey Medal for Distinguished Athletic Training Research in 2003 and of the Distinguished Merit Award from the Pennsylvania Athletic Trainers' Society in 2004.

Currently serving as the senior associate editor of the Journal of Athletic Training (JAT), Dr. Denegar also serves on the editorial boards of JAT, Journal of Strength Training and Conditioning Research, and Journal of Sport Rehabilitation. He received his PhD in education with a specialization in sports medicine and a master's degree in education with a specialization in athletic training from the University of Virginia. He earned a master's degree in physical therapy from the School of Physical Therapy, Slippery Rock, Pennsylvania.

In his spare time, Dr. Denegar enjoys playing soccer, cycling, and studying the history of the American West. He and his wife, Susan, live in State College, Pennsylvania.

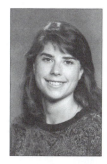

**Susan Foreman Saliba, PhD, ATC, PT** is a senior associate athletic trainer and a clinical instructor at the University of Virginia in Charlottesville, where she has taught therapeutic modalities for over 12 years. A certified athletic trainer and licensed physical therapist, Dr. Saliba also taught therapeutic modalities at James Madison University in Harrisonburg, Virginia. She is chairperson of the National Athletic Trainers' Association Clinical Education Committee and a member of its Education Executive Committee. She earned a master's degree in athletic training and a PhD in sports medicine from the University of Virginia.

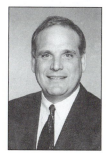

**Ethan Saliba, PhD, ATC, PT** has been teaching therapeutic modalities at the University of Virginia in Charlottesville for over 18 years. He is currently head athletic trainer, overseeing 24 varsity sports. Dr. Saliba is a certified athletic trainer, licensed physical therapist, and sport-certified specialist who has written extensively on various aspects of athletic injuries and rehabilitation. He earned a master's degree and PhD in sports medicine from the University of Virginia.

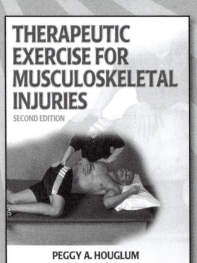
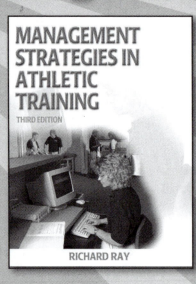
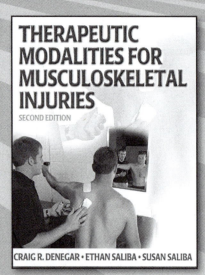
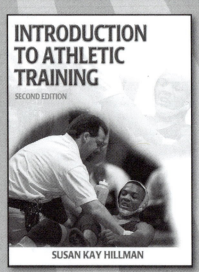
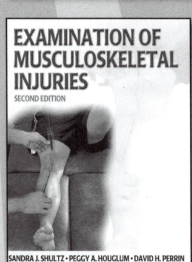